CRC SERIES IN AGING

Editors-in-Chief

Richard C. Adelman, Ph.D.
Executive Director
Institute on Aging
Temple University
Philadelphia, Pennsylvania

George S. Roth, Ph.D.
Research Chemist
Gerontology Research Center
National Institute on Aging
Baltimore City Hospitals
Baltimore, Maryland

HANDBOOK OF BIOCHEMISTRY IN AGING
Editor
James Florini, Ph.D.
Department of Biology
Syracuse University
Syracuse, New York

HANDBOOK OF PHYSIOLOGY IN AGING
Editor
Edward J. Masoro, Ph.D.
Department of Physiology
University of Texas
Health Science Center
San Antonio, Texas

HANDBOOK OF IMMUNOLOGY IN AGING
Editors
Marguerite M. B. Kay, M.D. and
Takashi Makinodan, Ph.D.
Geriatric Research Education and
Clinical Center
V.A. Wadsworth Medical Center
Los Angeles, California

IMMUNOLOGICAL TECHNIQUES APPLIED TO AGING RESEARCH
Editors
William H. Adler, M.D. and
Albert A. Nordin, Ph.D.
Gerontology Research Center
National Institute on Aging
Baltimore City Hospitals
Baltimore, Maryland

SENESCENCE IN PLANTS
Editor
Kenneth V. Thimann, Ph.D.
The Thimann Laboratories
University of California
Santa Cruz, California

CURRENT TRENDS IN MORPHOLOGICAL TECHNIQUES
Editor
John E. Johnson, Jr., Ph.D.
Gerontology Research Center
National Institute on Aging
Baltimore City Hospitals
Baltimore, Maryland

ALCOHOLISM AND AGING: ADVANCES IN RESEARCH
Editors
W. Gibson Wood, Ph.D.
Clinical Research Psychologist
Geriatric Research, Education, and
Clinical Center
VA Medical Center
St. Louis, Missouri
Merrill F. Elias, Ph.D.
Professor of Psychology
Department of Psychology
University of Maine at Orono
Orono, Maine

NUTRITIONAL APPROACHES TO AGING RESEARCH
Editor
Gairdner B. Moment, Ph.D.
Professor Emeritus of Biology
Goucher College
Guest Scientist
Gerontology Research Center
National Institute on Aging
Baltimore, Maryland

Additional topics to be covered in this series include Cell Biology of Aging, Microbiology of Aging, Pharmacology of Aging, Evolution and Genetics, Animal Models for Aging Research, Hormonal Regulatory Mechanisms, Detection of Altered Proteins, Insect Models, Lower Invertebrate Models, and Testing the Theories of Aging.

Nutritional Approaches to Aging Research

Editor

Gairdner B. Moment, Ph.D.
Professor Emeritus of Biology
Goucher College
Guest Scientist
Gerontology Research Center
National Institute on Aging
Baltimore, Maryland

CRC Series on Aging
Editors-in-Chief

Richard C. Adelman, Ph.D.
Executive Director
Institute on Aging
Temple University
Philadelphia, Pennsylvania

George S. Roth, Ph.D.
Research Chemist
Gerontology Research Center
National Institute on Aging
Baltimore City Hospital
Baltimore, Maryland

CRC Press, Inc.
Boca Raton, Florida

Library of Congress Cataloging in Publication Data

Main entry under title:

Nutritional approaches to aging research.

   (CRC series in aging)
   Includes bibliographies and index.
   Contents: Introduction -- Nutrition and age-
related changes of carbohydrate metabolism /
Jeffrey B. Halter and Mei Chen -- Lipids in
nutrition and aging / E. J. Masoro -- Human
aging : protein and amino acid metabolism and
implications for protein and amino acid
requirements / Vernon R. Young, Mitchell
Gersovitz, and Hamish N. Munro -- [etc.]
   1. Aging--Nutritional aspects. 2. Aged--
Nutrition. I. Moment, Gairdner Bostwich,
1905-   . II. Series.
QP86.N85   612'.67   81-9930
ISBN 0-8493-5831-0   AACR2

   Direct all inquiries to CRC Press, Inc., 2000 N.W. 24th Street, Boca Raton, Florida, 33431.

© 1982 by CRC Press, Inc.

International Standard Book Number 0-8493-5831-0

Library of Congress Card Number 81-9930
Printed in the United States

PREFACE

The general plan of this volume, *Nutritional Approaches to Aging Research* is for each chapter to present first a reasonably succinct state-of-the-art appraisal of present knowledge in the particular field or problem covered. This will vary considerably depending on the subject matter. Following this, each chapter will focus on the problems and pitfalls, both conceptual and technological, of work in that particular field and, no less important, present some of the opportunities and implications of work in that particular area.

The authors have been selected because of their expertise in each special field. Some of these authors are well known world wide, others are relative newcomers. It is our belief that this volume will be the stronger by virtue of this mix. It is an indication of the newly recognized importance of nutrition in the study of aging that only three of the authors invited to participate declined.

In today's world of increasing populations of both young and old and limited food supplies in many parts of this planet, this volume can not escape being an important one.

The editor wishes to thank the staff of CRC Press for their cooperation in many important areas of book making and for informing the authors in all matters of format and contractural arrangements.

Gairdner B. Moment
Professor Emeritus of Biology
Goucher College and
Guest Scientist, Gerontology Research Center,
National Institute on Aging,
Baltimore, Maryland

EDITORS-IN-CHIEF

Dr. Richard C. Adelman is currently Executive Director of the Temple University Institute on Aging, Philadelphia, Pa., as well as Professor of Biochemistry in the Fels Research Institute of the Temple University College of Medicine. An active gerontologist for more than 10 years, he has achieved international prominence as a researcher, educator, and administrator. These accomplishments span a broad spectrum of activities ranging from the traditional disciplinary interests of the research biologist to the advocacy, implementation, and administration of multidisciplinary issues of public policy of concern to elderly people.

Dr. Adelman pursued his pre- and postdoctoral research training under the guidance of two prominent biochemists, each of whom is a member of the National Academy of Sciences: Dr. Sidney Weinhouse as Director of the Fels Research Institute, Temple University, and Dr. Bernard L. Horecker as Chairman of the Department of Molecular Biology, Albert Einstein College of Medicine, Bronx, N.Y. His accomplishments as a researcher can be expressed in at least the following ways. He is the author and/or editor of more than 70 publications, including original research papers in referred journals, review chapters, and books. His research efforts have been supported by grants from the National Institutes of Health for the past 10 years, at a current annual level of approximately $300,000. He continues to serve as an invited speaker at seminar programs, symposiums, and workshops all over the world. He is the recipient of the IntraScience Research Foundation Medalist Award, an annual research prize awarded by peer evaluation for major advances in newly emerging areas of the life sciences. He is the recipient of an Established Investigatorship of the American Heart Association.

As an educator, Dr. Adelman is also involved in a broad variety of activities. His role in research training consists of responsibility for pre- and postdoctoral students who are assigned specific projects in his laboratory. He teaches an Advanced Graduate Course on the Biology of Aging, lectures on biomedical aspects of aging to medical students, and is responsible for the biological component of the basic course in aging sponsored by the School of Social Administration. Training activities outside the University include membership in the Faculty of the National Institute on Aging summer course on the Biology of Aging; programs on the biology of aging for AAA's throughout Pennsylvania and Ohio; and the implementation and teaching of Biology of Aging for the Nonbiologist locally, for the Gerontology Society of America and other national organizations, as well as for the International Association of Gerontology.

Dr. Adelman has achieved leadership positions across equally broad areas. Responsibilities of this position include the integration of multidisciplinary programs in research, consultation and education, and health service, as well as advocacy for the University on all matters dealing with aging. He coordinates a city-wide consortium of researchers from Temple University, the Wistar Institute, the Medical College of Pennsylvania, Drexel University, and the Philadelphia Geriatric Center, conducting collaborative research projects, training programs, and symposiums. He was a past President of the Philadelphia Biochemists Club. He serves on the editorial boards of the *Journal of Gerontology, Mechanisms of Ageing and Development, Experimental Aging Research,* and *Gerontological Abstracts.* He was a member of the Biomedical Research Panel of the National Advisory Council of the National Institute on Aging. He chairs a subcommittee of the National Academy of Sciences Committee on Animal Models for Aging Research. As an active Fellow of the Gerontological Society of America, he is a past Chairman of the Biological Sciences section; a past Chairman of the Society Public Policy Committee for which he prepared Congressional testimony and represented the Society on the Leadership Council of the Coalition of National Aging Organizations; and is Secretary-Treasurer of the North American Executive

Committee of the International Association of Gerontology. Finally, as the highest testimony of his leadership capabilities, he continues to serve on National Advisory Committee which impact on diverse key issues dealing with the elderly. These include a 4-year appointment as a member of the NIH Study Section on Pathobiological Chemistry; the Executive Committee of the Health Resources Administration Project on publication of the recent edition of *Working with Older People — A Guide to Practice;* a recent appointment as reviewer of AOA applications fo Career Preparation Programs in Gerontology; and a 4-year appointment on the Veterans Administration Long-Term Care Advisor Council responsible for evaluating their program on Geriatric Research, Education, and Clinical Centers (GRECC).

Dr. George S. Roth is a Research Chemist with the Gerontology Research Center of the National Institute on Aging in Baltimore, Md., where he has been affiliated since 1972. Dr. Roth received his B.S. in Biology from Villanova University in 1968 and his Ph.D. in Microbiology from Temple University School of Medicine in 1971. He received postdoctoral training in Biochemistry at the Fels Research Institute in Philadelphia, Pa. Dr. Roth has also been associated with the Graduate Schools of Georgetown University and George Washington University where he has sponsored two Ph.D. students.

He has published more than 70 papers in the area of aging and hormone/neurotransmitter action, and has lectured, organized meetings, and chaired sessions throughtout the world on this subject.

Dr. Roth's other activities include Fellowship in the Gerontological Society of America, where he has served in numerous capacities, including Chairmanship of the 1979 Mid-Year Conference on "Functional Status and Aging". He is presently Chairman of the Biological Sciences Section and a Vice President of the Society. He has twice been selected as an exchange scientist by the National Academy of Sciences and in this capacity has established liasons with gerontologists, endocrinologists, and biochemists in several Eastern European countries. Dr. Roth serves as an editor of *Neurobiology of Aging* and is a frequent reviewer for many other journals including *Mechanisms in Aging and Development, Life Sciences, The Journal of Gerontology, Science,* and *Endocrinology.* He also serves as a grant reviewer for several funding agencies, including the National Science Foundation. In 1981 Dr. Roth was awarded the Annual Research Award of the American Aging Association.

THE EDITOR

Gairdner B. Moment, Ph.D., is Professor Emeritus of Biology at Goucher College and Guest Scientist at the Gerontology Research Center of the National Institute on Aging, both in Baltimore, Maryland.

Dr. Moment received his A.B. from Princeton University in 1928 and his Ph.D. in Zoology from Yale University in 1932. He has been on the staff of Goucher College since 1932, serving as Chairman of the Biology Department from 1945 to 1958 and becoming Professor Emeritus of Biology in 1970. Dr. Moment is the Editor-in-Chief of *Growth,* a journal devoted to problems of normal and abnormal growth.

Dr. Moment is a member of the Government Science Advisory Council, Fel AAAS, American Society of Zoologists, Society of Developmental Biology, Society of General Physiology, and the American Institute of Biological Science. His research interests include animal development, and behavior; biochemical, electrical, and anatomical study of animal growth; general biology; annelids; protein electrophoresis; regeneration, and tissue culture.

CONTRIBUTORS

Charles H. Barrows, Sc.D.
Gerontology Research Center
National Institute on Aging
Baltimore City Hospital
Baltimore, Maryland

Mei Chen, M.D.
Assistant Professor of Medicine
University of Washington
Staff Physician
Seattle Veteran's Administration
  Hospital
Seattle, Washington

Arthur V. Everitt, Ph.D.
Associate Professor of Physiology
University of Sydney
Sydney, New South Wales
Australia

Barbara B. Fleming, Ph.D.
Staff Fellow
National Institute on Aging
Baltimore City Hospitals
Baltimore, Maryland

Mitchell Gersovitz, Ph.D.
McGaw Laboratories
Santa Ana, California

Jeffrey B. Halter, M.D.
Associate Professor of Medicine
University of Washington
Associate Director
Geriatric Research
Education and Clinical Center
Seattle Veterans Administration
  Medical Center
Seattle, Washington

Peter R. Holt, M.D.
Director
Division of Gastroenterology
St. Luke's Roosevelt Hospital Center
Professor of Medicine
College of Physicians and Surgeons
Columbia University
New York, New York

Jeng M. Hsu, Ph.D.
Medical Research
Veteran's Administration Hospital
Bay Pines, Florida

Frank L. Iber, M.D.
Professor of Medicine
Chief
Gastroenterology Division
University of Maryland Hospital
Baltimore Veteran's Administration
  Hospital
Baltimore, Maryland

Gertrude C. Kokkonen, B.A.
Gerontology Research Center
National Institute on Aging
Baltimore City Hospital
Baltimore, Maryland

Edward J. Masoro, Ph.D.
Professor and Chairman
Department of Physiology
University of Texas Health Science
  Center
San Antonio, Texas

Gairdner B. Moment, Ph.D.
Guest Scientist
Gerontology Research Center
National Institute on Aging
Baltimore City Hospital
Baltimore, Maryland

Hamish N. Munro, D.Sc.
Director
USDA Human Nutrition Research
  Center on Aging at Tufts University
Boston, Massachusetts

Agatha A. Rider, Sc.M.
Assistant Professor
Department of Biochemistry
School of Hygiene and Public Health
The Johns Hopkins University
Baltimore, Maryland

J. Cecil Smith, Jr., Ph.D.
Chief
Vitamin and Mineral Nutrition
  Laboratory
Beltsville Human Nutrition Research
  Center
Beltsville, Maryland

Albert Y. Sun, Ph.D.
Associate Professor
Department of Biochemistry
University of Missouri
Columbia, Missouri

Grace Y. Sun, Ph.D.
Associate Professor
Department of Biochemistry
University of Missouri
Columbia, Missouri

Vernon R. Young, Ph.D.
Professor of Nutritional Biochemistry
Massachusetts Institute of Technology
Cambridge, Massachusetts

TABLE OF CONTENTS

Chapter 1

INTRODUCTION

G. B. Moment

TABLE OF CONTENTS

I. OBJECTIVES OF GERONTOLOGICAL RESEARCH

The stated aim of the National Institute on Aging is to gain the knowledge necessary to alleviate "the physical infirmities resulting from advanced age (and) the economic, social and psychological factors associated with aging which operate to exclude millions of older Americans from a full life and place in our society." The importance of this in the U.S. where the proportion of older individuals continues to grow at the expense of younger must be clear to all. The cost of Social Security for those who have retired either by choice or from necessity is staggering, even excluding nursing home care. To make it possible for people everywhere to age well, both physically and mentally so that a satisfying old age can be the good fortune of us all is not only a humane goal but a realistic one.

What is not a realistic goal is the discovery of the Fountain of Ponce de Leon, the fountain of eternal youth, or perhaps of eternal middle age. However astronomically removed such a possibility, it cannot be excluded absolutely. Helmholtz, as a brash young man, measured the speed of a nervous impulse after the leading physiologists of Europe had declared that it would be forever impossible. Moreover, the truly shattering surprises in the history of knowledge have not been either foreseen or searched for. Roentgen did not intend to discover X-rays. He was as surprised as everyone else. Columbus did not set sail to discover a new world but to reach India by a shorter route.

It is conceivable that an aging chronometer process of some kind exists in every cell of the body or in the hypothalamus, the limbic, or some other region of the brain, and that this biochronometer could be slowed or even stopped. The discoverer might be investigating the cause of jet lag, or the timing mechanism of circadian rhythms which exist throughout most if not perhaps the entire living world. It might be, of course, that the biochemical machinery of the aging timepiece does not lie in the nervous system. Plants possess a circadian "clock" and no nervous system.

Three salient facts demand attention. The probability of stopping the hypothetical aging clock appears all but infinitely removed, while the benefits from age-related research are real. Secondly, if an aging process of whatever sort could be stopped, it would result in a watershed in human history fully comparable to the discovery of the use of fire or how to domesticate plants and animals. Unimagined population problems would arise at once, along with vast psychological, personal, and social problems. Strehler[24] has discussed these issues in the fields of physical health and survivorship curves from ancient times to the present, of mental health, of social effects, and of economic effects and polycareers. Lastly, for better or for worse, the only way to be sure of escaping such a discovery would be to halt most medical and physiological research, even on the plants. Serendipity in science is rare but very real.

We are left with the conclusion that gerontological research will provide a continuing flow of beneficial discoveries and that the hazard of a mega-breakthrough to permanent control of aging is as remote as the possibility of the existence of a single well somewhere that yields molasses. Only someone considerably more competent in Neo-Bayesian statistics than Lewis Carroll's Alice or the present writer could say how remote that is.

II. THE NEWLY DISCOVERED IMPORTANCE OF NUTRITIONAL RESEARCH

One of the most remarkable and probably one of the most important facts so far discovered in the field of gerontology is that the maximum life span of certain warm-blooded (endothermic or homoiothermic) animals can be extended by 50% or more by dietary restriction. This dramatic result has so far been tested only in rats and mice, but there is a high probability amounting almost to certainty that it could be replicated in all mammals including humans, a point to which we will return later.

This surprising result of what is often called "underfeeding" was recorded first by Osborne et al.[18] in 1917. It was further investigated by McCay[8] and associates in the 1930s, and Berg and Simms[2] in the 1960s; but even after Ross,[20] Barrows (this volume) and Goodrick[9] began their contemporary work on this apparently paradoxical phenomenon, very few additional investigators have entered the field.

Nevertheless, the possible implications of dietary restriction studies are enormous on both the theoretical and practical sides. On the theoretical side it is quite possible that food restriction studies will prove to be a very useful probe to assist in understanding the biochronometer of animal development, whatever it may turn out to be, from sometime prior to reproductive maturity through the final stages of senescence. The mechanism or mechanisms by which food restriction extends lifespan are unknown. However, they appear to act at a very deep level because the 50% or more extension of life span is far greater than can be explained by the elimination or postponement of the diseases characteristic of the aging rodent, although dietary restriction does that.

There is some evidence cited by Everitt (this volume) and by others that dietary restriction results in a form of hypophysectomy which is the underlying cause of aging extension. Wurtman et al.[29] and Lytle and Altar[12] among others have shown that diet can influence brain catechol amines involved in the neuroendocrine system and even influence the choice of food. In this series, Ross[20] and associates have shown that self-selection of foods by rats influences the age of onset of renal, pulmonary, and other diseases of aging as well as the time of incidence of tumors. Restriction of food lowers basal metabolism somewhat so it is conceivable that specific metabolic rate is reduced more than the specific activity of superoxide dismutase and other enzymes protective against the destructive effect of oxidation. But whether the rate of aging is determined by some form of Orgelian wear and tear from radiation, thermal agitation or chemical accidents on the genetic material, or by some as yet unguessed process, dietary restriction will remain one of the probes in helping to distinguish between the multiplicity of aging theories.

On the practical side, the data now available present new research opportunities in the field of nutrition which promise new vistas for a future in which human life will be healthier and more productive and satisfying over the full 3 score and 10 years and probably a bit more.

Entirely aside from whether or not food restriction extends life span beyond the natural limit characteristic of the species, a reevaluation of the traditional nutritional guidelines is in order. The fact alone that the age of onset of specific diseases and of specific types of tumors of several organs is very significantly postponed justifies an investigative program not presently in sight.

A first order of business is to confirm and perhaps extend the studies of dietary restriction on mammals other than rats and mice. That food restriction would increase the health and longevity in all mammals seems extremely probable on general physiological principles, but there is at least one specific study on the human which supports such an extrapolation from the rat and mouse.

Ross,[20] Barrows, and Goodrick[9] have each found that alternate feeding and fasting results in marked life extension in these laboratory rodents. Ross cites a study where E. A. Vallejo divided some institutionalized subjects (number unspecified) all over 65 years of age into two groups. One group was given the regular institutional food every day. The other was given the same food one day and on alternate days only milk and raw fruit. The caloric intake on the "lactopomaceous" days was 60% less and the protein intake 28% lower than on the standard diet days. During the 3 years of this study, the length of time spent in the infirmary by those fully fed was twice that of those fed every other day. Twice as many of those fed the standard diet every day died.

This is a single study and the details apparently are not available. Clearly, additional studies should be made and it should not be difficult to find volunteers if they are given the proper motivation.

Life span extension by dietary restriction has been known for many years in a number of invertebrates, insects, a crustacean (Daphina) and in rotifers. Neither this, nor the case cited by Ross, is enough to justify neglecting taking a hard look at the results of dietary restriction in some mammal other than the mouse and rat. The guinea pig comes to mind as a relatively short-lived animal having a life span of about 7 years. Although a rodent, it requires an outside source of vitamin C like the human but unlike rats and mice. Dogs would be especially interesting first because they are not rodents but also because of the puzzling way large dogs have a shorter life span than small ones.

The present data about the results of restriction indicate that a number of standard ideas about nutrition, at least human nutrition, will need to be reexamined. The long-held belief, for example, that the best of all possible diets is simply a well-balanced one may turn out to be only part of the story. Quantitative considerations may take on a new dimension. As far as protein is concerned, more may actually be worse for the best health and longest active life. It has been known for over 80 years through the pioneering work described by Matthews[13] of Chittenden and his associates that a man can satisfactorily carry out "ordinary exertions" on less than an ounce of protein per day. Because in restriction studies it is uncertain whether reduction of calories or of protein or both is most effective in postponing diseases and increasing healthy life span, the whole question of the role and the amount of protein in the diet stands to be reexamined.

Before any restriction diet can be safely used for people, there is a host of questions which spring to mind and require answers. An important caveat to keep always in mind is that severe quantitative and qualitative protein deficiencies result in mental retardation and in kwashiorkor in children. That the mental retardation, as shown by the work of Brasel,[3] Winick and others, can be at least partially reversed and kwashiorkor cured does not remove that caveat. Moreover, on some restriction diets the rats have been stunted in growth, undeveloped sexually, and, in some, scrawny. How are these undesirable effects to be avoided? The differences between restriction of calories and of amino acids remains to be clarified. When should the restriction begin? Soon after weaning, sometime before reproductive maturity, well after that event? Is alternate fasting and feeding more effective biologically and psychologically than level restriction? What role does exercise play? How can vitamin and trace element requirements be met? What is the role and significance of self-selection of diet? The number of variations, combinations, and permutations of these different approaches to the problem is certainly very large, even only counting those which appear especially significant.

After there are reasonably firm answers to questions of this sort, tests should begin on some of the smaller, i.e., shorter lived, primates and on human volunteers. Obviously this is an investigative program which can be undertaken only by workers in a large university or research institute able to make a firm commitment extending over several decades.

Meanwhile it appears highly important to begin at once a study of several quite different groups of people living on a low subsistence level along with a parallel study of control groups on what is considered an ample diet. How does the average life span of two sets of such groups compare? Do they die of the same diseases? How does their general level of physical and mental energy compare? Such a study could provide data unattainable in any other way.

In conclusion, there would appear to be no area with any greater potential than the study of restriction dietary programs for achieving the goal of gerontological research to extend the years of healthy, productive, and self-sufficient life.

III. PRESENT THEORIES OF AGING

Gerontology, in the effort to gain the knowledge that will enable everyone to continue in active good health throughout the entire life span, is very much in the position of medicine before the germ theory of diseases was established. It is only possible to look at the symptoms. In aging studies it is often impossible to be certain which of several events are causal and which are effects, or if they are all the results of a single prior event.

The current state of knowledge about growth theories has been presented with increasing frequency within the past few years. Such accounts can be found in Behnke, Finch, and Moment,[1] in Dietz,[7] in Finch and Hayflick,[8] in Oata et al.,[17] in Rockstein,[19] in Thornbecke,[25] and in others. It seems of value here only to present a brief statement of some of the more general concepts and to mention a few that are relatively new or neglected.

The ecological-evolutionary theory of aging attributes a long life span to K-selection which favors large size, few young at birth, and occurs when a population is close to the carrying capacity of the environment. At the opposite end of the selection spectrum is r-selection which favors a short life span, small size, many young at a birth, and occurs when the carrying capacity has not been closely approached or is subject to great fluctuations. While this widely accepted theory may furnish an evolutionary frame-work for the study of aging, so far it has offered few clues about physiological or biochemical mechanisms.

Sacher's[21] predictive formula relating brain weight, body weight, resting metabolism, and body temperature to life span does seem to point toward possible mechanisms. $L = 8B^{0.6} S^{-0.4} M^{-0.5} 10^{0.025T_b}$ where L = lifespan in months, B = brain weight in grams, S = bodyweight in grams, M = resting metabolic rate (cal/g-hr) and T_b = body temperature in °C. This formula works well for various rodents, carnivores, ungulates, and primates.

Probably the most long-standing dichotomy of views about aging is between the "extrinsic" or "epi-phenomenal" theory and the "intrinsic", programmatic, or "biochronometer" theory. The first has been supported on the level of organ physiology by Shock and on the cellular level by Szilard, Orgel, and many others. Put in simplistic terms, this view holds that aging is due to some form of wear or damage either by the use of structures, or by injuries to the genetic or protein-forming mechanisms from radiation, thermal agitation, or some other source. However, it is impossible to believe that anyone really thought that living organisms wore out like automobiles (or Oliver Wendell Holmes' "wonderful one horse shay"). The "mortality" curve for glass beakers which become more brittle as they age does resemble a mortality curve for a population of aging animals. What the automobile and glass beaker analogy overlooks is the fact which everyone knows: a characteristic feature of living things is their ability for repair. Mammals, amphibians, and even earthworms possess many well-known mechanisms for the repair of wounds and for many kinds of continuous replacement, e.g., in skin and blood systems. The compensatory proliferation of the remaining portion of the mammalian liver after partial hepatectomy is another example indicating that there is more to the story of aging that just wear and tear.

The other view looks to an intrinsic biochronometer of some kind. Finch and Everitt are among those who have shown evidence that such a pace-maker process may reside in a neuroendocrine mechanism in the brain, specifically in the hypothalamus. Denckla and Bolla[6] have postulated an aging hormone produced by the pituitary-thyroid system. Recent work in Finch's laboratory has shown that if a rat is ovarectomized before ovarian cycling begins and then, after the age at which cycling would have ceased, receives an implant of an ovary from a very young rat, the young implanted ovary will cycle. This is in contrast to the well-known failure of ovaries from young rats implanted into post-cycling females to begin to function. This result strongly suggests that the aging of the female reproductive system is regulated by some sort of "counting" mechanism for the interaction between the alternation of stimulating tropic hormones of the pituitary and feedback inhibitory hormones from the ovary. Whether such a mechanism can be generalized remains to be determined.

As more and more data are accumulated, it begins to appear that these two classical concepts of aging, the extrinsic and the intrinsic, may not be as different as was once thought. Both extrinsic and intrinsic hypotheses meet in the idea that aging is due to the interaction of damage to the DNA-RNA-enzyme-protein mechanism from radiation, thermal agitation and oxidation, and the ability of repair and protective enzymes to compensate for this "wear and tear". The importance of repair enzymes for nucleic acids has been recognized for some years. More recently, Cutler[5,26] and associates have found a very close correlation between the ratio of the specific activity of superoxide dismutase to specific metabolic rate and the life span of many mammals particularly primates. Superoxide dismutase, it will be recalled, is one of the enzymes which protects cells from the toxicity of active oxygen involved in metabolism.

In cold-blooded (exothermic or poikilothermic) animals, life span is well known to be dependent on temperature. The higher the temperature, the higher the oxidative respiration and the shorter the life. In earthworms it has recently been found by Moment[14] and colleagues that as temperature is increased not only does oxidative metabolism increase, but so does the specific activity of superoxide dismutase, although not to the same extent. Thus it would appear that at higher temperatures a cold blooded animal like an earthworm has proportionally less and less enzymatic protection against oxygen which results in the shorter life span.

The recent discovery of Finch, cited above, of the relationship of the ovary and the pituitary can be interpreted as an accumulation of wear on the pituitary, essentially not very different from the interacting wear on organ systems postulated in the classical "wear and tear" view.

One old idea about aging which is only recently coming into its own was proposed by Minot in 1908. He held that the aging process begins during the cleavage of the egg and is a continuous developmental process through the final stages of senescence. One of the clearest examples of the truth of this idea is found in the regular decline with age in the egg production of domestic hens. Because of the economic importance of the poultry industry, this decline has been carefully studied in a number of agricultural stations associated with universities. The results have always been the same with only very slight differences in rate, perhaps attributable to extrinsic factors such as diet and intrinsic factors such as breed. Hens first lay when they are approximately 1 year old. The number of eggs laid that first year is the maximum number a hen will ever lay. On each succeeding year for the next 12 to 15 years, i.e., during the life span of the hen, the number of eggs laid will be about 80% of the number laid the previous year[10] (Figure 1).

The famous "Baltimore longitudinal" study of Shock[8] shows the same steady, if not quite as regular, decline with age in a variety of physiological parameters in men measured from age 30 to 85 (Figure 2). For practical reasons the Shock study began at age 30 and the mean values at that age were designated as 100% from which all

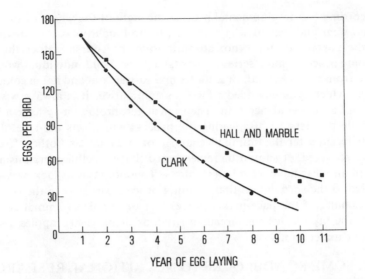

FIGURE 1. The annual decline of egg production in domestic hens in two different laboratories, indicating that the "biochronometer" for aging begins almost at the start of life. (From Hall, G. O. and Marble, D. R., *Poultry Sci.*, 10, 194, 1931. With permission.)

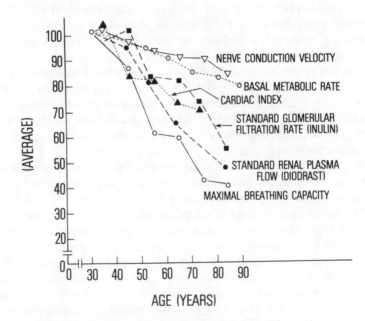

FIGURE 2. The decline with age in six physiological parameters beginning with age 30, at which time the values found were designated as 100%. (Adapted from Shock, N. W., in Progress and Papers, Conference on Gerontology, Duke University Council on Gerontology, Durham, N.C., November 19-21, 1959.)

parameters declined. It would be extremely interesting to begin tracing the history of these and other parameters from infancy. No doubt adjustments would have to be made in a number of parameters because of size differences. Maximum breathing capacity, for example, surely increases during childhood. Does it increase relative to size?

There is, of course, an impelling logical reason why the aging timepiece or timepieces must be recording the developmental process throughout the whole of the life span. If there was no wear and tear of whatever sort, or no biochronometer of whatever sort, recording the passage of time (not absolute time, of course, rather the cumulative action of some process, some series of events) a 20-year-old individual would be indistinguishable from a 30-year-old, or a 30- from a 40-year-old and aging could not occur.

In science, which is open-ended as well as cumulative, it is always wise to reserve judgment until all the evidence is in. Theoretical gerontology may have a long way to go. The whole problem of discovering the process which sets the rate of aging may look very different after the timing mechanism of circadian and other "free-running" rhythms is discovered. It should be remembered that unicellular organisms as well as plants and plant parts have circadian rhythms. These organisms lack nervous systems, which has led to the speculation that a timing process can exist in the cell membrane. On the other hand, if the pace-maker process for the whole of animal development is understood, the mystery of the circadian rhythms of harvested apples and migrating birds might be understood also.

IV. SOME ROADBLOCKS TO NUTRITIONAL RESEARCH

The most visible impediment is what Broad,[4] in a recent indepth review, terms the "gingerly" approach of the National Institutes of Health (NIH) to any exploration of possible diet-disease linkage. Unfortunately this is nothing new. When the NIH research programs went into high gear after Sputnik I in 1957, research in nutrition was left behind. In cold fact even the small already-existing program was allowed to atrophy. There was a reason for this in the existing state of the science of nutrition at that time a quarter of a century ago, but there were surely other reasons which are fully operative today.

The first is the financial force of the food-processing industries and what is now called agribusiness. The cattle industry, for example, has been particularly strident in pressing for the acceptance of its views and possibly more dogmatic than the tobacco industry, and there is a flock of others. These special interests make their influence felt through pressures on congressmen on key committees and financial contributions to their election campaigns.

In addition, there is the politics that always exists in any large organization whether it be the armed services, a business corporation, or a governmental agency. In this particular case there is well-documented public rivalry between the NIH and the USDA. There are also intra-agency vested interests and professional establishments. In the clash of views about nutritional guidelines, the arguments have fallen to such a low level that one group is calling the recommendations of another "trash" but refusing to be specific! All this indicates the need for a week-long symposium in some serene environment with a salubrious climate, or at least outside of the pressure cooker of Washington, where the issues could be brought into some sort of useful focus.

The fear of making a whale of an error by throwing precious research funds to the winds in supporting work on some new and controversial idea that may not pan out acts as a powerful break on administrators and scientists of peer review groups. No one wants to make his or her institute appear either spend-thrift or ridiculous. One is reminded of the day when Ernest Rutherford's superior at McGill University in Montreal tried to dissuade him from publishing his results on the structure of the atom because he didn't want this young instructor in physics to make a fool of himself, not to mention the university.

One solution to this very difficult problem might lie in assigning a certain percent of the total budget to what might be termed "risk capital for ideas". Without the testing of radically new ideas, science stagnates. In nutrition it would seem appropriate to include "cost effectiveness" and feasibility among the several criteria for judging a project. The benefits to be obtained from important new knowledge about human nutrition would outweight by several orders of magnitude the foreseeable benefits from, to use an example from another field, saving the snail darter of which there are over a dozen very closely similar species.

Hard dogmatisms, especially those held with passionate conviction, are also an impediment to research in the field of nutrition whether it be a refusal to admit that food allergies could possibly be involved in arthritis without conducting thorough testing or a belief that red meat is the food par excellence for health and vigor.

A further impediment to nutritional research, especially in relation to aging, is the apparent fact that there is no certain theory, not even an agreed-upon, most likely hypothesis, about the nature of the timing mechanism or mechanisms which set the pace for aging. The fact that Strehler in Dietz[7] can very easily list seven major "alternative theories" of biological aging, with many variations under some of these headings, indicates how confused and baffling the situation is. Small wonder then that it is extremely difficult to form rational hypotheses and design experiments in nutrition and age changes.

One further handicap for nutrition studies needs to be mentioned. For several decades research in nutrition has been a very unfashionable field. When the age of discovering new vitamins and determining their chemical structure and the symptomatology brought on by their deficiency in a diet was over, the excitement and rewards of biological research lay elsewhere. Able and zealous young students and young investigators turned to more promising fields. The policy of granting agencies such as the National Institutes of Health reinforced this movement away from nutrition. The general attitude was that a balanced diet with ample vitamins was the whole story. The U.S. Department of Agriculture had promulgated the "Basic Four Food Groups" for such a diet: meat, milk, bread and cereal, and fruit and vegetables. What more was there? "Not much" was the answer given some 25 years ago.

Credit for the change in outlook goes to many factors. The widespread interest of the association, whether directly causal or not, of cholesterol with cardiovascular diseases and the newer knowledge of the importance of diet in the control of diabetes were major influences in bringing about the change. A measure of credit should be assigned to the food faddists who believe that only "natural" foods are wholesome and that if it's natural it has to be good, forgetting completely that toadstool and rattlesnake toxins are both highly deadly and entirely natural. It should be said in their defense that they rival some of the representatives of the meat and dairy industries in their devotion to an idea. They are just more ignorant. Lastly, the remarkable discoveries of Wurtman[29] and others that diet directly influences how the brain functions in adults has added a new dimension of scientific importance and respectability to nutritional research.

V. SOME NEGLECTED BUT IMPORTANT PROBLEMS

The intention of each of the following chapters is to present, along with an account of the present state of knowledge in each special field covered, some indication of the unsolved problems in that field and additional areas awaiting exploration.

We will mention here only four areas which, in the judgment of the editor, have not received the attention they deserve.

The remarkable effects of dietary restriction in postponing diseases characteristic of the second portion of the rodent life span and apparently prolonging healthy life beyond the normal life span of the species is a problem that has been intensively studied so far by only three investigators — Ross, Barrows and Goodrick. Yet these results, which open up many unanswered questions, are surely as new and challenging a discovery as the finding of Chittenden in 1905, described by Mathews,[13] that a man can carry on "ordinary exertions" on less than an ounce of protein per day while maintaining his weight and general health. It is to be hoped that the work on dietary restriction will be better utilized than that of Chittenden and his associates here and abroad. That discovery set off a violent controversy which spread as far as India. Some writers argued that only meat eaters were vigorous enough to maintain a high civilization or be effective soldiers. They overlooked a tribe of vegetarian but fierce warriors and the well-known fact that the most belligerent of bulls are strict vegetarians. If the discovery of the effects of the various modes of dietary restriction is pursued, it may turn out to be the most important nutritional discovery in the second half of this century.

A possible relationship of diet to arthritis was investigated extensively a decade and more ago. The results were negative. However, these studies, although involving many different diets, high versus low protein for example, were not designed to test for allergies. As is pointed out in a subsequent chapter where this subject is discussed, there is now a lot of data suggesting very strongly that food allergies are involved. Many and perhaps all of the "old guard" specialists in arthritis and allergies have met this suggestion with a hard dogmatism entirely out of place in any scientific problem, especially one with a multibillion dollar price tag annually, according to the literature of the Arthritis Association.

The importance for the aged of flavorful food, food which tastes good, is well recognized. So also is the sad fact that in many people certain flavors seem to disappear with age. It may be that something of the sort applies also to taste in the strict sense of bitter, sweet, sour, and salt, but ignorance is great in both these areas. Taste is not difficult to measure but the whole problem of olfaction and flavor is complicated by the collapse of the attractive molecular lock-and-key theory. Some progress has been possible without any adequate theory.

As in the case of dietary restriction, the investigators in this field are few indeed. Wolstenholme and Knight have a useful review.[28] Henkin and Schiffman[22,23] are almost alone, and neither of them are devoting full time to investigation in this field despite its not inconsiderable importance. John N. Labows, Jr., and others at the Monell Chemical Senses Center in Philadelphia are active in the field of olfaction, but their work centers on medical diagnostic uses of odor, on perfumes, and on human and animal body odors and their possible significance, and apparently not at all on changing abilities to detect the flavor of foods with human aging.

The possibility that the various food dyes, preservatives, and flavor enhancers may have especially deleterious effects on some of the elderly seems to have been overlooked. There now seems little doubt that they do work harm on some children and occasional adults. There are two reports,[15,16] sponsored by the National Academy of Sciences, on such substances, but this is only a beginning though a good one. It would seem that this is an entirely appropriate field for gerontological research, but here we again enter an area where administrators tend to walk "gingerly".

REFERENCES

1. Behnke, J. A., Finch, C. E., and Moment, G. B., Eds., *The Biology of Aging*, Plenum Press, New York, 1978.
2. Berg, B. N. and Simms, H. S., Nutrition and longevity in the rat. III. Food restriction beyond 800 days, *J. Nutr.*, 74, 23, 1961.

3. Brasel, J. A., Impact of malnutrition on reproductive endocrinology in *Nutrition and Human Reproduction*, W. H. Mosley, Ed., Plenum Press, New York, 1978.

4. Broad, W. J., NIH deals gingerly with diet-disease link, *Science*, 204, 1175, 1979.

5. Cutler, R. G., On the evolution of aging, in *The Biology of Aging*, Behnke, J. A., Finch, C. E., and Moment, C. B., Eds., Plenum Press, New York, 1978.

6. Denckla, W. D., Scott, M., and Bolla, R., Age-related changes in immune function of rats and the effect of long-term hypophysectomy, *Mechanisms of Aging and Development*, 11, 127, 1979.

7. Dietz, A. A., Ed., *Aging — Its Chemistry*, American Association for Clinical Chemistry, Washington, D.C., 1979.

8. Finch, C. E. and Hayflick, L., Eds., *Handbook of the Biology of Aging*, D Van Nostrand Reinhold, New York, 1977.

9. Goodrick, C. I., Fasting fosters longevity in rats: a preliminary account before the Gerontological Society, *Sci. News*, 116(22), 375, 1979.

10. Hall, G. O. and Marble, D. R., The relationship between the first year egg production and the egg production of later years, *Poultry Sci.*, 10, 194, 1931.

11. Henkin, R. I. and Bradley, D. F., Hypogensta corrected by Ni and Zn, *Life Sci.*, 9, 701, 1970.

12. Lytle, L. D. and Altar, A., Diet, central nervous system, and aging, *Fed. Proc.*, 38, 2017, 1979.

13. Mathews, A. P., *Physiological Chemistry*, 4th ed., W. Wood & Co., New York, 1927.

14. Moment, G. B., Tolmasoff, J. M., and Cutler, R. G., Superoxide dismutase, thermal respiratory acclimation, and growth in an earthworm, *Eisenia foetida*, *Growth*, 44, 230, 1980.

15. The Use of Chemicals, in *Food Production, Processing, Storage, and Distribution*, National Research Council Committee on Food Protection, National Academy of Sciences, Washington, D.C., 1973.

16. *Toxicological Evaluation of Some Food Additives, Including Food Colors, Enzymes, Flavor Enhancers, Thickening Agents and Others*, Nutrition Meetings Report Food and Agriculture Organization, Series No. 54, Unipublishers, New York, 1976.

17. Oata, K. T., Makinodan, Iriki, M., and Baker, L. S., *Aging Phenomena: Relationships Among Different Levels of Organization*, Plenum Press, New York, 1980.

18. Osborne, T. B., Mendel, L. B., and Ferry, E. L., The effect of retardation of growth upon the breeding period and duration of life in rats, *Science*, 40, 294, 1917.

19. Rockstein, M., *The Biology of Aging*, Academic Press, New York, 1979.

20. Ross, M. H., Nutritional regulation of longevity in *The Biological Basis of Aging*, Behnke, J. A., Finch, C. E., and Moment, G. B., Eds., Plenum Press, New York, 1978.

21. Sacher, G. A., Longevity, aging and death: an evolutionary perspective, *Gerontologist*, 18, 112, 1978.

22. Schiffman, S., Changes in taste and smell with age: psychophysical aspects in *Sensory Systems and Communications in the Elderly*, Ordy, J. M. and Brizzee, K., Eds., Raven Press, New York, 1979.

23. Schiffman, S., Orlandi, M., and Erickson, R. P., Changes in taste and smell with age: biological aspects, in *Sensory Systems and Communications in the Elderly*, Ordy, J. M. and Brizzee, K., Eds., Raven Press, New York, 1979.

23a. Shock, N. W., The science of gerontology, Progress and Papers, Conference on Gerontology, Duke University Council on Gerontology, Durham, N.C., November 19—21, 1959.

24. Strehler, B. L., Implications of aging research for society in *Biology of Aging and Development*, Thornbecke, G. J., Ed., Plenum Press, New York, 1975.

25. Thornbecke, G. J., Ed., *Biology of Aging and Development*, Plenum Press, New York, 1975.

26. Tolmasoff, J. M., Ono, T., and Cutler, R. G., Superoxide dismutase: correlation with life span and specific metabolic rate in Primate species, *Proc. Natl. Acad. Sci. U.S.A.*, 77, 2777, 1980.

27. Winick, M. and Brasel, J. A., Early malnutrition and subsequent brain development in *Food and Nutrition in Health and Disease*, Vol. 300, Moss, S. O., Mayer, H., and Mayer, J., Eds., New York Academy of Sciences, New York.

28. Wolstenholme, G. E. W. and Knight, J., *Taste and Smell in Vertebrates: A Ciba Foundation Symposium*, Longman, London, 1970.

29. Wurtman, R. J., Cohen, E. L., and Fernstrom, J. D., Control of brain neurotransmitter synthesis by precursor availability and food consumption, in *Neuro-Regulators and Psychiatric Disorders*, Usidin, E., Hambur, D. A., and Barchas, J. D., Eds., Oxford University Press, Oxford, 1977.

Chapter 2

NUTRITION AND AGE-RELATED CHANGES OF CARBOHYDRATE METABOLISM

Jeffrey B. Halter and Mei Chen

TABLE OF CONTENTS

I. INTRODUCTION

Noninsulin-dependent diabetes mellitus, or maturity-onset diabetes, is a condition of unknown etiology characterized by markedly abnormal carbohydrate metabolism that most often becomes clinically apparent in middle-aged or elderly people. A more subtle abnormality of carbohydrate metabolism, glucose intolerance, can be identified in a large proportion of apparently healthy elderly people. Since dietary factors can have a major influence on carbohydrate metabolism, the nutritional aspects of both noninsulin-dependent diabetes mellitus and glucose intolerance have received considerable attention, both from an etiological and a therapeutic standpoint. This chapter will review the alterations of carbohydrate metabolism occurring with age, the relationship between nutritional factors and carbohydrate metabolism, and the potential interaction between age-related nutritional changes and alterations of carbohydrate metabolism. The chapter will conclude with a discussion of current research problems in this area.

II. ALTERATIONS OF CARBOHYDRATE METABOLISM IN AGING

Aging in man is associated with a marked increase of both overt hyperglycemia and of glucose intolerance. The relationship between these two findings has been the subject of some debate and is discussed in detail below. However, from a clinical point of view a distinction between overt hyperglycemia and glucose intolerance is important. At the present time the diagnosis of diabetes mellitus is generally applied only to patients with overt hyperglycemia, and therapeutic interventions are limited to this group of patients.[1,2]

A. Diabetes Mellitus in the Elderly

Diabetes mellitus is a clinical syndrome characterized by a number of alterations of metabolic homeostasis which eventually are associated with neurovascular abnormalities in most patients. It is a common disorder, affecting 1 to 5% of the population, and is particularly common in the elderly.[2-4] Approximately ten times as many cases of overt diabetes are diagnosed in people over the age of 45 as in people under the age of 45. The most widely accepted marker for diabetes mellitus is the presence of hyperglycemia, i.e., an elevated circulating glucose level. However, the circulating glucose level in normal subjects varies considerably during the course of a day in relationship to meals and activity. Therefore, it has been difficult to precisely define the key term "hyperglycemia".

The most reproducible physiological circulating plasma glucose level is the level after an overnight fast (fasting plasma or serum glucose). People who have a clearly elevated fasting plasma glucose concentration (greater than 140 mg/dℓ) have a gross abnormality of carbohydrate metabolism. In the absence of a coexistent stressful illness, which can result in hyperglycemia in otherwise normal subjects, patients with fasting hyperglycemia meet even the most rigorous criteria for a diagnosis of diabetes mellitus.

The National Diabetes Data Group of the National Institutes of Health (NIH) has recently reclassified patients with fasting hyperglycemia into two general categories based on clinical, autoimmune, and genetic findings.[1] One group is ketosis-prone in the absence of insulin treatment, has an increased frequency of certain histocompatibility antigens, and tends to have islet cell antibodies. This condition has been termed insulin-dependent diabetes mellitus (IDDM) and tends to occur in young people, although occasional elderly patients will have similar characteristics. The other major category is patients who are stable metabolically in the absence of insulin therapy, are usually overweight, and have been termed noninsulin-dependent diabetics (NIDDM).

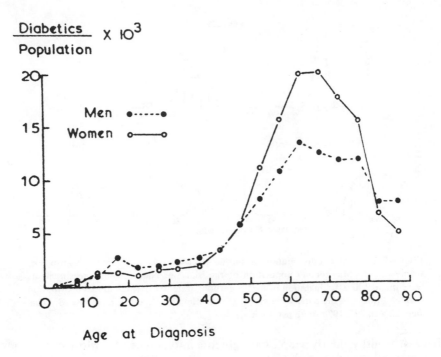

FIGURE 1. Increased incidence of diabetes mellitus in people over age 50. The relative incidence of diabetes was determined from newly diagnosed cases referred to a hospital clinic. (From Fitzgerald, M. G., *Textbook of Geriatric Medicine and Gerontology*, Brocklehurst, J. C., Ed., Churchill Livingstone, Edinburgh, 1978, 497. With permission.)

Although this condition may occur at any age (as shown in Figure 1), there is a marked increase in the incidence of NIDDM in people over the age of 50. Thus there appears to be an age-related factor which either directly or indirectly contributes to the development of NIDDM.

B. Carbohydrate Intolerance in the Elderly

The presence of fasting hyperglycemia identifies patients with grossly abnormal carbohydrate metabolism. However, there are other people who do not have fasting hyperglycemia, but who do have a more subtle alteration of glucose homeostasis. Although a number of provocative tests have been devised to identify such individuals, the most commonly used test has been the oral glucose tolerance test (OGTT). This procedure involves oral administration of a given amount of glucose, generally 50 to 100 g, and serial measurement of the circulating glucose level. A number of criteria for normality of the OGTT have been devised, based on tests in large populations of healthy people.[1,2,5,6] However, this procedure has limited usefulness in the early diagnosis of diabetes mellitus because of its lack of specificity. Long term follow-up studies of patients with abnormal OGTTs have demonstrated a low rate of progression to overt diabetes, generally in the range of 1 to 5%/year.[1,6-8] All such studies have found that the majority of patients with glucose intolerance have either an unchanged or actually an improved OGTT on follow-up testing. In addition, development of microvascular disease, which is part of the diabetes mellitus syndrome, has not been observed in longitudinal studies of people with impaired glucose tolerance, although there may be some increase in the incidence of large vessel atherosclerosis.[1,6,7]

A number of studies have demonstrated an age-related decline of glucose tolerance in man, as assessed by the OGTT. Depending on the specific criteria used, 10 to 50%

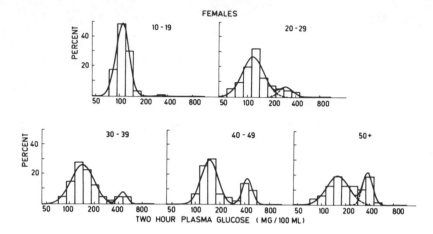

FIGURE 2.   Bimodal distribution of plasma glucose levels in different age groups of women of the Micronesian population of the island of Nauru. These measurements were made 2 hr after ingestion of a 75 g carbohydrate load. The bimodal distribution is most evident in the older age groups. (From Zimmet, P. and Whitehouse, S., *Diabetes*, 27(8), 793, 1978. With permission.)

of otherwise healthy elderly people have glucose intolerance.[5,8-11] Most studies in which glucose tolerance has been assessed by measurement of the rate of disposal of plasma glucose after intravenous glucose administration have also documented an age-related decline.[8-12] An effect of age on carbohydrate metabolism has been found in experimental animals as well as in man. Studies in rats have demonstrated an age-related increase of fasting plasma glucose levels as well as a decline of both oral and intravenous glucose tolerance. All of these findings have been reviewed in detail by Davidson.[8]

An important question that has been asked is whether the decline of glucose tolerance with aging observed in cross-sectional studies represents the appearance of mild diabetes in some people, while others are unaffected, or whether it represents a direct or indirect effect of aging in everyone. Studies in two small populations with a high incidence of diabetes mellitus, the Pima Indians and the Micronesian population on the island of Nauru, have demonstrated a bimodal distribution of plasma glucose levels (see Figure 2). These findings have been interpreted to be indicative of the presence of two populations, one with diabetes mellitus and one without.[13,14] Most of the age-related increases of glucose levels observed in these studies in the population as a whole could be ascribed to relatively large increases in the subpopulation with diabetes. However, smaller increases of glucose levels also occurred with age in the nondiabetic subpopulation. A similar interpretation has been made of a study of a U.S. population (Tecumseh, Mich.): the largest age effect occurred in the most hyperglycemic people; but an age effect was present, though less dramatic, in the entire population.[15,16]

In addition to an age-related decline of glucose tolerance, a number of studies have also reported that the fasting plasma glucose level increases with age, even when people with fasting hyperglycemia are excluded.[8] As shown in Figure 3, the age-related increase of fasting glucose levels is accompanied by an increase of levels of glycosylated hemoglobin.[17] Hemoglobin is glycosylated by a nonenzymatic reaction in which the glucose molecule attaches to the N terminal valine of the beta chain.[18] This process occurs slowly in vivo over the life span of the red blood cell. Thus the percentage of glycosylated hemoglobin reflects the average glucose level to which the red blood cell has been exposed over an extended period of time and has been used as an integrated measure of the circulating glucose level.[19-21] The finding of an age-related increase of glycosylated hemoglobin suggests that the mean glucose level over a period of weeks

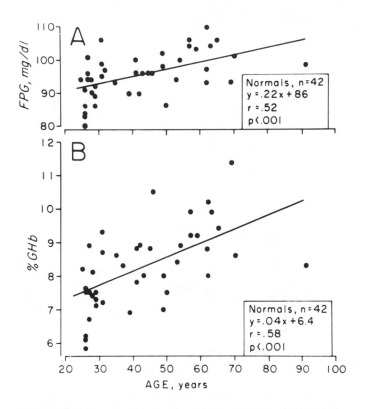

FIGURE 3. Age-related increases of levels of (A) fasting plasma glucose and (B) glycosylated hemoglobin, expressed as a percentage of total hemoglobin, in healthy volunteers. (From Graf, R. J., Halter, J. B., and Porte, D., Jr., *Diabetes,* 27, 834, 1978. With permission.)

is higher in older subjects, thereby confirming the physiological significance of the elevated fasting glucose levels and abnormal OGTTs that have been observed.

C. Aging and Insulin Secretion

One potential mechanism for hyperglycemia in the elderly is diminished insulin secretion. There is considerable evidence that islet function is impaired in all patients with overt diabetes mellitus, i.e., patients with fasting hyperglycemia.[22] However, as reviewed in detail by Davidson, studies in man and animals of insulin secretion with aging when overt hyperglycemia is not present have provided conflicting results — some showing increased insulin levels, others decreased insulin levels, and yet others showing no change with aging.[8] There are several reasons why studies to date have not provided a clear-cut answer to the question of whether there is an effect of aging per se on insulin secretion.

A major confounding variable in the interpretation of insulin secretion studies is the presence of obesity. An increased fat cell mass is associated with resistance to the action of insulin (see below). Most obese subjects are able to compensate for this insulin resistance by increasing insulin secretion so that glucose homeostasis is maintained, but at higher rates of insulin secretion.[22] As indicated above, many people who have overt diabetes or who have impaired glucose tolerance are overweight. Bagdade et al. have clearly demonstrated that proper interpretation of insulin secretion studies requires that body weight be eliminated as a variable.[23] They compared plasma insulin levels during OGTT in subjects age 40 to 60 of varying body weight who had normal or abnormal glucose tolerance. As shown in Figure 4, normal obese subjects had much

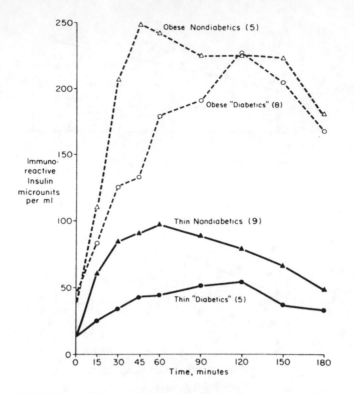

FIGURE 4.   Effect of obesity on plasma insulin responses during a 3-hr oral glucose tolerance test (100 g glucose). The "diabetics" all had glucose intolerance, but most did not have fasting hyperglycemia. The "diabetics" have lower plasma insulin responses than normal subjects of comparable body weight. (From Bagdade, J. D., Bierman, E. L., and Porte, D., Jr., *J. Clin. Invest.*, 46, 1549, 1967. With permission.)

higher insulin levels throughout the test than thin subjects. Obese patients with glucose intolerance ("diabetics") also had higher insulin levels than thin normals, but had *lower* insulin levels than the obese normals during the first 90 min. of the test. Thus the impairment of insulin secretion in the patients with glucose intolerance is only apparent in comparison to appropriately weight matched controls.

Such findings are pertinent to the question of whether insulin secretion is affected by aging, since adiposity increases with age. The increase of adipose mass in the elderly can at times be overlooked because of the concurrent fall of lean body mass in some people. As a result, as shown in Figure 5, net body weight may remain relatively normal, despite an increase of fat mass.[12,24-26] A comparison then of insulin secretory responses of old people with glucose intolerance (who are relatively obese and, therefore, have insulin resistance) with insulin responses of thin young people may result in a misleading interpretation. In order to properly compare insulin secretion in groups of old and young people, every effort should be made to match the groups for degree of adiposity. Ideally such matching should not be done on the basis of body weight alone, but should be based on some more direct measure of body fat mass.

An additional problem in the interpretation of insulin secretory responses during a test like the OGTT is the complexity of the pancreatic stimulus. Oral ingestion of glucose results in activation of neural signals to the islets as well as release of gastrointestinal hormones that can affect insulin release. The overall islet response is a complex function of integration of multiple neurohumoral signals plus the glucose stimulus

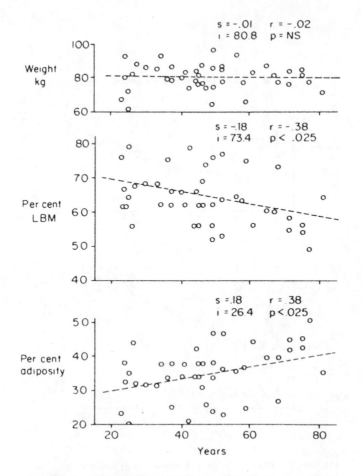

FIGURE 5.   Decline of lean body mass (LBM) and increase of percent adiposity with age in healthy male volunteers. Note that total body weight does not change with age in these subjects. Lean body mass was estimated from measurement of endogenous radioactive ^{40}K. s = slope; i = intercept; r = correlation coefficient. (From Ensinck, J. W. and Dudl, R. J., *Metabolism,* 26(1), 33, 1977. With permission.)

itself. Thus variable insulin responses can result from variation of any of these islet signals as well as from variation in the rate of glucose absorption from the GI tract.

In order to avoid these problems with the OGTT, a number of investigators have used the intravenous route to provide a glucose challenge. The insulin secretory response to an i.v. glucose challenge is multiphasic in normal human subjects as well as in isolated pancreas in vitro.[22] There is a rapid spike of insulin release (first phase) that occurs immediately after a glucose challenge and is over within 10 to 15 min. despite continued hyperglycemia. Subsequently, there is a gradual increase of insulin release (second phase) that continues as long as the stimulus of hyperglycemia persists. In old subjects with noninsulin dependent diabetes (patients who have fasting hyperglycemia), there is a gross impairment of the first phase insulin response to i.v. glucose.[27] Not only is the first phase response markedly impaired in such patients, but a paradoxical inhibition of insulin secretion has also been observed.[28] The second phase insulin responses of these patients are variably diminished, depending on the severity of the islet defect.[22]

Insulin responses to i.v. glucose in old subjects with glucose intolerance have been reported to be low, normal, or high.[8] The problem of adiposity, as discussed above in

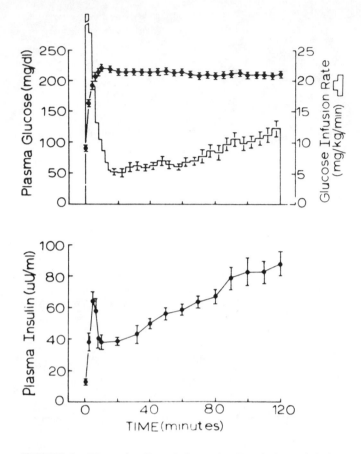

FIGURE 6.   Plasma insulin and glucose levels and glucose infusion rates during the hyperglycemic glucose clamp technique in healthy volunteers. This procedure can be used to assess both first phase and second phase insulin secretion in response to a constant glucose stimulus. (From DeFronzo, R. A., Tobin, J. A., and Andres, R., *Am. J. Physiol.*, 237(3), E214, 1979. With permission.)

interpretation of the OGTT, also applies to interpretation of the i.v. glucose tolerance test. In addition, patients with glucose intolerance have (by definition) higher plasma glucose levels during these tests. Thus the glucose stimulus to the pancreas will be different in young subjects with normal glucose tolerance than in old glucose-intolerant people.

In order to study insulin responses to a comparable glucose stimulus in different patient groups, the hyperglycemic glucose clamp technique has been developed.[29] In this procedure a pulse of glucose is administered i.v. to rapidly elevate the glucose level and a variable glucose infusion is given to maintain a constant level of hyperglycemia (see Figure 6). Using this procedure, Andres and Tobin compared the insulin responses of groups of young and old subjects at clamped glucose levels of 140, 180, 220, and 300 mg/dℓ.[10] They found decreased insulin responses in the old group at the three lower glucose levels, but normal responses at the highest glucose concentration. They concluded that β cell sensitivity to glucose was decreased in the elderly, but the response to a maximal challenge was unaffected. However, using the same technique, DeFronzo found no difference of insulin responses between old and young subjects at a clamped glucose level of approximately 220 mg/dℓ, and only a borderline impairment of insulin secretion in the old group at a lower glucose level.[30] However, DeFronzo also provided

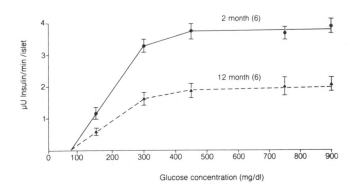

FIGURE 7. Decreased insulin secretion by isolated pancreatic islets obtained from 12 month-old rats compared to islets from 2 month-old rats. The figures in parentheses are the number of studies conducted for each age group. Decreased insulin secretion per islet was observed in the islets of the older rats even at maximal stimulatory glucose concentrations. (From Reaven, E. P., Gold, G., and Reaven, G. M., *J. Clin. Invest.,* 64, 591, 1979. With permission.)

evidence that these older patients had insulin resistance (see below). If this insulin resistance of aging is like the insulin resistance of obesity, a compensatory increase of insulin secretion would be expected (see Figure 4). Thus, the lack of such an increase in old subjects with insulin resistance could be interpreted to be indicative of an impairment of islet function.

Studies in experimental animals have also documented an age-related decline of glucose tolerance.[8] Just as in the human studies discussed above, several animal studies have not found evidence for an alteration of islet function with aging. However, these animal studies suffer from some of the same problems as the human studies — effects of adiposity and insulin resistance have not been separately evaluated, and insulin secretion has not usually been studied at comparable glucose levels in old and young animals.[8] More recently, insulin secretion by isolated islets of old rats has been reported to be markedly decreased compared to that of islets from young rats,[31,32] particularly since the total β cell mass was greater in the pancreases of old animals[31] (see Figure 7). On the basis of these findings, it was hypothesized that β cell dysfunction is an important factor in the glucose intolerance of aging rats. The development of hyperglycemia might obscure this deficit in vivo by stimulating an increase of β cell number which would tend to compensate for the insulin secretory defect of each cell.

D. Aging and Insulin Resistance

Resistance to the action of insulin could contribute to the development of hyperglycemia in the elderly. However, it should be emphasized that carbohydrate metabolism should remain relatively normal despite the presence of insulin resistance if there is a sufficient compensatory increase of insulin secretion.[22] Studies of tissue sensitivity to insulin with aging in man and in experimental animals have generally supported the idea that older populations have less tissue sensitivity to insulin than younger populations.

An age-related decrease of insulin effects on functions such as glucose uptake, glucose oxidation, and amino acid transport of fat and muscle cells in vitro has been reported in experimental animals by a number of investigators.[8] In addition, decreased binding of insulin to cell surface membrane receptors from liver, muscle, and fat cells has been demonstrated in older animals.[33-35] However, a number of these changes have been observed during the early rapid growth phase of animals, so have more relevance to the physiology of growth and development than to the aging process.[8]

An additional problem in interpretation of these studies has been to separate the effects of aging from the effects of increases of body weight. As mice and rats get older, they tend to become more obese and to have larger fat cells. Large fat cells have both reduced numbers of insulin receptors and post receptor defects of glucose metabolism.[36,37] These latter defects appear to be the major explanation for the insulin resistance of obesity. Attempts to separately evaluate effects of aging from effects of obesity have involved comparison of fat cells of different sizes from the same animal, comparison of fat cells of equal size from animals of different ages, and use of dietary manipulations to equalize body weights of animals of different ages. However, all of these approaches have limitations, particularly diet alterations which, as indicated in more detail below, can have major direct effects on metabolism.

Studies in man using relatively insensitive procedures such as determining the rate of glucose disappearance following i.v. insulin administration have provided conflicting evidence about whether tissue sensitivity to insulin decreases in the elderly.[8] Several more elaborate procedures have subsequently been devised to assess insulin sensitivity in man. One of these tests involves administration of constant infusions of insulin and glucose while suppressing endogenous insulin secretion by alpha adrenergic stimulation with epinephrine plus propranolol. The resulting steady state level of plasma glucose is then used as an index of the total body sensitivity to the level of insulin achieved by the insulin infusion. When this procedure was performed in a large group of nonobese men aged 22 to 69 who did not have fasting hyperglycemia, no age effect on the steady state plasma glucose level was observed.[38] However, the young group in this study population included a rather high percentage of people with glucose intolerance so that there was no overall age-related decline of glucose tolerance in the subjects of this study.

An alternative procedure not involving use of adrenergic drugs, which may be handled differently in old than young subjects, has been to use a variation of the glucose clamp technique described above, the euglycemic clamp.[29] In this procedure the circulating insulin level is raised to a certain concentration by a priming dose plus a constant infusion of exogenous insulin for 120 min. Glucose is then infused as needed to prevent the basal glucose level from changing. Total body glucose utilization during this procedure is then assumed to be equal to the amount of glucose infused plus endogenous glucose production. Endogenous glucose production can be estimated by using a constant infusion of radiolabelled glucose as a tracer, allowing glucose turnover to be calculated based on an isotope dilution principle. Subjects who are more sensitive to insulin will presumably utilize more glucose at a given insulin level and require a greater rate of glucose infusion to maintain euglycemia. DeFronzo has used this procedure to compare tissue sensitivity to insulin in weight-matched groups of young and old subjects.[30] The plasma insulin level was raised to approximately 100 μU/mℓ, resulting in almost complete suppression of hepatic glucose production in both groups. The amount of glucose infused to maintain euglycemia was approximately 25% less in the older group, suggesting that these subjects were less sensitive to exogenous insulin than the younger group.

The amount of glucose infused during the hyperglycemic clamp technique has also been used to assess tissue sensitivity to endogenously secreted insulin.[29] However, interpretation of the amount of glucose infused during this procedure is made difficult because the amount and time course of insulin secretion may vary considerably among subjects and because endogenous glucose production is not measured. DeFronzo has reported an age-related decrease of the amount of glucose infused during the hyperglycemic clamp (see Figure 8).[30] However, the major age effect occurred between ages 20 to 40 with no further decline in subjects over age 40. This finding is somewhat surprising, since glucose intolerance is unusual under age 40, but occurs with increasing fre-

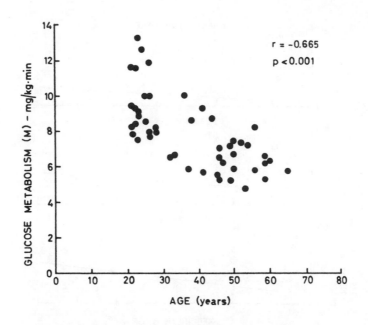

FIGURE 8. Correlation between age and the estimated amount of glucose metabolized during a hyperglycemic clamp study. The lower amount of glucose metabolized in older subjects is interpreted to reflect diminished tissue sensitivity to insulin in these people. (From DeFronzo, R. A., *Diabetes*, 28, 1095, 1979. With permission.)

quency in older populations. In contrast to this finding of DeFronzo, Andres et al. interpreted the results of their hyperglycemic clamp studies to show no effect of age on tissue sensitivity to insulin.[10]

As in animal studies, it may be difficult to separate age-related effects in man from findings secondary to increased adiposity. People who were obese by body weight criteria were excluded from the glucose clamp studies summarized above. However, as indicated previously and shown in Figure 5, the older subjects probably had relative increases of body fat. A number of studies have provided evidence for insulin resistance in human obesity. Binding of insulin by mononuclear cells and by isolated fat cells is reduced in obese people.[39-44] In addition diminished insulin-mediated glucose utilization has been reported in obese people using the euglycemic glucose clamp technique.[43] When euglycemic clamp studies were done at multiple insulin infusion rates,[44] impaired suppression of hepatic glucose production was demonstrated in obese subjects at lower rates of insulin infusion, but glucose production was fully suppressed in all subjects at higher insulin levels. In contrast, the impairment of glucose utilization in most obese subjects persisted even at maximal insulin levels. Since the capacity of cells to bind insulin greatly exceeds the amount of insulin that needs to be bound for maximal insulin effects,[45] it has been reasoned that insulin resistance due to diminished cellular insulin binding should be overcome by maximal doses of insulin. Thus, the impaired suppression of hepatic glucose production by insulin in obese patients has been felt to be compatible with an insulin receptor deficit. However, the impairment of glucose utilization is more likely to be due to a post receptor defect of glucose metabolism, as has been observed in isolated fat cells of obese rats,[36 37] than due solely to the receptor deficiency. It is of interest that there has been a report of an age-related increase of insulin binding to cultured human fibroblasts.[46] However, such an age effect has not been reported in a more physiological setting.

In addition to being a result of a primary alteration of tissue responsiveness to in-

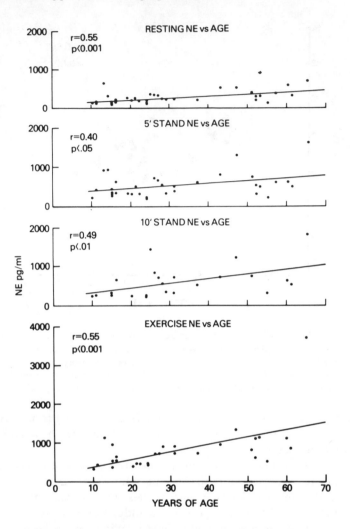

FIGURE 9.   Increase of plasma norepinephrine (NE) levels as a
function of age in men. Samples were obtained in the supine position,
during upright posture, and after a short period of isometric hand
exercise. (From Ziegler, M. G., Lake, C. R., and Kopin, I. J., *Nature,*
261, 333, 1976. With permission.)

sulin, insulin resistance can occur due to release of hormones which have anti-insulin
effects on carbohydrate metabolism. The corticosteroids, growth hormone, glucagon,
and catecholamines can cause increased glucose production by the liver and/or diminished glucose utilization by tissues, thereby potentially leading to glucose intolerance.[2]
There is no evidence that secretion of corticosteroids, growth hormone or glucagon
increases with age in man.[11,12] However, there is a report of an age-related loss of
glucagon suppression after glucose administration in anesthetized rats.[47] Circulating
levels of norepinephrine are increased in the elderly both in the supine position and
with upright posture or mild exercise[48-52] (see Figure 9). These increases appear to be
due to increased production, since the removal rate of infused catecholamines has been
reported to be either increased or unchanged, rather than decreased, in old subjects.
[52-53] Larger and more prolonged increases of plasma norepinephrine levels have also
been reported in a group of elderly subjects following oral administration of glucose.[53]
Whether the age-related increase of plasma norepinephrine is related to the glucose
intolerance of aging remains unknown.

III. NUTRITION AND CARBOHYDRATE METABOLISM

The nutritional state of an individual has been shown to have effects on several aspects of carbohydrate metabolism including circulating glucose levels, insulin secretion, and tissue sensitivity to insulin. Although short-term dietary manipulations can clearly affect glucose tolerance, there is no convincing evidence that overt diabetes mellitus can be precipitated by any specific dietary factor. Nevertheless, appropriate dietary intervention can markedly improve levels of hyperglycemia in many older patients with NIDDM.

A. Diet and Glucose Tolerance

Dietary preparation is part of the standard procedure for performance of an OGTT. Because of the recognized effects of carbohydrate restriction to impair glucose tolerance, a diet containing at least 300 g of carbohydrate per day should be followed for at least 3 days before an OGTT.[2,54] Although some OGTT preparatory diets require only 150 g of carbohydrate per day, Seltzer has pointed out that this amount may be inadequate.[5]

1. Caloric Restriction

Acute caloric restriction or starvation will result in a fall of basal glucose levels, but an impaired ability to regulate glucose levels following an intravenous or oral challenge. This carbohydrate intolerance of caloric restriction is likely to be a result of both an impairment of insulin secretion and of resistance to insulin action.

During total starvation basal plasma insulin levels fall, and insulin secretory responses to oral or intravenous glucose are impaired. These findings have been demonstrated in man as well as in both in vivo and in vitro studies in experimental animals.[55-59] Marked dietary restriction of carbohydrate, without a reduction of total calories, has also been reported to result in decreased basal and stimulated insulin levels in man.[60,61] However, the precise relationship between total caloric intake, carbohydrate content, and islet function has not been defined.

There is also evidence that starvation is associated with diminished tissue sensitivity to insulin. Insulin-mediated glucose uptake by forearm muscle in man is reduced during starvation.[62,63] In addition, in vivo resistance to insulin action during starvation has been demonstrated in man using the euglycemic glucose clamp technique.[43] However, binding of insulin to cellular insulin receptors has been reported to be increased during starvation in fat and muscle cells of experimental animals,[64,65] and in fat cells and circulating mononuclear cells in man.[40,43,66] This increase of insulin binding is presumably a response to the decrease of circulating insulin levels during starvation. Despite these increases of insulin binding, there is evidence of a decrease of insulin-mediated glucose transport and oxidation by rat adipocytes during starvation,[64] suggesting that effects of starvation on post receptor events may predominate over effects on insulin receptor binding. The effect of starvation on insulin-mediated glucose oxidation by isolated rat adipocytes is illustrated in Figure 10. Dietary carbohydrate restriction, in the absence of caloric restriction, is also associated with diminished glucose uptake and oxidation by isolated rat adipocytes.[67] In contrast to these findings in rat adipocytes, the sensitivity of isolated mouse or rat muscle to insulin effects on glucose uptake has been reported to be increased during starvation.[65,68] These findings raise the possibility that muscle insensitivity to insulin observed in vivo during starvation may be due to circulating antagonists of insulin action such as counter-regulatory hormones or products of lipolysis (free fatty acids or ketones).

2. High Carbohydrate Diet

The effect of a high carbohydrate diet to improve glucose tolerance has been recog-

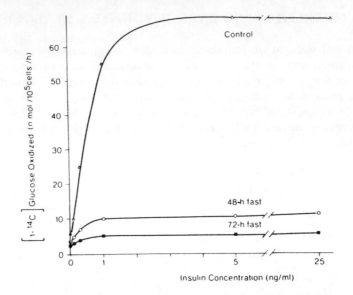

FIGURE 10.   Inhibition of glucose oxidation by isolated rat adipocytes during starvation. Cells from fed rats (control) were compared
with cells from rats fasted for 48 or 72 hr. The inhibitory effect of
fasting is observed even with maximal stimulatory insulin concentrations. (From Olefsky, J. M., *J. Clin. Invest.*, 58, 1450, 1976. With
permission.)

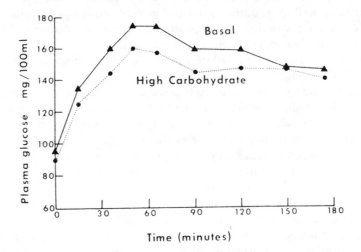

FIGURE 11.   Improvement of glucose tolerance by a high carbohydrate diet. Oral glucose tolerance tests were performed in 12 subjects
on a weight-maintaining basal formula diet (45% carbohydrate) and
on a high carbohydrate formula (85% carbohydrate). Plasma glucose
levels were significantly lower after the high carbohydrate diet both
in the fasting state and after oral glucose ingestion. (From Brunzell,
J. D., Lerner, R. L., Hazzard, W. L., Porte, D., Jr., and Bierman,
E. L., *N. Engl. J. Med.*, 284, 521, 1971. With permission.)

nized for many years.[5,69] An example of this effect is shown in Figure 11. Despite the
lower plasma glucose levels during OGTT on a high carbohydrate diet, plasma insulin
levels are quite similar.[70] This finding could be due to an enhancement of islet respon-

siveness to glucose by high carbohydrate feeding, to increased tissue sensitivity to insulin action, or to a combination of both effects. Although plasma glucose levels during a standard OGTT are lower when people are maintained on a high carbohydrate diet than when they are on a low carbohydrate diet, postprandial plasma glucose levels are higher when the carbohydrate content of a meal is high. As a result, postprandial insulin levels are higher when people are eating high carbohydrate meals than when they are on a regular diet.[71,72]

Isolated fat cells from both humans and rats maintained on high carbohydrate diets have increased rates of insulin-mediated glucose metabolism.[67,72,73] This increased sensitivity to insulin has been observed despite the findings that insulin binding to human and rat adipocytes is decreased by high carbohydrate feeding, presumably secondary to the increased insulin levels to which these cells are exposed in vivo. As in starvation, this dissociation of insulin binding from insulin responsiveness suggests that the effect of high carbohydrate diet on post receptor actions of insulin predominates over effects on insulin binding. Increased in vivo insulin sensitivity in man on a high carbohydrate diet is also suggested by the finding of a lower steady state plasma glucose level during infusion of insulin, glucose, epinephrine, and propranolol.[72]

3. Other Dietary Factors

Considerable evidence has been presented recently which indicates that the addition of plant fiber will attenuate increases of blood glucose levels following ingestion of glucose or a mixed meal in normal subjects and in patients with diabetes mellitus.[74-78] An example of this effect is shown in Figure 12. There is little evidence that the attenuation of postprandial hyperglycemia by plant fiber is due to enhancement of either insulin secretion or of tissue sensitivity to insulin. The most likely mechanism for this effect is a delay in absorption of nutrients.[79] Based on epidemiological evidence indicating a relatively low incidence of diabetes mellitus in an African population which routinely ingests a high fiber, high carbohydrate diet, Trowell has hypothesized that a diet low in fiber may contribute to the pathogenesis of diabetes mellitus.[80,81] However, there are a number of other genetic and cultural differences between such an African population and other groups which can contribute to a different incidence of a variety of diseases.

Experimental evidence has been presented that chromium, in a biologically active form found in brewer's yeast and known as the glucose tolerance factor (GTF), is necessary for maintenance of normal glucose homeostasis. A diet deficient in chromium leads to glucose intolerance in experimental animals, and severe chromium deficiency in rats has been reported to cause overt hyperglycemia and glycosuria.[82,83] These abnormalities can be reversed by chromium supplementation. Chromium deficiency has been reported in man during total parenteral nutrition and was associated with glucose intolerance, which improved with administration of chromium salts.[84,85] It has been suggested that GTF improves tissue sensitivity to insulin. When GTF was administered to mice with genetic diabetes, the blood glucose lowering effect of exogenous insulin was enhanced.[86] In addition, GTF has been reported to augment insulin-mediated glucose utilization by adipose tissue and muscle in vitro.[83] However, there is little evidence for a role of chromium deficiency in the pathogenesis of human diabetes mellitus.[87]

B. Dietary Therapy of Diabetes

Obesity is a very common finding in older people with NIDDM. As indicated above, obesity is associated with tissue insensitivity to insulin, a finding that is reversible with weight loss.[39,40,73] Since a reduction of insulin resistance would be expected to improve glucose homeostasis in an obese patient with NIDDM, weight reduction is a widely

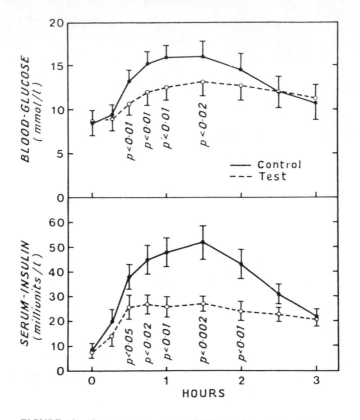

FIGURE 12.   Decrease of postprandial hyperglycemia in eight non-insulin dependent diabetic patients by addition of fiber to a standard meal (test) compared to hyperglycemia after the meal alone (control). Serum insulin levels were also lower after the test meal containing fiber. (From Jenkins, D. J. A., et al., *Lancet,* 2, 172, 1976. With permission.)

accepted therapeutic goal for such patients.[2,88] There is, in fact, substantial evidence that plasma glucose levels can fall considerably after weight reduction by obese patients with NIDDM[89-92] (see Figure 13). This beneficial effect can occur even with modest amounts of weight loss. Unfortunately, significant long term weight reduction is a therapeutic goal that is not often achieved with current dietary interventions.[93-97]

There is less evidence that dietary modifications other than caloric restriction for obese patients have any long-term beneficial effects on diabetes control. Diabetics are, by definition, intolerant to a glucose challenge and have greater and more prolonged plasma glucose elevations after an acute carbohydrate load. Therefore, in the past a restriction of carbohydrate intake was often recommended as part of the therapeutic regimen for diabetics.

However, two factors have caused this apparently rational approach to be reevaluated. First, diets low in carbohydrate calories are almost invariably high in fat calories. Since accelerated atherosclerosis is the leading cause of death in patients with NIDDM[2] and since high fat diets may be atherogenic, there has been great reluctance in recent years to recommend this type of dietary regimen. Second, a critical evaluation of the effects of high carbohydrate feeding to diabetics has not supported the concept that such a diet will cause deterioration of diabetes control. In fact, as indicated above, there is substantial evidence that high carbohydrate diets lead to enhancement of tissue sensitivity to insulin. Thus even an extremely high carbohydrate diet (85%) does not lead in short-term studies to worsening of hyperglycemia either in patients who have

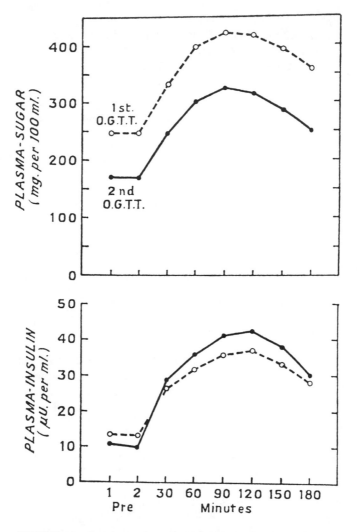

FIGURE 13. Improvement of plasma sugar levels of 118 diabetics during diet therapy. The first oral glucose tolerance test was performed before treatment and the second after 2 months of treatment with diet alone. The amount of weight lost during the diet period was a predictor of the plasma sugar response during the second OGTT. (From Doar, J. W. H., Wilder, C. E., Thompson, M. E., and Sewell, P. F. J., *Lancet*, 1, 1263, 1975. With permission.)

only glucose intolerance[70] or in treated overt diabetics.[98] Furthermore, long term treatment with a clinically practical high carbohydrate (55 to 60%), low fat diet does not result in worsening of diabetes control. Modest sustained improvement of both fasting plasma glucose levels and glucose tolerance has been reported in diabetics on a long term high carbohydrate diet.[99-101]

However, it should be reemphasized that total caloric restriction is the most effective dietary approach to diabetes management in patients who are overweight. For this reason, caloric restriction to achieve normal body weight is the major therapeutic recommendation for overweight diabetics in the most recent report of the Committee on Food and Nutrition of the American Diabetes Association.[88] Caloric restriction is not indicated in diabetics of normal body weight, most of whom have IDDM. For these patients a relatively high carbohydrate, low fat diet has been recommended. Since sev-

TABLE 1
COMPARISON OF EFFECTS OF NORMAL AGING
AND DIETARY FACTORS ON VARIOUS ASPECTS OF
CARBOHYDRATE METABOLISM

	Normal aging	Caloric restriction	High carbohydrate diet
Glucose tolerance	↓[a]	↓	↑[b]
Insulin secretion	[c]		
Basal	− or ↓	↓	− or ↓
Stimulated	− or ↓	↓	− or ↓
Tissue sensitivity to insulin			
Total body	− or ↓	↓	↑
Insulin receptors	−	↑	↓
Post receptor events (e.g., glucose uptake or oxidation)	?[d]	↓	↑

[a]   ↓ = decreased
[b]   ↑ = increased
[c]   − = no reported change
[d]   ? = no data reported

eral studies have demonstrated that postprandial hyperglycemia is attenuated in diabetics with addition of plant fiber to meals, it has also been recommended that natural foods containing unrefined carbohydrate and fiber be substituted for refined carbohydrate when possible. However, the long term effects of high fiber intake on diabetes management are not known.

IV. INTERACTION OF NUTRITION AND AGING ON CARBOHYDRATE METABOLISM

As indicated in the above discussion, it is clear that aging is associated with an alteration of carbohydrate metabolism and that carbohydrate metabolism can be influenced in a major way by the nutritional state of the organism. An obvious question which follows is whether there are nutritional changes occurring in older populations which contribute to the age-related changes of carbohydrate metabolism.

Dietary studies in the U.S. have found that the caloric intake is diminished in older populations.[102-103] Such studies have generally utilized the Recommended Daily Allowances of the National Research Council as a standard. Most of these studies have relied upon 24-hr dietary recall data, which may tend to underestimate calorie number. However, similar findings have been reported in other studies in which more reliable estimates of calorie intake have been used, including dietary histories and food records. Although not specifically studied, it seems likely that when total caloric intake is reduced, carbohydrate calories will be reduced proportionately.

A comparison of the effects of aging, caloric restriction, and high carbohydrate diets on several aspects of carbohydrate metabolism is presented in Table 1. Calorie restriction (generally starvation studies) has been found to have many effects on carbohydrate metabolism that are qualitatively similar to some of the findings in aging. High carbohydrate feeding has opposite effects. Therefore, it is tempting to postulate that some of the age-related changes of carbohydrate metabolism are due, at least in part, to diminished caloric intake. This hypothesis has been supported by Seltzer's findings that abnormal OGTTs reverted to normal after 300 g carbohydrate diet preparation in 11 of 16 elderly subjects.[5] However, there have been no studies comparing glucose tolerance in people of various ages in whom caloric intake has been carefully matched.

Since addition of fiber to meals has been shown to improve carbohydrate tolerance, it is possible that glucose intolerance in the elderly could be related to diminished dietary intake of fiber. However, there is little information on dietary fiber content in general and no information about possible changes with aging. No studies have been done of glucose tolerance in different age groups in whom dietary fiber intake has been controlled. Similarly, dietary chromium deficiency could theoretically lead to glucose intolerance in the elderly. There is one report of diminished excretion of volatile chromium in old men.[104] However, the relationship between this finding and glucose intolerance has not been defined.

V. RESEARCH PROBLEMS AND FUTURE DIRECTIONS

Much remains to be learned about the relationship between dietary changes in the elderly and age-related effects on carbohydrate metabolism. As indicated in Table 1, the effects of age on specific aspects of carbohydrate metabolism such as insulin secretion and tissue sensitivity to insulin remain relatively undefined. In addition, there is virtually no information on the effects of various dietary manipulations on these aspects of carbohydrate metabolism in the elderly. The problems to be dealt with in this area include the currently available methods for assessing glucose tolerance, islet function, and tissue sensitivity to insulin; and the effects of variables other than age and diet, such as obesity and exercise, which can also affect carbohydrate metabolism. In addition, there is the general problem with aging studies which, because of practical considerations, often must be done as cross-sectional rather than longitudinal investigations.

Dietary studies are, in general, rather difficult and expensive to do in humans. Such studies require highly motivated and cooperative subjects and generally must be done in a sheltered inpatient setting in order to assure compliance. The length of time that a test diet is used may be an important variable. For example, the time course of effects of high carbohydrate feeding on carbohydrate tolerance and tissue sensitivity to insulin could be different in old and young subjects. Failure to assess this possible effect might lead to misinterpretation of study results. Dietary manipulations are much easier to accomplish in experimental animals. However, extrapolation of the results of such studies to human physiology is particularly difficult because the "normal" diet of many experimental animals is vastly different from human diets.

A. Methods of Assessing Carbohydrate Metabolism

The OGTT has been the standard test utilized to assess glucose tolerance in man. However, this test has major limitations. As indicated above, oral glucose ingestion provides a complex islet stimulus. The size of the islet stimulus also varies with time, since glucose levels change during the test and presumably gastrointestinal and neural signals change as well. Thus it is virtually impossible to quantitatively compare insulin secretion in different age groups with this procedure. Although there is little evidence that glucose absorption is affected by age, there is virtually no information on whether there is an age effect on gastrointestinal hormone and/or neural responses to glucose ingestion. Because of the complex time-related changes of both glucose and insulin levels, as well as the neural and gastrointestinal factors, the OGTT provides little useful information about tissue sensitivity to insulin.

As indicated above, the hyperglycemic and the euglycemic glucose clamp techniques have been devised to deal with many of the problems with interpretation of the OGTT. However, both of these procedures must be performed in order to assess in a given individual both islet function (hyperglycemic clamp) and tissue sensitivity to insulin (euglycemic clamp). Each of these procedures is rather elaborate, requiring continuous bedside monitoring of arterialized plasma glucose levels to adjust glucose infusion rates over a period of at least two hours. In addition, the euglycemic clamp study provides an estimate of tissue sensitivity to only a single insulin level and the hyperglycemic clamp provides an estimate of islet responsiveness to only a single level of hyperglycemia. Expanding such studies to include the full dose-response relationship adds even more complexity.[44] Investigation of the effect of a particular dietary intervention would then require repetition of these studies.

Measurement of cell membrane receptor binding of insulin is another potential method of assessing insulin sensitivity, since insulin receptors are reduced in some insulin resistant states. Insulin receptor measurements can be made on blood cells, so such studies are feasible in vivo. However, interpretation of insulin binding assays is complex because insulin binding curves cannot be accommodated by a homogeneous class of receptor sites.[45] Furthermore, insulin binding appears to be primarily related to the circulating insulin level, and does not necessarily reflect tissue sensitivity to insulin. As indicated above, starvation is associated with tissue insensitivity to insulin despite an increase of insulin binding to tissues. Under these circumstances, impairment of insulin action on post-receptor events predominates over the increase of insulin receptor binding. Thus use of insulin binding measurements as the sole index of tissue sensitivity to insulin may lead to misleading conclusions.

An alternative approach to the assessment of tissue sensitivity to insulin and islet responsiveness to glucose stimulation has been proposed by Bergman et al.[105,106] They have developed mathematical models of the dynamic pattern of plasma glucose levels following an intravenous glucose injection in relationship to the time course of plasma insulin. One model analyzes the insulin levels as a function of the glucose levels during the test, providing an estimate of islet sensitivity to glucose. A second model independently analyzes glucose levels after glucose injection as a function of the insulin levels, providing an estimate of tissue sensitivity to insulin. Thus, it is potentially possible to simultaneously obtain an estimate of islet function and of tissue sensitivity to insulin from blood samples obtained after a simple intravenous injection of glucose. If this type of data analysis can be validated by comparison with more laborious procedures, such as the glucose clamp studies, it would provide a relatively simple way of studying the effects of various dietary interventions on carbohydrate metabolism in people of different ages.

In experimental animals it is possible to eliminate a number of the variables involved in studies in vivo by removing the tissues and studying them in vitro. Thus islet responsiveness in animals of different ages can be studied under comparable conditions in vitro, and effects of various diet manipulations can be assessed. Similarly, insulin responsiveness of specific tissues can be studied in vitro. Of course, the physiological relevance of such studies and their relationship to findings in man must ultimately be confirmed in vivo.

B. Other Variables Affecting Carbohydrate Metabolism

As indicated above, obesity is associated both with tissue insensitivity to insulin and an increase of insulin secretion (presumably compensatory for the insulin resistance). Thus a comparison of obese old people with thin young people will not provide information about age effects alone. The major problem involves the definition of obesity in the elderly, since the proportion of body weight that is fat increases with age (See Figure 5). Increased body fat is associated with increased fat cell size, and fat cell size appears to be closely related to fat cell sensitivity to insulin. Thus matching of such subjects on the basis of body fat rather than total body weight may be crucial. Interpretation of animal studies has also been complicated by the increase of body weight that accompanies increased age.

Exercise training is an additional variable which can affect carbohydrate metabolism and may be difficult to control in different groups of study subjects. There is now evidence that exercise training can alter insulin receptors and tissue sensitivity to insulin.[107] Caloric intake may also be different in groups of subjects whose daily exercise regimen differs. It is possible to estimate the physical training status of individuals by performing standardized exercise tolerance procedures. However, no studies of the effects of aging on carbohydrate metabolism have attempted to control for possible differences of physical conditioning among study subjects. Exercise regimens have been used in some animal studies in order to help maintain comparable body weight in old and young animals. However, the interpretation of a comparison between older, exercise-trained rats with younger, untrained rats becomes rather complex.

As indicated above, a variety of neuroendocrine glucose counter regulatory hormones can have major effects on glucose homeostasis. During acute illnesses the increased levels of these hormones contribute to the development of stress hyperglycemia.[2] However, circulating levels of norepinephrine are increased with age even in apparently unstressed healthy people (see Figure 9). The role of nutritional factors in this age-related increase of sympathetic nervous activity has not been explored, and the contribution of elevated catecholamine levels to the hyperglycemia of aging is unknown. It is clear, however, that studies of mechanisms by which nutritional factors influence the age-related changes of carbohydrate metabolism should include evaluations of glucose counterregulatory hormones.

VI. SUMMARY

The incidence of overt diabetes mellitus is markedly increased in older populations. In addition, there is a more general decline of glucose tolerance with aging both in man and experimental animals. Although impaired pancreatic islet function is an important feature of overt diabetes mellitus, the specific mechanisms underlying the glucose intolerance of aging remain poorly understood. This lack of understanding is primarily due to the complex interaction of multiple endogenous factors that determine glucose tolerance. These factors include pancreatic islet function, tissue sensitivity to insulin, and counterregulatory hormones which can affect both islet function and sensitivity to insulin as well as having direct effects on glucose production and utilization. The nutritional state of the organism is one of several environmental influences that can, in turn, affect the endogenous factors to alter glucose homeostasis. Thus, carbohydrate restriction appears to cause both an impairment of islet function and diminished tissue sensitivity to insulin. In order to define the role of nutritional factors such as low carbohydrate dietary intake in the glucose intolerance of aging, quantitative measurements of islet function, tissue sensitivity to insulin, and glucose counterregulatory hormones are needed in subjects of different ages in whom diet is tightly controlled. In addition, such studies must control for other influences which can affect these measures of carbohydrate metabolism such as body adiposity, exercise status, and stressful illnesses.

REFERENCES

1. National Diabetes Data Group, Classification and diagnosis of diabetes mellitus and other categories of glucose intolerance, *Diabetes,* 28, 1039, 1979.

2. **Porte, D., Jr., and Halter, J. B.,** The endocrine pancreas and diabetes mellitus, in *Textbook of Endocrinology,* 6th ed., Williams, R. H., Ed., in press, 1981.

3. **Fitzgerald, M. G., Malins, J. B., O'Sullivan, D. J., and Wall, M.,** The effect of sex and parity on the incidence of diabetes mellitus, *Q. J. Med.,* 15, 57, 1961.

4. **Fitzgerald, M. G.,** Diabetes, in *Geriatric Medicine and Gerontology,* Brocklehurst, J. C., Ed., Churchill Livingston, Edinburgh, 1978, 495.

5. **Seltzer, H. S.,** Diagnosis of diabetes, in *Diabetes Mellitus: Theory and Practice,* Ellenberg, M. and Rifkin, H., Eds., McGraw-Hill, New York, 1970, 1070.

6. **Keen, H., Jarrett, R. J., and Alberti, K. G. M. M.,** Diabetes mellitus: a new look at diagnostic criteria, *Diabetologia,* 16, 283, 1979.

7. **Jarrett, F. J. and Keen, H.,** Hyperglycaemia and diabetes mellitus, *Lancet,* 2, 1009, 1976.

8. **Davidson, M. B.,** The effect of aging on carbohydrate metabolism: a review of the English literature and a practical approach to the diagnosis of diabetes mellitus in the elderly, *Metabolism,* 28, 688, 1979.

9. **Andres, R.,** Aging and diabetes, *Med. Clin. N.A.,* 55, 835, 1971.

10. **Andres, R. and Tobin, J. D.,** Aging and the disposition of glucose, *Adv. Exp. Med. Biol.,* 61, 239, 1975.

11. **Andres, R. and Tobin, J. D.,** Endocrine systems, in *Handbook of the Biology of Aging,* Finch, C. E. and Hayflick, L., Eds., D Van Nostrand, New York, 1977, 357.

12. **Dudl, R. J. and Ensinck, J. W.,** Insulin and glucagon relationships during aging in man, *Metabolism,* 26, 33, 1977.

13. **Rushforth, N. B., Bennett, P. H., Steinberg, A. G., Burch, T. A., and Miller, M.,** Diabetes in the Pima Indians: evidence of bimodality in glucose tolerance distributions, *Diabetes,* 20, 756, 1971.

14. **Zimmet, P. and Whitehouse, S.,** The effect of age on glucose tolerance: studies in a Micronesian population with a high prevalence of diabetes, *Diabetes,* 28, 617, 1979.

15. **Hayner, N. S., Kjelsberg, M. O., Epstein, F. H., and Francis, T.,** Carbohydrate tolerance and diabetes in a total community, Tecumseh, Michigan, *Diabetes,* 14, 413, 1965.

16. **O'Sullivan, J. B.,** Age gradient in blood glucose levels: magnitude and clinical implications, *Diabetes,* 23, 713, 1974.

17. **Graf, R. J., Halter, J. B., and Porte, D., Jr.,** Glycosylated hemoglobin in normal subjects and subjects with maturity-onset diabetes, *Diabetes,* 27, 834, 1978.

18. **Bunn, H. F., Haney, D. N., Kamin, S., Gabbay, K. H., and Gallop, P. M.,** The biosynthesis of human hemoglobin A_{Ic}: slow glycosylation of hemoglobin in vivo, *J. Clin. Invest.,* 57, 1652, 1976.

19. **Koenig, R. H., Peterson, C. N., Jones, R. L., Saudek, C., Lehrman, M., and Cerami, A.,** Correlation of glucose regulation and hemoglobin A_{Ic} in diabetes mellitus, *New Engl. J. Med.,* 295, 417, 1976.

20. **Gabbay, K. H., Hasty, K., Breslow, J. L., Ellison, R. C., Bunn, H. F., and Gallop, P. M.,** Glycosylated hemoglobins and long-term blood glucose control in diabetes mellitus, *J. Clin. Endocrinol. Metab.,* 44, 859, 1977.

21. **Dunn, P. J., Cole, R. A., Soeldner, J. S., and Gleason, R. E.,** Reproducibility of hemoglobin A_{Ic} and sensitivity to various degrees of glucose intolerance, *Ann. Intern. Med.,* 91, 390, 1979.

22. **Pfeifer, M. A., Halter, J. B., and Porte, D., Jr.,** Insulin secretion in diabetes mellitus, *Am. J. Med.,* 70, 579, 1981.

23. **Bagdade, J. D., Bierman, E. L., and Porte, D., Jr.,** The significance of basal insulin levels in the evaluation of the insulin response to glucose in diabetics and nondiabetic subjects, *J. Clin. Invest.,* 46, 1549, 1967.

24. **Novak, L. P.,** Aging, total body potassium, fat-free mass, and cell mass in males and females between age 18 and 85 years, *J. Gerontol.,* 27, 438, 1972.

25. **Rossman, I.,** Anatomic and body composition changes with aging, in *Handbook of the Biology of Aging,* Finch, C. E. and Hayflick, L., Eds., D Van Nostrand, New York, 1977, 189.

26. **Lesser, G. T. and Markofsky, J.,** Body water compartments with human aging using fat-free mass as the reference standard, *Am. J. Physiol.,* 236, R215, 1979.

27. **Brunzell, J. D., Robertson, R. P., Lerner, R. L., Hazzard, W. R., Ensinck, J. W., Bierman, E. L., and Porte, D., Jr.,** Relationships between fasting plasma glucose levels and insulin secretion during intravenous glucose tolerance tests, *J. Clin. Endocrinol. Metab.,* 42, 222, 1976.

28. **Metz, S. A., Halter, J. B., and Robertson, R. P.,** Paradoxical inhibition of insulin secretion by glucose in human diabetes mellitus, *J. Clin. Endocrinol. Metab.,* 48, 827, 1979.

29. **DeFronzo, R. A., Tobin, J. A., and Andres, R.,** Glucose clamp technique: a method for quantifying insulin secretion and resistance, *Am. J. Physiol.,* 237(3), E214, 1979.

30. **DeFronzo, R. A.,** Glucose intolerance and aging: evidence for tissue insensitivity to insulin, *Diabetes,* 28, 1095, 1979.

31. **Reaven, E. P., Gold, G., and Reaven, G. M.,** Effect of age on glucose stimulated insulin release by the β-cell of the rat, *J. Clin. Invest.,* 64, 591, 1979.

32. Kitihara, A. and Adelman, R. C., Altered regulation of insulin secretion in isolated rat islets to different sizes in aging rats, *Biochem. Biophys. Res. Commun.*, 87, 1207, 1979.

33. Freeman, C., Karoly, K., and Adelman, R. C., Impairments in availability of insulin to liver in vivo and in binding of insulin to purified hepatic plasma membrane during aging, *Biochem. Biophys. Res. Commun.*, 54, 1573, 1973.

34. Soll, A. H., Kahn, C. R., Nevill, D. N., Jr., and Roth, J., Insulin receptor deficiency in genetic and acquired obesity, *J. Clin. Invest.*, 56, 769, 1975.

35. Olefsky, J. N. and Reaven, G. M., Effects of age and obesity on insulin binding to isolated adipocytes, *Endocrinology*, 96, 1486, 1975.

36. Czech, M. P., Richardson, D. K., and Smith, C. J., Biochemical basis of fat cell insulin resistance in obese rodents and man, *Metabolism*, 26, 1057, 1977.

37. Crettaz, M. and Jeanrenaud, B., Postreceptor alterations in the states of insulin resistance, *Metabolism*, 29, 467, 1980.

38. Kimmerling, G., Javorski, C., and Reaven, G. M., Aging and insulin resistance in a group of nonobese male volunteers, *J. Am. Geriatr. Soc.*, 25, 349, 1977.

39. Archer, J. A., Gorden, P., and Roth, J., Defect in insulin binding to receptors in obese man: amelioration with calorie restriction, *J. Clin. Invest.*, 55, 166, 1975.

40. Bar, R. S., Gorden, P., Roth, J., Kahn, C. R., and De Meyts, P., Fluctuations in the affinity and concentration of insulin receptors on circulating monocytes of obese patients: effects of starvation, refeeding and dieting, *J. Clin. Invest.*, 58, 1123, 1976.

41. Harrison, L. C., Marin, F. I. R., and Melick, R. A., Correlation between insulin receptor binding in isolated fat cells and insulin sensitivity in obese human subjects, *J. Clin. Invest.*, 58, 1435, 1976.

42. Olefsky, J. M., Decreased insulin binding to adipocytes and circulating monocytes from obese subjects, *J. Clin. Invest.*, 57, 1165, 1976.

43. DeFronzo, R. A., Soman, V., Sherwin, R. S., Hendler, R., and Felig, P., Insulin binding to monocytes and insulin action in human obesity, starvation and refeeding, *J. Clin. Invest.*, 62, 204, 1978.

44. Kolterman, O. G., Insel, J., Saekow, M., and Olefsky, J., Mechanisms of insulin resistance in human obesity: evidence for receptor and postreceptor defects, *J. Clin. Invest.*, 65, 1272, 1980.

45. Pollet, R. J. and Levey, G. S., Principles of membrane receptor physiology and their application to clinical medicine, *Ann. Intern. Med.*, 92, 664, 1980.

46. Rosenbloom, A. L., Goldstein, S., and Yip, C. C., Insulin binding to cultured human fibroblasts increases with normal and precocious aging, *Science*, 193, 412, 1976.

47. Klug, T. L., Freeman, C., Karoly, K., and Adelman, R. C., Altered regulation of pancreatic glucagon in male rats during aging, *Biochem. Biophys. Res. Commun.*, 89, 907, 1979.

48. Ziegler, M. G., Lake, C. R., and Kopin, I. J., Plasma noradrenaline increases with age, *Nature*, 261, 333, 1976.

49. Palmer, G. J., Ziegler, M. G., and Lake, C. R., Response of norepinephrine and blood pressure to stress increases with age, *J. Gerontol.*, 33, 482, 1978.

50. Prinz, P. N., Halter, J., Benedetti, C., and Raskind, M., Circadian variation of plasma catecholamines in young and old men: relation to rapid eye movement and slow wave sleep, *J. Clin. Endocrinol. Metab.*, 49, 300, 1979.

51. Rowe, J. W. and Troen, B. R., Sympathetic nervous system and aging in man, *Endocrine Rev.*, 1, 167, 1980.

52. Pfeifer, M. A., Halter, J. B., Wilkie, F., Cook, D. L., Brodsky, J., and Porte, D., Jr., Autonomic nervous system function and age related increases of blood pressure and heart rate (HR) in man, *Clin. Res.*, 28, 335A, 1980.

53. Young, J. B., Rowe, J. W., Pallotta, J. A., Sparrow, D., and Landsberg, L., Enhanced plasma norepinephrine response to upright posture and oral glucose administration in elderly human subjects, *Metabolism*, 29, 532, 1980.

54. Conn, J. W., Interpretation of the glucose tolerance test: the necessity of a standard preparatory diet, *Am. J. Med. Sci.*, 199, 555, 1940.

55. Cahill, G. F., Jr., Herrera, M. B., Morgan, A. P., Soeldner, J. S., Steinke, J., Levy, P. L., Reichard, G. A., Jr., and Kipnis, D. M., Hormone-fuel interrelationships during fasting, *J. Clin. Invest.*, 45, 1751, 1966.

56. Grey, N. J., Goldring, S., and Kipnis, D. M., The effect of fasting, diet, and actinomycin D on insulin secretion in the rat, *J. Clin. Invest.*, 49, 881, 1970.

57. Misbin, R. I., Edgar, P. J., and Lockwood, D. H., Influence of adrenergic receptor stimulation on glucose metabolism during starvation in man: effects on circulating levels of insulin, growth hormone, and free fatty acids, *Metabolism*, 20, 544, 1971.

58. Fink, G., Butman, R. A., Cresto, J. C., Selawry, H., Lavine, R., and Recant, L., Glucose-induced insulin release patterns: effect of starvation, *Diabetologia*, 10, 421, 1974.

59. Misbin, R. I., Edgar, P. J., and Lockwood, D. H., Influence of adrenergic receptor stimulation on glucose metabolism during starvation in man: effects on circulating levels of insulin, growth hormone, and free fatty acids, *Metabolism,* 20, 554, 1971.
60. Muller, W. A., Faloona, F. R., and Unger, R. H., The influence of the antecedent diet upon glucagon and insulin secretion, *N. Engl. J. Med.,* 285, 1450, 1971.
61. Anderson, J. W. and Herman, R. H., Effects of carbohydrate restriction on glucose tolerance of normal men and reactive hypoglycemic patients, *Am. J. Clin. Nutr.,* 28, 748, 1975.
62. Zierler, K. L. and Rabinowitz, D., Roles of insulin and growth hormone, based on studies of forearm metabolism in man, *Medicine,* 42, 385, 1963.
63. Owen, O. E. and Reichard, G., Human forearm metabolism during prolonged starvation, *J. Clin. Invest.,* 50, 1536, 1971.
64. Olefsky, J. M., Effects of fasting on insulin binding, glucose transport, and glucose oxidation in isolated rat adipocytes: relationships between insulin receptors and insulin action, *J. Clin. Invest.,* 58, 1450, 1976.
65. Le Marchand-Brustel, Y. and Freychet, P., Effect of fasting and streptozotocin diabetes on insulin binding and action in the isolated mouse soleus muscle, *J. Clin. Invest.,* 64, 1505, 1979.
66. Kolterman, O. G., Saekow, M., and Olefsky, J. M., The effects of acute and chronic starvation on insulin binding to isolated human adipocytes, *J. Clin. Endocrinol. Metab.,* 48, 836, 1979.
67. Olefsky, J. M. and Saekow, M., The effects of dietary carbohydrate content on insulin binding and glucose metabolism by isolated rat adipocytes, *Endocrinology,* 103, 2252, 1979.
68. Goodman, M. N. and Ruderman, N. B., Insulin sensitivity of skeletal muscle: effects of starvation and aging, *Am. J. Physiol.,* 236, E619, 1979.
69. Himsworth, H. P., The dietetic factor determining the glucose tolerance and sensitivity to insulin of healthy men, *Clin. Sci.,* 2, 67, 1935.
70. Brunzell, J. D., Lerner, R. L., Hazzard, W. R., Porte, D., Jr., and Bierman, E. L., Improved glucose tolerance with high carbohydrate feeding in mild diabetes, *New Engl. J. Med.,* 284, 521, 1971.
71. Reaven, G. M. and Olefsky, J. M., Increased plasma glucose and insulin responses to high-carbohydrate feedings in normal subjects, *J. Clin. Endocrinol. Metab.,* 38, 151, 1974.
72. Kolterman, O. G., Greenfield, M., Reaven, G. M., Saekow, M., and Olefsky, J. M., Effect of a high carbohydrate diet on insulin binding to adipocytes and on insulin action in vivo in man, *Diabetes,* 28, 731, 1979.
73. Salans, L. B., Bray, G. A., Cushman, S. W., Danforth, E., Jr., Glennon, J. A., Horton, E. S., and Sims, E. A. H., Glucose metabolism and the response to insulin by human adipose tissue in spontaneous and experimental obesity: effects of dietary composition and adipose cell size, *J. Clin. Invest.,* 53, 848, 1974.
74. Jenkins, D. J. A., Lees, A. R., Wolever, T. M. S., Hockaday, R. D., Goff, D. V., Alberti, K. G. M. M., and Gassull, M. A., Unabsorbable carbohydrates and diabetes: decreased post-prandial hyperglycaimia, *Lancet,* 2, 172, 1976.
75. Kiehm, T. G., Anderson, J. W., and Ward, K., Beneficial effects of a high carbohydrate, high fiber diet on hyperglycemic diabetic men, *Am. J. Clin. Nutr.,* 29, 895, 1976.
76. Jenkins, D. J. A., Leeds, A. R., Gassull, M. A., Cochet, B., and Alberti, K. G. M. M., Decrease in postprandial insulin and glucose concentrations by guar and pectin, *Ann. Intern. Med.,* 86, 20, 1977.
77. Miranda, P. M. and Horwitz, D. L., High-fiber diets in the treatment of diabetes mellitus, *Ann. Intern. Med.,* 88, 482, 1978.
78. Anderson, J. W., Midgley, W. R., and Wedman, B., Fiber and diabetes, *Diabetes Care,* 2, 369, 1979.
79. Anderson, J. W. and Chen, W. J. L., Plant fiber. Carbohydrate and lipid metabolism, *Am. J. Clin. Nutr.,* 32, 346, 1979.
80. Trowell, H. D., Dietary-fiber hypothesis of the etiology of diabetes mellitus, *Diabetes,* 24, 762, 1975.
81. Trowell, H., Diabetes mellitus and dietary fiber of starchy foods, *Am. J. Clin. Nutr.,* 31, S53, 1978.
82. Schroeder, H. A., Chromium deficiency in rats: a syndrome simulating diabetes mellitus with retarded growth, *J. Nutr.,* 88, 439, 1966.
83. Mertz, W., Chromium occurrence and function in biological systems, *Physiol. Rev.,* 49, 163, 1969.
84. Jeejeebhoy, K., Chur, R., Marliss, E., Greenbery, G., and Bruce-Robertson, A., Chromium deficiency, glucose tolerance, and neuropathy reversed by chromium supplementation, in a patient receiving long-term total parenteral nutrition, *Am. J. Clin. Nutr.,* 39, 531, 1977.
85. Freund, H., Atamian, S., and Fischer, J., Chromium deficiency during total parenteral nutrition, *JAMA,* 241, 496, 1979.
86. Tuman, R. W. and Doisy, R. J., Metabolic effects of the glucose tolerance factor (GTF) in normal and genetically diabetic mice, *Diabetes,* 26, 820, 1977.
87. Rabinowitz, M. B., Leven, S. R., and Gonick, H. C., Comparisons of chromium status in diabetic and normal men, *Metabolism,* 29, 355, 1980.

88. Committee on Food and Nutrition of the American Diabetes Association, Principles of nutrition and dietary recommendations for individuals with diabetes mellitus, *Diabetes,* 28, 1027, 1979.

89. Doar, J. W. H., Wilder, C. E., Thompson, M. E., and Sewell, P. F. J., Influence of treatment with diet alone on oral glucose-tolerance test and plasma sugar and insulin levels in patients with maturity-onset diabetes mellitus, *Lancet,* 1, 1263, 1975.

90. Hadden, D. R., Montgomery, A. D., Skelly, R. J., Trimble, E. R., Weaver, J. A., Wilson, E. A., and Buchanan, K. D., Maturity onset diabetes mellitus: response to intensive dietary management, *Br. Med. J.,* 3, 276, 1975.

91. Savage, P. J., Bennion, L. J., Flock, E. V., Nagulesparan, M., Mott, D., Roth, J., Unger, R. H., and Bennett, P. H., Diet-induced improvement of abnormalities in insulin and glucagon secretion and in insulin receptor binding in diabetes mellitus, *J. Clin. Endocrinol. Metab.,* 48, 999, 1979.

92. Stanik, S. and Marcus, R., Insulin secretion improves following dietary control of plasma glucose in severely hyperglycemic obese patients, *Metabolism,* 29, 346, 1980.

93. Stunkard, A. and McLaren-Hume, M., The results of treatment for obesity. A review of the literature and report of a series, *Arch. Intern. Med.,* 103, 79, 1959.

94. Bray, G. A., The myth of diet in the management of obesity, *Am. J. Clin. Nutr.,* 23, 1141, 1970.

95. Penick, S. B., Filion, R., Fox, S., and Stunkard, A. J., Behavior modification in the treatment of obesity, *Psychosom. Med.,* 33, 49, 1971.

96. Asher, W. L. and Dietz, R. E., Effectiveness of weight reduction involving "diet pills", *Curr. Ther. Res.,* 14, 510, 1972.

97. West, K. N., Diet therapy of diabetes: an analysis of failure, *Ann. Intern. Med.,* 79, 425, 1973.

98. Brunzell, J. D., Lerner, R. L., Porte, D., Jr., and Bierman, E. L., Effect of a fat free, high carbohydrate diet on diabetic subjects with fasting hyperglycemia, *Diabetes,* 23, 138, 1974.

99. Weinsier, R. L., Seeman, A., Herrera, G., Assal, J. P., Soeldner, J. S., and Gleason, R. E., High-and low-carbohydrate diets in diabetes mellitus, *Ann. Intern. Med.,* 80, 332, 1974.

100. Farinaro, E., Stamler, J., Upton, M., Mojonnier, L., Hall, Y., Moss, D., and Berkson, D., Plasma glucose levels: long-term effect of diet in the Chicago Coronary Prevention Evaluation Program, *Ann. Intern. Med.,* 86, 147, 1977.

101. Hockaday, T. D. R., Hockaday, J. N., Mann, J. I., and Turner, R. C., Prospective comparison of modified-fat-high-carbohydrate with standard low-carbohydrate dietary advice in the treatment of diabetes: one year follow-up study, *Br. J. Nutr.,* 39, 357, 1978.

102. O'Hanlon, P. and Kohrs, M. B., Dietary studies of older Americans, *Am. J. Clin. Nutr.,* 31, 1257, 1978.

103. Barrows, C. H. and Roeder, L. M., Nutrition, in *Handbook of the Biology of Aging,* Finch, C. E. and Hayflick, L., Eds., D Van Nostrand, New York, 1977, 561.

104. Canfield, W. and Doisy, R., Chromium and diabetes in the aged, in *Biomedical Role of Trace Elements in Aging,* Hsu, J., Davis, R., and Neithamer, R., Eds., Gerontology Center, Eckerd College, St. Petersburg, Fla., 1976, 119.

105. Bergman, R. N., Ider, Y. Z., Bowden, C. R., and Cobelli, C., Quantitative estimation of insulin sensitivity, *Am. J. Physiol.,* 236(6), E667, 1979.

106. Bergman, R. N. and Cobelli, C., Minimal modeling, partition analysis, and the estimation of insulin sensitivity, *Fed. Proc.,* 39, 110, 1980.

107. Vranic, M. and Berger, M., Exercise and diabetes mellitus, *Diabetes,* 28, 147, 1979.

Chapter 3

LIPIDS IN NUTRITION AND AGING

E. J. Masoro

TABLE OF CONTENTS

Much of the intense interest in lipids during the last quarter century relates to the possible role that adiposity plays in the pathogenesis of diabetes mellitus, hypertension, and atherosclerosis[1-6] and in the relationship between serum lipids and atherosclerosis.[7,8] Focus has been placed on nutrition as a major way of modifying body lipids and the related disease processes.[9] Since adiposity, hyperlipemia, and the related diseases are also age-associated events,[10] the interactions between age and nutrition in relation to lipid metabolism is also of great interest to gerontologists and geriatricians. The following is a review of the current state of knowledge in regard to nutrition-lipid interactions with the aging process.

I. ADIPOSE TISSUE MASS AND STRUCTURAL CHARACTERISTICS

It is established that in human populations of the developed nations fat mass makes up an increasing fraction of total body mass with increasing age at least until late middle age.[11,12] However, whether fat mass in humans continues to increase into old age or actually decreases at this stage of life is not clear from available evidence.[13-15] Although hypertension, diabetes mellitus, and atherosclerosis appear to relate to the amount of fat mass,[10] there is a lack of agreement as to whether fat content moderately above the so-called ideal level increases the mortality risk.[16]

An extensive study utilizing both longitudinal and cross-sectional designs on age and adipose tissue in male Fischer 344 rats has recently been carried out by Bertrand and her collaborators.[17] This study involved rats allowed to eat *ad libitum* and rats fed 60% of the *ad libitum* intake from 6 weeks of age on. The rats allowed to eat *ad libitum* had a median length of life of 24 months and a maximum length of life of 32 months while those fed the restricted diet had a median length of life of 36 months and a maximum length of life of 48 months. The longitudinal studies reveal that in the case of both the *ad libitum* fed rats and those fed the restricted amount of food, fat mass increased until about 75% of the rat's life span after which it decreased. Moreover, this late in life loss of fat mass did not relate to a general loss in body mass but occurred in some instances without a loss in body mass and in most of the other instances with a percent decline of body mass that was far less than the percent loss in fat mass. The cross-sectional studies on the perirenal and epididymal fat depots yielded results which fully support the conclusions drawn from the longitudinal study of total fat mass. Although the restricted rats have a lower fat mass than the rats fed *ad libitum,* this does not seem to be a factor in the life-prolonging action of food restriction for the following reason: since each rat of the population of rats fed *ad libitum* has a different amount of fat, it was possible to statistically analyze the relationship in this population between fat mass and length of life. There is no significant correlation between the amount of fat and length of life. Moreover, a similar analysis of rats fed the restricted diet revealed a significant positive correlation between maximum amount of fat attained and length of life ($r = 0.63$, $p < 0.001$).

It has been generally believed that adipocyte number is fixed in adults and that changes in depot mass in the adult involve increases or decreases in volume of existing fat cells. The validity of this concept which was based on studies involving only brief periods of the life span[18-21] has recently been questioned.[22] The studies that have caused a reevaluation involved the feeding of high fat diets in adult rats,[23,24] regeneration after lipectomy in adult rats,[25] and human obesity.[26] The study of Bertrand et al.[17] which did not involve high fat diets or surgical manipulations or obesity shows that the marked growth in the perirenal depot in *ad libitum* fed rats between young adulthood and late middle age occurred solely by increasing the number of adipocytes in this depot. In these same rats, the epididymal depot grew during this same portion of the life span solely by hypertrophy of existing cells. It is also of note that from late middle age to old age, even though there was a fall in epididymal mass due to a marked reduction of the size of the fat cells, a significant increase occurs in the number of adipocytes in the epididymal depot. The latter finding is in agreement with the work of Stiles et al.[27] who in addition showed that this increase in adipocyte number is not due to the early death of rats with smaller numbers of adipocytes in this depot.

Bertrand et al.[17] also found that the number of adipocytes were less throughout the life span in the depots of the rats fed the life-prolonging restricted diet than in those fed *ad libitum*. This clearly shows that food restriction can influence adipocyte number at times other than during the preweaning period.

II. SERUM LIPIDS

In human populations, most investigators have found that serum lipids increase with age.[28-30] A major focus has been the serum cholesterol levels. Studies on American, Northern European, and New Zealand men show that serum cholesterol rises from young adulthood until late middle age after which it declines.[31-34] Keys et al.[35] did not find this age-related change in serum cholesterol in Neopolitan men and suggested this might be due to the fact that Italians living in Naples eat a low fat diet. The work of Walker and Arvidsson[36] on South African Bantus provides further evidence that a low-fat intake may prevent the age-related increase in serum cholesterol. American and Northern European women also show an age-related rise in serum cholesterol which is less marked than in men, but continues until late in life.[37,38]

Serum triglyceride levels also increase with age in American and European men until middle age after which they fall.[39,40] In women, this rise is less pronounced early in the life span but is more prolonged.[39-41] South African Bantu men show no age-related trend in serum triglyceride levels.[41] In men, serum phospholipid levels rise during early adult life and appear to remain relatively constant thereafter while in women there is a gradual increase at least until late middle age.[42]

Carlson et al.[43] found that serum cholesterol, phospholipid, and triglyceride levels markedly increase with age in male Sprague-Dawley rats. Since these changes are similar to those occurring in men, Carlson et al.[43] suggest that the rat is a good model to investigate age-related changes in lipid metabolism in relation to man. Liepa et al.[44] found age-related changes in serum lipids of male Fischer 344 rats to be similar to those reported by Carlson et al.[43] for male Sprague-Dawley rats.

Liepa et al.[44] also studied the effects of life-prolonging food restriction on serum lipids. Food restriction started at 6 weeks of age did not influence serum cholesterol or phospholipid levels in young adults which shows that food restriction does not acutely affect the serum concentrations of these lipids. However, food restriction delays the age-related increase in these serum lipids. Serum phospholipid and cholesterol levels, which are reached by 18 months of age in *ad libitum* fed rats, do not occur until 30 months of age in rats fed the life-prolonging restricted diet.

It seems clear from the available data that there is an age-nutrition interaction in regard to serum lipid levels. However, much further work is needed to further define and to mechanistically understand this interaction.

III. LIPOLYTIC ACTIVITY IN ADIPOCYTES

Fat mobilization involves the hydrolysis of stored triglyceride to FFA (free fatty acids) and glycerol in the adipocyte and the release of these hydrolysis products to the blood.[45] One or more lipolytic enzyme(s) is or are involved; one of these which is called the hormone-sensitive lipase is regulated by hormones such as insulin and glucagon and by catecholamines.[45]

In 1972, Manganiello and Vaughan[46] reported that there is an inverse relationship between the body weight of rats and the responsiveness of their adipocytes to the lipolytic action of glucagon. They suggested that the loss in responsiveness might be due to an increase in size of the adipocytes which accompanies the increase in body weight. Since then, Holm et al.[47] showed that the marked lipolytic responsiveness to glucagon of adipocytes from 4-week-old rats is lost by 15 weeks of age, a change found to be unrelated to the dimensions of the adipocytes. Bertrand et al.[48] found that adipocytes from *ad libitum* fed male Fischer 344 rats of 6 months of age and older do not have any lipolytic response to glucagon. However, adipocytes from rats fed a life-prolonging restricted diet have full responsiveness to glucagon through 12 months of age and do not completely lose this response even when isolated from 36-month-old rats. It was also shown that the action of food restriction on glucagon-promoted lipolysis is not an acute one, but rather a long-term effect of this dietary regimen.

The molecular or cellular basis for this age-related loss in glucagon-promoted lipolysis has been the subject of study. Livingston et al.[49] found that this loss in lipolytic responsiveness to glucagon is accompanied by reduced glucagon binding by adipocytes. Cooper and Gregerman[50] found that glucagon did not activate adenylate cyclase in adipocyte ghosts obtained from 6-month-old rats. De Santis et al.[51] showed that elevated phosphodiesterase activity in the adipocytes occurred with increasing age. Voss and Masoro[52] found that in *ad libitum* fed rats there is a marked loss in the response of adipocytes to glucagon between 6 and 15 weeks of age of rats and that this loss is totally prevented by life-prolonging food restriction. Moreover, the changes with age in adenylate cyclase activity of adipocyte ghosts was found to parallel the changes in lipolytic responsiveness. Specifically, a marked loss in glucagon-promoted adenylate cyclase activity occurred between 6 and 15 weeks of age in the case of *ad libitum* fed rats but not with rats fed the restricted amount of diet. Although phosphodiesterase activity increased from 6 to 15 weeks of age, this progressive increase in phosphodiesterase activity was not associated with a loss in lipolytic responsiveness to glucagon in rats fed restricted amounts of food. Voss and Masoro[52] concluded that the major reason for the age-related loss in lipolytic response to glucagon in *ad libitum* fed rats is due to either a loss or change in the glucagon receptors or a derangement of the system coupling these receptors with adenylate cyclase and that food restriction delays and partially prevents this change.

Yu et al.[53] found that the effects of age on the response of the lipolytic system of fat cells to epinephrine differs from that observed for glucagon. At 6 months of age, fat cells from *ad libitum* fed rats are very responsive to epinephrine and food restriction from 6 weeks of age on has no effect on this response to catecholamines. With increasing age, however, the fat cells from *ad libitum* fed rats progressively lose responsiveness to epinephrine until by 24 months of age epinephrine has little effect. In contrast, adipocytes from rats fed the restricted diet show no loss in responsiveness to epinephrine until after 18 months of age and the extent of loss even at very old age (e.g., 36 months of age) is not great.

Although Giudicelli and Pecquery[54] also find that responsiveness of rat adipocytes to catecholamine declines with age, Miller and Allen[55] and Gonzales and De Martinis[56] do not. In analyzing the reasons for this difference, it appears that the difference in diet is probably the major reason. For example, Yu et al.[53] fed a diet containing 10% corn oil while Miller and Allen[55] and Gonzales and De Martinis[56] fed low fat diets. When it is further recognized that food restriction can greatly prevent the age-related loss in responsiveness to catecholamines, it seems reasonable to conclude that there is a nutrition-aging interaction that leads to the loss in the responsiveness of adipocytes to the fat-mobilizing action of catecholamines.

That this age-nutrition interaction observed in the in vitro studies with adipocytes also occurs in the intact rat, i.e., under in vivo circumstances, is shown by the work of Liepa et al.[44] They found that the postabsorptive serum FFA levels in rats fed *ad libitum* (10% corn oil containing diet) and those fed the restricted diet were the same at 6 months of age. However, with increasing age, the postabsorptive FFA levels fell in *ad libitum* fed rats but in rats fed restricted diets, this fall is delayed and much less marked. Since serum FFA levels are a good index of the rate of fat mobilization,[45] it seems likely that the ability to mobilize fat declines with age and that this decline can be modulated by dietary manipulations.

IV. LIPID BIOSYNTHESIS

Both in rat and man, increasing age reduces the ability to biosynthesize saturated and monounsaturated fatty acids.[57-59] Moreover, the response of the adipocytes to insulin, which increases glucose metabolism including fatty acid biosynthesis, is blunted with increasing age.[58] These changes in fatty acid biosynthesis may be of little physiological significance, however, since in adult rats and man, eating the usual mixed diet containing significant amounts of fat, fatty acid biosynthesis does not and need not occur at appreciable rates.[45] Although it has been shown that cholesterol biosynthesis decreases with age,[60] there is no information on how nutrition is involved in this age-related change.

V. UTILIZATION AND DEGRADATION OF LIPIDS

Lipoprotein lipase is involved in the utilization of triglycerides present in the blood in the form of chylomicrons (the transport form of dietary fat) or of very low-density lipoproteins. Huttenen et al.[61] have found that in both men and women lipoprotein lipase activity decreases with increasing age. Chlouverakis[62] found that as rats age the lipoprotein lipase activity of the adipose tissue declines, but not that of muscle and aortic tissue. Recently, Reaven[63] found that with increasing age the ability of rats of both sexes to remove triglycerides from plasma decreases. The activity of the metabolic systems involved in the degradation of cholesterol also decreases with increasing age.[60] However, the role that nutrition plays in these age-related changes in lipoprotein lipase activity and in triglyceride and cholesterol degradation remains to be explored.

VI. SUMMARY

Fat mass increases with age in man and in rats until late middle age. In rats, there is a decrease in fat mass from late middle age throughout old age. Reliable data on fat mass for this late part of the life span are not available for man. In rats, the number of fat cells increases throughout most of the life span in certain depots while in other depots this increase in adipocyte number does not occur until old age. The life span characteristics of adipose tissue of rats are markedly affected by life-prolonging food restriction. However, the life-prolonging effect of food restriction is not a result of the reduction in fat mass caused by this dietary manipulation.

In both men and rats, there is an age-related increase in serum lipids. In rats, life-prolonging food restriction does not influence serum cholesterol or phospholipid levels in young adults but markedly delays the age-related increase in these serum lipids.

The response of isolated rat adipocytes to the lipolytic hormones (glucagon and epinephrine) decreases with increasing age. This age-related loss in responsiveness can be delayed and partially prevented by life-prolonging food restriction. Evidence is presented which indicate that these findings also are true of fat mobilization in rats under in vivo conditions. It seems clear that there is a strong nutrition-aging interaction in regard to the fat mobilization system of rats. Further work is needed to know if this is also true of other mammals.

Lipid biosynthesis and lipid utilization and degradation are also influenced by age. However, there is no information on the role of nutrition on these age-related changes.

The conclusion to be drawn is that there is a strong nutrition-aging interaction on lipid metabolism. However, further research is needed to fully define the nutritional aspects of this interaction.

REFERENCES

1. Weinsier, R. L., Fuchs, R. J., Kay, T. D., Triebwasser, J. H., and Lancaster, M. C., Body fat: its relationship to coronary disease, blood pressure, lipids and other risk factors measured in a large male population, *Am. J. Med.,* 61, 815, 1976.
2. Medalie, J. H., Papier, C. M., Goldbourt, V., and Hernan, J. B., Major factors in the development of diabetes mellitus in 10,000 men, *Arch. Intern. Med.,* 135, 811, 1975.
3. Sims, E. A. H., Goldsmith, R. F., Gluck, C. M., Horton, E. S., Kelleher, P. C., and Rowe, D. W., Experimental obesity in man, *Trans. Assoc. Am. Physicians,* 81, 153, 1968.
4. Drenick, E. J. and Johnson, D., Evaluation of diabetic ketoacidosis in gross obesity, *Am. J. Clin. Nutr.,* 28, 264, 1975.
5. Tran, M. H., Lellouch, J., and Richard, J. L., Fat body mass. II. Its relationships with some biological parameters, blood pressure and physical training in a population of 8,660 men aged 20 to 55, *Biomedicine,* 18, 499, 1973.
6. Mann, G. V., Diet and diabetes, *Diabetologia,* 18, 89, 1980.
7. Kannel, W. B., Dawber, T. R., Kagan, A., Revotskie, N., and Stokes, J., III, Factors of risk in the development of coronary heart disease — six year follow up experience. The Framingham study, *Ann. Intern. Med.,* 55, 33, 1961.
8. Kagan, A., Kannel, W. B., Dawber, T. R., and Revotskie, N., The coronary profile, *Ann. N. Y. Acad. Sci.,* 97, 883, 1962.
9. Goodman, D. S. and Smith, F. R., Hyperlipidemia, arteriosclerosis, and ischemic heart disease in *Nutrition & Aging,* Winick, M., Ed., John Wiley & Sons, New York, 1976, 177.
10. Bierman, E. L., Atherosclerosis and aging, *Fed. Proc.,* 37, 2832, 1978.
11. Brozek, J., Changes in body composition in man during maturity and their nutritional implications, *Fed. Proc.,* 11, 784, 1952.
12. Malina, R. M., Quantification of fat, muscle and bone in man, *Clin. Orthoped. Relat. Res.,* 65, 9, 1969.
13. Novak, L., Aging, total body potassium, fat-free mass and cell mass in males and females between the ages of 18 and 85 years, *J. Gerontol.,* 27, 438, 1972.
14. Parizkova, J. and Eiselt, E. A., A further study on changes in somatic characteristics and body composition of old men followed longitudinally for 8 to 10 years, *Hum. Biol.,* 43, 318, 1971.
15. Myhre, L. G. and Kessler, W. V., Body density and potassium 40 measurements of body composition as related to age, *J. Appl. Physiol.,* 21, 1251, 1966.
16. Bray, G. A., Obesity in Perspective, No. (NIH) 75-708, U.S. Department of Health, Education and Welfare, Washington, D.C., 1975.
17. Bertrand, H. A., Lynd, F. T., Masoro, E. J., and Yu, B. P., Changes in adipose mass and cellularity through adult life of rats fed *ad libitum* or a life prolonging restricted diet, *J. Gerontol.,* 35, 827, 1980.
18. Knittle, J. L. and Hirsch, J., Effect of early nutrition on the development of rat epididymal fat pads: cellularity and metabolism, *J. Clin. Invest.,* 47, 2091, 1968.
19. Hirsch, J. and Han, P. W., Cellularity of rat adipose tissue: effects of growth, starvation, and obesity, *J. Lipid Res.,* 10, 77, 1969.
20. Salans, L. B., Horton, E. S., and Sims, E. A. H., Experimental obesity in man. Cellular character of the adipose tissue, *J. Clin. Invest.,* 50, 1005, 1971.
21. Greenwood, M. R. C. and Hirsch, J., Postnatal development of adipocyte cellularity in the normal rat, *J. Lipid Res.,* 15, 474, 1974.
22. Bulfer, J. M. and Allen, C. E., Fat cells and obesity, *BioScience,* 29, 736, 1979.
23. Lemmonier, D., Effect of age, sex, and site on the cellularity of adipose tissue in mice and rats rendered obese by high fat diet, *J. Clin. Invest.,* 51, 2907, 1972.

24. Faust, J. M., Johnson, P. R., Stern, J. S., and Hirsch, J., Diet-induced adipocyte number increases in adult rats: a new model of obesity, *Am. J. Physiol.,* 235, E279, 1978.

25. Faust, J. M., Johnson, P. R., and Hirsch, J., Adipose tissue regeneration in adult rats, *Proc. Soc. Exp. Biol. Med.,* 161, 111, 1979.

26. Ashwell, M., Durrant, M., and Garrow, J. S., How a "fat cell pool" hypothesis could account for the relationship between adipose tissue cellularity and the age of onset of obesity, *Proc. Nutr. Soc.,* 36, 111A, 1977.

27. Stiles, J. A., Francendese, A. A., and Masoro, E. J., Influence of age on size and number of fat cells in the epididymal depot, *Am. J. Physiol.,* 229, 1561, 1975.

28. Milch, L. J., Redmond, R. F., and Chinn, H. I., Serum lipoproteins during aging of Air Force flying personnel, *J. Aviat. Med.,* 23, 589, 1952.

29. Carlson, L. A., Serum lipids in normal men, *Acta Med. Scand.,* 167, 377, 1960.

30. Woldow, A., Hyperlipidemia and its significance in the aged population, *J. Am. Geriatr. Soc.,* 23, 407, 1975.

31. Keys, A., Mickelson, O., Miller, E. O., Hayes, E. R., and Todd, R. I., The concentration of cholesterol in the blood serum of normal man and its relation to age, *J. Clin. Invest.,* 29, 1347, 1950.

32. Montoye, H. J., Epstein, F. H., and Kjelsberg, M. O. P., Relationship between serum cholesterol and body fat mass, *Amer. J. Clin. Nutr.,* 18, 397, 1966.

33. Schaefer, L. E., Adlersberg, D., and Steinberg, A. G., Heredity, environment and serum cholesterol, *Circulation,* 17, 537, 1958.

34. Hunter, J. D. and Wong, L. C. K., Plasma cholesterol levels in New Zealand, *Brit. Med. J.,* 2, 486, 1961.

35. Keys, A., Fidanzia, F., Scardi, V., Bergami, G., Keys, M. H., and Di Lorenzo, F., Studies on serum cholesterol and other characteristics of clinical healthy men in Naples, *Arch. Intern. Med.,* 93, 328, 1954.

36. Walker, A. R. P. and Arvidsson, U. B., Fat intake, serum cholesterol concentration and atherosclerosis in the South African Bantu. I. Low fat intake and the age trend of serum cholesterol concentration in the South African Bantu, *J. Clin. Invest.,* 33, 1358, 1954.

37. Lewis, L. A., Olmsted, F., Page, I. H., Lawry, E. Y., Mann, G. U., Stare, F. J., Honig, M., Lauffler, M. A., Gordon, T., and Moore, F. E., Serum lipid levels in normal persons, *Circulation,* 16, 227, 1957.

38. Lawry, E. Y., Mann, G. U., Peterson, A., Wysocki, A. P., O'Connell, R., and Stare, F. J., Cholesterol and beta lipoproteins in serums of Americans, *Am. J. Med.,* 22, 605, 1957.

39. Schilling, F. J., Christakis, G., Orbach, A., and Becker, W. H., Serum cholesterol and triglyceride: an epidemiological and pathogenetic interpretation, *Am. J. Clin. Nutr.,* 22, 133, 1969.

40. Schaeffer, L. E., Serum cholesterol-triglyceride distribution in a "normal" New York City population, *Am. J. Med.,* 36, 262, 1964.

41. Antonis, A. and Bersohn, I., Serum-triglyceride levels in South Africans, Europeans and Bantu and in ischaemic heart disease, *Lancet,* 1, 998, 1960.

42. Schaeffer, L. E., Adlersberg, D., and Steinberg, A. G., Serum phospholipids, genetic and environmental influence, *Circulation,* 18, 341, 1958.

43. Carlson, L. A., Froberg, S. O., and Nye, E. R., Effect of age on blood and tissue lipid levels in the male rat, *Gerontologia,* 14, 65, 1968.

44. Liepa, G. U., Masoro, E. J., Bertrand, H. A., and Yu, B. P., Food restriction as a modulator of age-related changes in serum lipids, *Am. J. Physiol.,* 238, E253, 1980.

45. Masoro, E. J., Lipids and lipid metabolism, *Ann. Rev. Physiol.,* 39, 301, 1977.

46. Manganiello, V. and Vaughan, M., Selective loss of adipose cell responsiveness to glucagon with growth in the rat, *J. Lipid Res.,* 13, 12, 1972.

47. Holm, G., Jacobsson, B., Bjorntorp, P., and Smith, U., Effects of age and cell size on rat adipose metabolism, *J. Lipid Res.,* 16, 461, 1975.

48. Bertrand, H. A., Masoro, E. J., and Yu, B. P., Maintenance of glucagon promoted lipolysis in adipocytes by food restriction, *Endocrinology,* 107, 591, 1980.

49. Livingston, J. M., Cuatrecasas, P., and Lockwood, D. H., Studies of glucagon resistance in large rat adipocytes: ^{125}I-labeled glucagon binding and lipolytic activity, *J. Lipid Res.,* 15, 26, 1974.

50. Cooper, B. and Gregerman, R. I., Hormone-sensitive fat cell adenylate cyclase in the rat: influences of growth, cell size, and aging, *J. Clin. Invest.,* 57, 161, 1976.

51. De Santis, R. A., Gorenstein, T., Livingston, J. N., and Lockwood, D. H., Role of phosphodiesterase in glucagon resistance of large adipocytes, *J. Lipid Res.,* 15, 33, 1974.

52. Voss, K. H. and Masoro, E. J., An analysis of age-related loss of glucagon-stimulated lipolysis, *Fed. Proc.,* 38, 1027, 1979.

53. Yu, B. P., Bertrand, H. A., and Masoro, E. J., Nutrition-aging influence of catecholamine-promoted lipolysis, *Metabolism,* 29, 438, 1980.

54. Giudicelli, Y. and Pecquery, R., β-adrenergic receptors and catecholamine-sensitive adenylate cyclase in rat fat-cell membranes: influence of growth, cell size and aging, *Eur. J. Biochem.*, 90, 413, 1978.
55. Miller, E. A. and Allen, D. O., Hormone stimulated lipolysis in isolated fat cells from young and old rats, *J. Lipid Res.*, 14, 331, 1973.
56. Gonzales, J. and De Martinis, F. D., Lipolytic response of rat adipocytes to epinephrine: effect of age and cell size, *Exp. Aging Res.*, 4, 455, 1978.
57. Di Girolamo, M. and Rudman, D., Variations in glucose metabolism and sensitivity to insulin of the rat's adipose tissue in relation to age and body weight, *Endocrinology*, 82, 1133, 1968.
58. Gries, F. A. and Steinke, J., Comparative effects of insulin on adipose tissue segments and isolated fat cells of rat and man, *J. Clin. Invest.*, 46, 1413, 1967.
59. Gellhorn, A. and Benjamin, W., Effects of aging on the composition and metabolism of adipose tissue in the rat in *Handbook of Physiology, Section 5,* Renold, A. E. and Cahill, G. F., Jr., Eds., American Physiological Society, Washington, D.C., 1975, 399.
60. Kritchevsky, D., Diet, lipid metabolism and aging, *Fed. Proc.*, 38, 2001, 1979.
61. Huttunen, J. K., Ehnholm, C., Kekki, M., and Nikkila, E. A., Postheparin plasma lipoprotein lipase and hepatic lipase in normal subjects and in patients with hypertrigeridaemia: correlations to sex, age and various parameters of triglyceride metabolism, *Clin. Sci. Mol. Med.*, 50, 249, 1976.
62. Chlouverakis, C., Lipoprotein lipase activity in adipose, muscle and aortic tissue from rats of different age and in human subcutaneous adipose tissue, *Proc. Soc. Exper. Biol. Med.*, 119, 775, 1965.
63. Reaven, G. M., Effect of age and sex on triglyceride metabolism in the rat, *J. Gerontol.*, 33, 368, 1978.

Chapter 4

HUMAN AGING: PROTEIN AND AMINO ACID METABOLISM AND IMPLICATIONS FOR PROTEIN AND AMINO ACID REQUIREMENTS

Vernon R. Young, Mitchell Gersovitz, and Hamish N. Munro

TABLE OF CONTENTS

I. INTRODUCTION

The gradual loss of body cell mass[1,2] and even greater erosion of the skeletal musculature[3,4] that occurs during passage of the adult years reflects fundamental changes in the status of protein and amino acid metabolism in cells and organs,[5-7] modified by the influence of various environmental factors, including diet and nutritional status of the host. In turn, these various changes may affect the utilization of and requirements for dietary proteins and their constituent amino acids in elderly subjects and/or the capacity to resist unfavorable nutritional conditions or other stressful stimuli, such as infection and physical trauma. Thus it is pertinent to review here aspects of human protein and amino acid metabolism, with particular reference to aging, and then to examine them in relation to dietary requirements for protein and indispensable (essential) amino acids. Because we have reviewed this topic on a number of occasions,[4,8-11] the purpose of this chapter will be to present an update of the field, giving particular emphasis to recent studies carried out in our laboratories. An objective will be to identify areas in which further research is needed, in order to improve upon approaches that might be taken in the evaluation of protein nutritional status and quantitative determination of protein requirements in aging humans. No attempt will be made to review the molecular and cellular events of protein metabolism or the extensive work dealing with animal models, except where it might help describe observations obtained from direct human studies.

The discussion will begin with an account of methods used to study whole body protein and amino acid metabolism and their application in human adults. This will be followed by a brief review of specific organ and tissue protein metabolism in the aging human. The responses of body protein and amino acid metabolism to changes in dietary protein and energy intakes will be described in order to establish a metabolic basis for assessing methods and approaches used for estimating the dietary requirements for protein in human adults. Finally, current estimates of protein needs will be reviewed with an account of uses made of these estimates in relation to food and nutrition concerns in the elderly population.

II. WHOLE BODY PROTEIN AND AMINO ACID METABOLISM

A. N Balance and Its Limitations

Viewed in general terms (Figure 1), amino acids represent the currency of body protein metabolism. Their major disposition upon entering the free amino acid pools in cells is incorporation into proteins, following activation as aminoacyl-tRNAs, or catabolism via transamination and oxidative metabolism to carbon dioxide, water, and nitrogen excretory products, principally urea and ammonia. In addition to the supply of amino acids by the diet, the continued breakdown of proteins[12-15] within compartments of cells also contributes amino acids to the free amino acid pools which undergo a fate similar to those obtained from the diet.

Thus measurements of the intake of amino acids or of dietary nitrogen and the output of nitrogen via the major excretory routes, urine, feces and integument, have been extensively applied in studies of whole body protein metabolism in human adults. This approach involves a determination of nitrogen balance, and although this technique has provided useful information, it does not allow a detailed picture of the status and integration of protein and amino acid metabolism within the body. Nitrogen (N) balance measurements reflect only the balance between overall body protein synthesis and breakdown rates and, in theory, a given N balance may be achieved within a wide range of protein synthesis and breakdown rates (Figure 2). For this reason and because of the technical problems associated with the conduct of balance determinations and

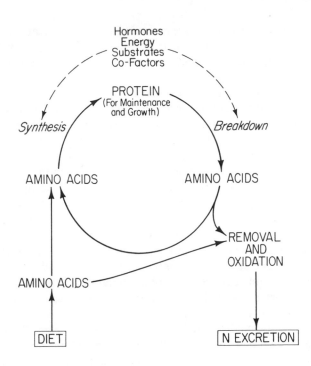

FIGURE 1. Schematic outline of the organization of amino acid metabolism in relation to protein turnover and the major fate of dietary amino acids. The difference between dietary intake (measured as N) and N excretion is a measure of body N balance.

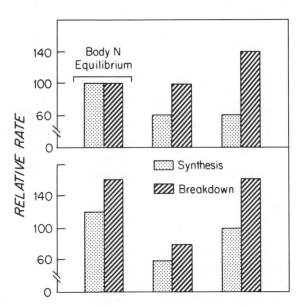

FIGURE 2. Changes in the relative rates of body protein synthesis and breakdown that may account for the development of a reduced or negative body nitrogen balance.

difficulties faced in the interpretation of N balance data,[11,16] recent research concerned with identifying the impact of aging on whole body protein and amino acid metabolism has focused on dynamic aspects of nitrogen and amino acid metabolism, studied with the aid of tracer techniques. Hence, before reviewing this area, it might be useful to discuss briefly the methodology involved in studies with human subjects.

B. Isotopes in Tracer Studies with Human Adults

The various phases of the economy of whole body nitrogen and amino acid metabolism that support body protein maintenance or bring about changes in body protein (nitrogen) balance, have been explored and quantified by use of isotopically-labeled proteins and amino acids and other N-containing compounds such as ammonia, urea, and creatinine. An extensively used label has been radiocarbon, ^{14}C. However, with increased ethical concerns regarding studies in humans and the regulation of human and clinical investigations, the nonradioactive tracers, such as ^{15}N and ^{13}C, offer a particularly attractive tool for study of in vivo protein and amino acid metabolism in adults. Furthermore, these stable isotope tracers enable comparative study in humans of all ages, thus the opportunity to examine protein and amino acid metabolism before reproductive maturity and during the onset of senescence. Indeed, there has been a rapidly growing use of stable isotopes in human metabolic research during the past 10 years, although discovery of stable isotopes and their potential for use in human investigations dates back about 50 years.[17]

The studies of Schoenheimer,[18] together with those of Sprinson, Rittenberg, and San Pietro,[19-23] utilizing ^{15}N-labeled compounds to explore whole body protein turnover and N metabolism established an earlier interest in the dynamic aspects of protein and amino acid metabolism in humans. The extensive work conducted during the past 10 years or so by Waterlow and his colleagues,[24] first in Jamaica and more recently in London, has advanced significantly the use of tracer techniques for study of the physiology of human protein and amino acid metabolism. These workers[24] have reviewed in detail the measurement of protein and amino acid turnover in mammals. The reader should consult this comprehensive survey for additional information about approaches used to study protein and amino acid metabolism in the intact host, especially men.

The increased production of stable isotopes,[25] coupled with analytical advances permitting convenient, practical determination of isotope enrichment in biological samples by coupled gas-chromatography mass-spectrometry,[26-28] now offers the possibility of exploring many exciting and important problems of amino and protein metabolism during human aging. Although several analytical techniques are now available for determination of the composition of stable isotopes of carbon, hydrogen, oxygen, and nitrogen in biological samples, each technique has its advantages and limitations. Currently, isotope-ratio and/or combined gas chromatography-mass spectrometry with selected ion monitoring are suitable for routine analysis of the relatively large number of samples generated in human metabolic studies. We have made extensive use of these methods during the past few years and their applications in the study of aging and protein and amino acid metabolism will be considered below.

C. Survey of Stable Isotope Approaches

The early studies with ^{15}N-labeled tracers in humans were conducted by giving a single, intravenous or oral dose of an isotopically labeled amino acid or precursor (e.g., ^{15}NH$_3$, [^{15}N]-glycine, [^{15}N]-aspartate), and measurement of isotope excretion as [^{15}N]-urea in the urine. Determination of the isotope enrichment in this end-product of N metabolism provided the means for estimating the rates of nitrogen turnover and protein synthesis in the body. Despite extensive use of this approach,[29] the single dose, end-product method involves several assumptions that are potential sources of error and these have been discussed in detail.[24] These assumptions include (1) the quantity of isotope administered must be a tracer amount in order to preserve metabolic homeostasis; (2) the distribution of the administered isotope in the metabolic pool is instantaneous and behaves metabolically as its unlabelled moiety. However, the distribution of an isotope, such as ^{15}N, throughout the metabolic pool involves separate finite processes due to factors related to rates of transamination, mixing of the labeled amino acids among organs and entry into cells. Thus instantaneous mixing is not likely to be achieved. Nevertheless, Waterlow et al.,[30] and Garlick et al.[31] have been shown that ^{15}N-glycine given as a single oral dose and measurement of ^{15}N in urinary ammonia offers a useful approach for comparative studies of whole body protein synthesis and breakdown rate under various pathophysiological conditions.

Following introduction of the single dose, end-product method, investigators then explored whole body protein and amino acid metabolism using a single tracer dose approach that was based on measurement of the enrichment of tracer in the plasma compartment.[29] This approach has been used recently to explore dynamic aspects of ^{15}N-glycine and ^{15}N-alanine metabolism in experimental animals[32,33] and human subjects.[34,35]

The method of continuous isotope infusion has been explored extensively and promoted by Waterlow and co-workers,[24] in order to overcome some of the difficulties inherent in the single isotope dose approaches. The continuous infusion of tracer may either be coupled with measurement of end products of N metabolism, as in the case of the Picou and Taylor-Roberts[36] model, or with determination of the enrichment of isotope (^{15}N or ^{13}C) in plasma following administration of a labeled amino acid or precursor.[37,38] Together with measurement of ^{13}C in expired CO_2 or ^{15}N in urinary urea or other excretory products, whole body amino acid flux can be examined for its major components as discussed below. This method, is, of course, applicable with radioisotopes.[38-41]

Although none of the current approaches gives a comprehensive picture of whole body protein dynamics, we believe that the most reliable and incisive first approach for estimating rates of whole body protein turnover and quantitative aspects of whole body protein and amino acid metabolism is the constant infusion technique, using a combined plasma and end-product analysis.[42] Our initial studies on protein metabolism in elderly subjects utilized the continuous isotope administration-end product method with ^{15}N-glycine, as described by Picou and Taylor-Roberts.[36] Some of the observations made with this latter approach (Figure 3) to examine the effects of adult age on protein metabolism will be discussed below.

The constant isotope infusion model of body amino acid and protein metabolism, involving measurement of stable isotope enrichment in plasma and in excretory products, views body N metabolism according to a metabolic pool from which amino acids leave via pathways of protein anabolism or via oxidative catabolism (Figure 4). The major inflow of nitrogen or amino acids into the metabolic pool is via the diet and/or via breakdown of cell and tissue proteins. These major routes of amino acid and N flow can be quantified by administration of labeled amino acids and measurement of the dilution of the stable isotope tracer in the free amino acid in blood plasma,[42,43] and its appearance in excretory products such as in expired air ($^{13}CO_2$) or in urinary nitrogen components (^{15}N in urea, ammonia or total N).[30,44] Thus, for example, the specific model (Figure 5) used for measurement of body leucine flux and its major components (rates of leucine oxidation, incorporation into body protein, and entry into the metabolic pool via protein breakdown and from dietary sources) represents a form of stochastic analysis in which the overall process is measured and not the intermediate pools and/or their exchanges. Briefly, the model assumes a single metabolic pool that serves as the source of leucine for protein synthesis and also the site of leucine oxidation. This extravascular, free leucine pool is in rapid isotopic equilibrium with plasma pool and so the latter is used for sampling to assess the isotope conditions in

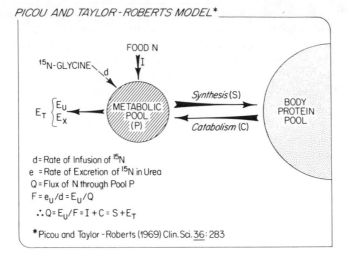

FIGURE 3.   The Picou and Taylor-Roberts model of whole body N metabolism, based on infusion of ^{15}N-glycine and the measurement of ^{15}N enrichment in urinary urea following an isotopic steady state. Q = N flux in the metabolic pool; E_u = total urinary urea N output; E_T = total N excretion. (From Picou, D. and Taylor-Roberts, T., *Clin. Sci.*, 36, 283, 1969. With permission.)

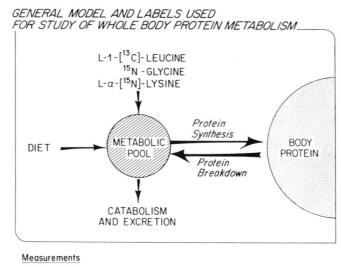

FIGURE 4.   General model of body protein and amino acid metabolism using a continuous infusion of amino acids labeled with ^{15}N or [13]C.

the metabolic pool. Movement of the isotopic tracer through the metabolic pool into pathways of protein synthesis and amino acid oxidation is taken to be unidirectional for the short duration of the experiment, an assumption that appears to be valid.[45] For labeled leucine (or other essential amino acids, such as lysine), this reflects the fact that label leaving the plasma compartment enters protein and thus is diluted by a

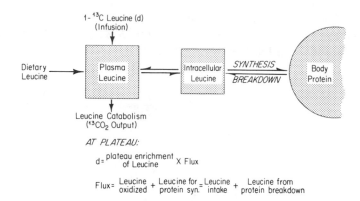

FIGURE 5. Model of whole body leucine metabolism, described initially by Waterlow and his colleagues[34] and with application of 1-^{13}C-leucine (From Matthews et al., *Am. J. Physiol.*, 238, E473, 1980. With permission.)

large nonisotopic "sink". Also, when leucine is catabolized in the metabolic pool, the labeled carboxyl carbon is lost as $^{13}CO_2$, further minimizing recycling. Thus with constant infusion of a stable state of isotope enrichment (plateau) of the free amino acid is achieved in the metabolic and excretory pools and this can be monitored by sampling blood, urine, and expired air ($^{13}CO_2$ only).[42] Furthermore, an isotopic steady state in expired $^{13}CO_2$ serves to confirm that there is isotopic equilibrium in the intracellular leucine pool. This model is, of course, an oversimplification of the complexity of whole body amino acid metabolism. Nonetheless, this stochastic approach provides a reliable means of exploring the dynamic status of whole body amino acid metabolism in the intact human subject under various physiological and pathological conditions.

We have also used this constant isotope infusion approach for the study of lysine metabolism, using ^{15}N-lysine as the tracer.[46] However, use of this particular label restricts investigation of whole body lysine metabolism to that of lysine flux and rate of lysine entry into the metabolic pool from endogenous and exogenous sources.

D. Whole Body Protein Turnover in Relation to Aging

During early growth and development in rats, and other experimental animals, the rates of whole body and muscle protein synthesis and breakdown are high initially and these fall with attainment of adulthood and reproductive maturity.[47,48] A similar pattern of change occurs in human subjects, and some published estimates of the rates of body protein synthesis during different phases of growth and development are summarized in Table 1. Although there is a wide variation in the reported estimates for the various age groups, due, in part, to differences and problems in the methodology, it seems clear that the rate of whole body protein synthesis and turnover during the neonatal period is high and declines to lower levels during the early years of life.

A more pertinent question, however, is the effect of advancement of the adult years in humans or of progressive aging in experimental animals on in vivo rates of tissue and whole body protein synthesis and breakdown. The report of Sharp et al.[56] suggests that the rate of whole body protein synthesis is lower in elderly people than in young adults. However, this study was limited to one young adult male and female and four older subjects, two males and two females.

Golden and Waterlow[44] and we have estimated rates of whole body protein synthesis and breakdown in young adults and healthy elderly subjects of both sexes, using the ^{15}N-glycine method of Picou and Taylor-Roberts.[36] The results of our cross-sectional studies show only small, but at times statistically significant, differences in these rates

Table 1

A SELECTED SURVEY OF ESTIMATES OF WHOLE BODY PROTEIN
SYNTHESIS RATES IN INFANTS, CHILDREN, ADOLESCENTS, AND
YOUNG ADULTS

Group	No. subjects	Age	Approach	Protein synthesis (g protein kg^{-1}day^{-1})	Ref.
Premature infants	3	42—68 days	^{15}N-glycine, PO	10—15.5	49
Premature infants	5	1—45 days	^{15}N-glycine, PO, infusion	26	50
Infants	5	10—20 months	^{15}N-glycine, infusion	6.1	36
Infants	5	15 months	^{15}N-glycine, infusion	6.4	51
Young children	5	[a]	^{15}N-glycine, infusion	6.9	52
Children	8	9—16 years	^{15}N-glycine, PO, infusion	3.7	53
Adolescents	5[b]	11—15 years	^{15}N-glycine, PO, infusion	5.7	54
Young adults	6	20—25 years	^{15}N-glycine, PO, infusion	3	55
Young adult men	40 studies	18—25 years	1-^{13}C-leucine, infusion	3.3	42

Note: PO = per os (by mouth).

[a] Not given.
[b] Obese subjects. Results expressed per ideal body weight.

between young adult and older subjects, when results are expressed per unit of body weight.[57,58] Because of the differences in body composition between young and elderly adults, we have examined rates of whole body protein synthesis and breakdown in relation to indices of body composition, namely, creatinine as an index of muscle mass, and body cell mass determined by whole body ^{40}K measurement. The results of a recent series of studies are summarized in Table 2. As can be seen, whole body protein synthesis and breakdown rates per unit of creatinine excretion were higher in the elderly than in young adults. Also these rates tended to be higher in the older subjects when expressed per unit of body cell mass. These findings may reflect a lower contribution by muscle to whole body protein synthesis and breakdown in the elderly than in young adults, since a reduced muscle mass would result in reduced creatinine excretion,[59] and because protein turnover is more rapid in visceral organs, including liver and intestines, than in muscle.[24]

E. Contribution Made by Skeletal Muscle to Whole Body Protein Turnover

The above interpretation can be explored by estimating rates of muscle protein breakdown in relation to whole body protein breakdown. This is accomplished in humans by measurement of urinary N^{τ}-methylhistidine (3-methylhistidine) excretion. We[60] have reviewed the evidence indicating that the output of this amino acid provides an index of the breakdown of muscle protein in vivo in both rats and human subjects.

Table 2
COMPARISION OF RATES OF
WHOLE BODY PROTEIN SYNTHESIS
IN YOUNG MEN AND ELDERLY
MALES

Parameter	Young men	Elderly men
Age (year)	21 ± 1[a]	72 ± 2
Body wt. (kg)	77 ± 5	69 ± 4
Body cell mass (kg)	37.6 ± 3.3	25.9 ± 1.4
BCM (% body wt.)	48 ± 1	38 ± 1
Creatinine excretion		
(g/day)	2.1 ± 0.2	1.3 ± 0.1
(mg/kgBCM/day)	55 ± 0.6	50 ± 1.6
Whole body protein synthesis (g)		
Per kg/day	3.1 ± 0.2	3.1 ± 0.2
Per kg BCM[b]	6.5 ± 0.3	8.1 ± 0.6
Per g creatinine	118 ± 6	165 ± 16
Whole body protein breakdown		
g/kg/day	3.0 ± 0.2	2.7 ± 0.2

[a]　Mean ± SEM for 5 young and 6 elderly men. Unpublished data of M. Gersovitz, H. N. Munro and V. R. Young.

[b]　BCM = Body cell mass determined from whole body ⁴⁰K.

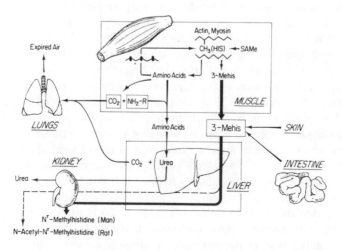
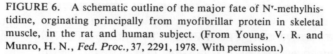

FIGURE 6.　A schematic outline of the major fate of Nᵗ-methylhistidine, orginating principally from myofibrillar protein in skeletal muscle, in the rat and human subject. (From Young, V. R. and Munro, H. N., *Fed. Proc.*, 37, 2291, 1978. With permission.)

Thus the major features of the metabolism of Nᵗ-methylhistidine are depicted in Figure 6, emphasizing that the daily excretion of the amino acid quantitatively related to its rate of release from the major myofibrillar proteins in skeletal muscle. Therefore, the urinary output reflects the breakdown rate of these proteins and if it accepted that there is 4.2 μmol Nᵗ-methylhistidine per gram mixed protein in adult human muscle,[61] the daily breakdown of protein within the skeletal musculature, can be computed from the measured output of Nᵗ-methylhistidine in urine. Finally, an additional reason for

Table 3
IN VITRO RATE OF PROTEIN SYNTHESIS
AND PROTEOLYTIC ACTIVITY IN TEASED
FIBERS OF RECTUS ABDOMINAL MUSCLE
OBTAINED FROM ADULT SUBJECTS OF
DIFFERENT AGES

Age group	Protein synthesis[a]	Proteolytic[b] activity
< 60 years	0.18	2.1
> 60 years	0.24	3.0
Significance (*P*)	<0.01	<.025

[a] ^{14}C-Leucine incorporation (μmol $h^{-1}g$ protein^{-1}).
[b]   Cathepsin D activity; nmol tyrosine release min^{-1} mg protein^{-1}.

From Lundholm, K. and Schersten, R., *Exp. Gerentol.*, 10, 155, 1975. With permission.

exploring the status of muscle protein metabolism in vivo is that Lundholm and Schersten[62] have concluded from studies of teased muscle fibers in vitro that rates of muscle protein synthesis and breakdown are enhanced in old age (Table 3).

The urinary excretion of N^τ-methylhistidine in small groups of young adult and elderly subjects, all consuming flesh-free diets free of sources of this amino acid, has been determined and some recent data are shown in Table 4. In addition, data for creatinine excretion are shown in the table for purposes of estimating the size of the muscle mass. The urinary output of the amino acid is lower for elderly men than for young adults. However, this appears to be due largely to the reduced muscle mass because N^τ-methylhistidine output per unit of creatinine output does not markedly differ between the two age groups (Table 4). The estimate of the amount of muscle protein breakdown, based on these findings, is about 68g daily in young men or 0.9 g protein kg^{-1} day^{-1}. In comparison total daily muscle protein breakdown approximates 36g daily or 0.5 g kg^{-1} day^{-1} in the elderly males. In relation to the rate of whole body protein breakdown (see Table 2), it can be seen that muscle accounts for 30% of whole body protein turnover in young men as compared to 20% in elderly men. These data confirm our previous findings,[58] and they indicate that during progression of the adult years there is a decline in the quantitaive contribution made by skeletal muscle to whole body protein metabolism.

The significance of this shift in the distribution of body protein metabolism during progressive aging in humans is not yet understood. However, if the major body organs exhibit different patterns in requirement for individual amino acids[63] and differences in the efficiency of re-utilization or recycling of amino acids,[64] it can be speculated that the efficiency of retention of dietary protein and amino acids would depend, in part, upon the relative contributions made by muscle and visceral organs to whole body protein turnover. Hence, it is possible that these changes in protein metabolism with aging would lead to alterations in the efficiency of dietary protein utilization and there is some evidence to support this speculation.[65] Furthermore, muscle contributes to the adaptations in body energy and amino acid metabolism during restricted dietary energy and protein intakes.[66,67] Therefore, a reduced contribution by muscle to whole body protein metabolism might restrict the capacity of the elderly individual to respond successfully to an unfavorable dietary situation or to other stressful conditions that depend upon adaptive changes in muscle protein and energy metabolism.

Because it is possible to estimate in adult subjects the size of muscle protein mass,

Table 4
MUSCLE MASS, URINARY N$^\tau$-
METHYLHISTIDINE EXCRETION
AND ESTIMATE OF MUSCLE
BREAKDOWN AS RELATED TO
ADULT AGE

	Young men	Elderly men
Mass		
Creatinine (Cr)		
g/day	2.1 ± 0.2[a]	1.3 ± 0.1
g/kg BCM[b]/day	55 ± 0.6	50 ± 1.6
N$^\tau$-Methylhistidine		
μ mol/day	287 ± 33	151 ± 9
μ mol/kg BCM	7.6 ± 0.3	5.6 ± 0.2
μ mol/g Cr	137 ± 6	118 ± 6
Muscle Protein		
Breakdown		
g/day	68 ± 8	36 ± 2
g/kg BCM	1.8 ± 0.06	1.4 ± 0.04
g/g Cr	33 ± 1.4	28 ± 1.6
% Whole body	30 ± 2	20 ± 1

[a]   Mean ± SEM for 5 young men and 6 elderly men.
    Unpublished data of M. Gersovitz, H. Munro and
    V. R. Young.
[b]   BCM = Body Cell Mass determined by whole
    body ^{40}K.

Table 5
ESTIMATION OF MEAN RATE OF
NON-MUSCLE (NM) PROTEIN
SYNTHESIS IN YOUNG ADULT AND
ELDERLY MEN

	Young adult	Elderly men
No. of subjects	5	6
Body protein		
Total (kg)	9.4	6.5 (70)[a]
Non-muscle (kg)	5.6	4.3 (77)
Muscle (kg)[b]	3.8	2.2 (56)
NM Protein Synthesis		
g/day	175	175 (100)
g/kg NM Protein	31	41 (132)

[a]   Figures in parentheses are percentage of value in
    young men. Unpublished data of M. Gersovitz, H.
    N. Munro and V. R. Young.
[b]   Muscle protein calculated by assuming 1.84 kg
    muscle protein equivalent to 1 g creatinine excre-
    tion (see text).

based on measurement of creatinine excretion,[68] and the magnitude of the total body
protein pool from the whole body ^{40}K measurements, a further exploration of possible
changes in body protein metabolism can be made with these data. As shown in Table
5, muscle protein mass is lower in the elderly males, accounting for a major proportion

of the difference (or decline) in total body protein mass between the two age groups of men. Utilizing data for whole body and muscle protein turnover discussed above (Tables 2 and 4) the amount of protein synthesis (and breakdown) in nonmuscle tissues can be computed. As also shown in Table 5, the daily amount of nonmuscle protein synthesis appears to be similar for the young adult and elderly men studied, but when expressed per unit of nonmuscle protein it appears that the fractional rate of synthesis may be increased as aging progresses.

It should be emphasized conclusions regarding changes in the amount and distribution of body protein synthesis and breakdown during passage of the adult years must be regarded as tentative. The data were based on cross-sectional studies in small groups of subjects and this poses problems.[69] Furthermore the methods used to quantify rates of whole body and muscle protein turnover are not without limitations and are open to criticism, including use of N^r-methylhistidine as an index of muscle protein breakdown.[70] New and improved noninvasive methods for quantifying dynamic aspects of protein metabolism in vivo will be required to establish the general validity of our findings.

III. ALBUMIN METABOLISM

In addition to studies of whole body and muscle protein metabolism in relation to human aging some attention has been given to the effects of increasing age on the metabolism of individual proteins, notably albumin. Findings in old rats suggest that they synthesize albumin at a faster rate than do young rats,[71,72] Chen et al.[73] found that albumin synthesis by isolated liver microsomes was 50% higher in old than in young rats, without a demonstrable difference in total protein synthesis in the liver. Obenrader et al.[72] isolated liver mRNA from old and young rats, and recovered more total mRNA from the liver polyribosomes of the old rats, and this was attributed to a greater recovery of albumin mRNA. Barrows[74] also concluded that the age-associated increase in liver protein synthesis was primarily due to increased serum albumin synthesis, responding to the proteinuria observed in aged animals. There is also evidence of age-dependent differences in the response of albumin synthesis to stimuli. Ove et al.,[71] showed that young rats increased their albumin synthesis rate by 40% in response to bleeding, whereas old rats did not show this response. It was concluded that albumin synthesis in old animals is already maximally stimulated and so unresponsive to the stress caused by blood loss. Recently, Van Bezooijen et al.,[75,76] measured total liver protein synthesis and albumin synthesis using isolated rat parenchymal cells, which in tissue culture achieved a level of albumin synthesis approximately equal to rates observed in vivo. With regard to the age of the donor, the capacity of the parenchymal cells to synthesize protein decreased between 3 and 12 months, remained constant between 12 and 24 months, and increased between 24 and 36 months.

While these studies favor an enhanced rate of albumin synthesis in senescent rats, other studies suggest that hepatic protein synthesis may be either unchanged[7] or reduced[77,78] during aging, including disaggregation of hepatic membrane-bound ribosomes, implying a reduced rate of synthesis of plasma proteins, and reduced rates of polypeptide chain initiation.[79] However, the rat may be an inappropriate model with respect to the aging human for comparisons of protein turnover.

Albumin is protein of particular interest in the biochemical evaluation of protein nutritional status in humans. In elderly humans, two studies[80,81] of the metabolism of albumin have been reported in which only catabolic rats were measured, using ^{131}I-albumin or ^{125}I-albumin. In a study of three men and three women aged 72 and 85 years, Yan and Franks[80] found no change in extravascular passage times and transcapillary flux compared with published findings for young subjects. They did observe a decrease in both the intravascular and interstitial albumin pools. Degradation rate was, however, not significantly affected by age. Misra et al.[81] investigated nine female and five male subjects aged 70 to 86 years, and found an increase in both the fractional and absolute catabolic rates compared to those of young adults. When they divided their elderly subjects according to those with plasma albumin concentrations below or above 3 g/dℓ, the "hypoalbuminemic" group had smaller albumin pools, although albumin degradation did not differ between the two groups. Consequently, although the "hypoalbuminemic" appeared to be degrading normal total quantities of albumin, this represented a higher proportion of their restricted pool of albumin. These latter authors postulate an impairment in control of degradation among the elderly. Both of these studies have limitations, including no evidence of control of dietary intake during the study and no direct comparison of results obtained in the elderly with those in young adults.

Whereas the catabolism of albumin has been measured relatively simply by injection of radioiodinated albumin, the rate of synthesis in man has been evaluated by a procedure involving administration of a pulse dose of ^{14}C-bicarbonate[82] or ^{14}C-guanidi-noarginine[83] which labels both the urea and the albumin synthesized in the liver. The labeling of urea was considered to provide a measure of the precursor free arginine pool in the liver, where albumin synthesis occurs. Also a stable isotope technique has been applied by Halliday and McKeran[37] for measuring albumin synthesis in man. These investigators infused [α-^{15}N] lysine for 36 hr and measured the change in ^{15}N-enrichment of the total N in albumin at two time intervals after the plasma free lysine pool had attained a constant ^{15}N-enrichment.

We have developed recently a stable isotope procedure for the estimation of albumin synthesis in relation to human aging, that involves labeling with ^{15}N-glycine administered orally every 3 hr as a donor of ^{15}N for liver free arginine.[84] This method follows the nitrogen enrichment of the guanidine group of albumin-bound arginine and monitors ^{15}N-urea in the urine at isotopic steady state, as an index of the enrichment of the liver free arginine pool. Thus, the progressive labeling of the arginine in serum albumin could be related to the plateau level of enrichment of urinary urea to provide a measure of the albumin synthesis rate. The concept behind this approach is depicted in Figure 7, and the various assumptions applied in the application of this model have been discussed in detail.[84] Because administration of radioiodinated albumin for the determination of the extravascular pool size could not be undertaken in our studies, fractional synthetic rates of albumin synthesis were converted to absolute synthetic rates assuming that the intravascular albumin pool comprises 40% of the total pool.[85]

Despite these limitations, the stable isotope method for the assessment of albumin synthesis in young adults receiving an adequate protein intake, namely 186 mg·kg^{-1} day^{-1}, (Table 6) that fall within the range obtained by the more widely used ^{14}C-carbonate method and are in good agreement with the fractional catabolic rate as measured with radioiodinate albumin, approximating 200 mg·kg^{-1} day^{-1}.[86] Furthermore, this new stable isotope method is sensitive in detecting a reduction in the rate of albumin synthesis (accompanied by a reduction in the proportion of albumin to whole body protein synthesis), when young adults receive a low protein diet (Table 6). Again, this observation is consistent with previous findings in the rat[87] and child.[88,89]

The ^{15}N-glycine method for in vivo measurement of albumin synthesis has also been applied in elderly subjects.[84] As also summarized in Table 6, our observations illustrate a lower concentration of albumin in the plasma of elderly people compared with young adults, but the fractional synthesis of the albumin pool is only slightly and insignificantly less in the elderly. This value in the elderly was not affected by dietary protein level, in contrast to the influence of protein intake in the young men. This implies that only the younger subjects are able to respond to increased protein intake. In this con-

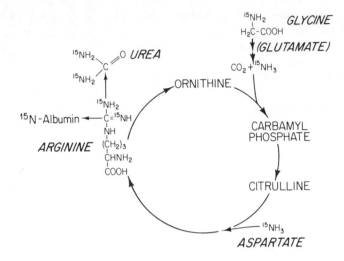

FIGURE 7.   Metabolic pathway for appearance of ^{15}N in urea and the guanidine group of albumin-bound arginine following administration of ^{15}N-glycine. This scheme indicate that the ^{15}N-enrichment of urea is a direct index of the level of ^{15}N in the guanidine group of arginine.

Table 6
PARAMETERS OF WHOLE BODY ALBUMIN METABOLISM IN *YOUNG ADULT AND ELDERLY MEN*, STUDIED WITH ^{15}N-GLYCINE AS PRECURSOR OF THE GUANIDINE N OF ALBUMIN-BASED ARGININE RECEIVING DIETS ADEQUATE OR LOW IN PROTEIN

| | Diet | | |
Parameter	Adequate	Low protein	P
Young men			
Serum albumin (g/dℓ)	4.5 ± 0.12	4.58 ± 0.05	NS
Intravascular albumin (g/kg body wt)	1.86 ± 0.04	2.22 ± 0.08	<0.01
Albumin synthesis			
% day^{-1}	3.97 ± 0.58	2.98 ± 0.31	<0.05
mg kg^{-1} day^{-1}	186 ± 30	140 ± 15	<0.025
% whole body synthesis	6.16 ± 1.22	4.57 ± 0.64	<0.05
Elderly men			
Serum albumin (g/dℓ)	4.22 ± 0.07	4.12 ± 0.13	NS
Intravascular albumin (g/kg body wt)	1.79 ± 0.15	1.90 ± 0.11	NS
Albumin synthesis			
% day^{-1}	3.35 ± 0.46	3.09 ± 0.49	NS
mg kg^{-1}day^{-1}	149 ± 22	147 ± 36	NS
% whole body synthesis	4.84 ± 0.68	5.56 ± 1.51	NS

Note: Mean ± SEM for 5 young men and 6 elderly men.

From Gersovitz, M., Munro, H. N., Udall, J., and Young, V. R., *Metabolism,* in press.

text, it has been pointed out by Munro et al.[90] that albumin synthesis in rats shows no consistent responses to increased consumption of protein when the animals already are receiving an adequate intake of protein, but became responsive when serum albumin concentration was first lowered by depletion.

From these findings, there appears to be an upper rate of albumin synthesis limited by a set-point beyond which amino acid supply cannot stimulate it further. Based on this conclusion, it would appear that the concentration of serum albumin in elderly subjects is maintained at a lower level than in younger subjects because of a lower set-point. This would explain why elderly subjects fail to show an increment in serum albumin synthesis in response to increasing dietary protein intake, whereas albumin synthesis in young subjects is responsive to this dietary change. Clearly, this hypothesis is based on a small population of elderly subjects, and it will be necessary to explore this further in large groups of subjects before the metabolic and clinical significance of these observations on albumin metabolism can be evaluated fully.

IV. METABOLISM OF INDIVIDUAL AMINO ACIDS

A. Plasma Amino Acid Levels

The economy of body nitrogen metabolism depends upon integration of the metabolism of the essential (indispensable) and nonessential (dispensable) amino acids. Thus it is important to know whether the age-dependent decline in muscle mass has any significant influence on the metabolism of individual amino acids and the dietary requirements for them. A reason for this is that the skeletal musculature exerts an influence on plasma amino acid levels and this tissue may act as a temporary biological reservoir for amino acids consumed in excess of immediate needs.[91] Furthermore, studies in dogs[92] and rats[93] have demonstrated that the liver modifies and regulates the level and pattern of free amino acids in blood plasma during the absorptive phase of the metabolism of protein-containing meals. Hence, the relative changes in muscle and liver mass and their changing contributions to whole body nitrogen metabolism, as described above, might be reflected by changes in plasma amino acid concentrations during advancement of the adult years.

Few investigations have been concerned with the determination of plasma amino acid levels in elderly subjects. Wehr and Lewis[94] concluded that 12 of 18 free amino acids measured in plasma samples taken from fasting elderly subjects were elevated, and Armstrong and Stave[95] have reported increased plasma levels of alanine, citrulline, cystine, and tyrosine together with a decrease in serine concentrations as man grows older. Möller et al.[96] found higher total essential amino acid concentrations in elderly subjects compared with a younger group, 20 to 36 years old, and for tyrosine, histidine, valine, and lysine, the differences were significant. These differences, although not large, were paralleled by comparable differences in the concentration of amino acids in muscle plasma amino acids. However, others have reported reduced levels for most amino acids.[97] Thus the available data do provide a consistent picture of the influence of aging on free amino acid patterns in plasma taken from subjects after an overnight fast.

Amino acid levels in blood plasma are sensitive to factors, including diet.[98-100] Thus the conditions under which blood samples are taken for measurement must be standardized in order to evaluate critically data for plasma amino acid levels between different age groups. For this reason, we have examined the comparative response of changes in plasma amino acids to alterations in the intake of individual essential amino acids in young adult and elderly subjects.

When young men receive an amino acid diet providing graded reductions in leucine, the concentration of this amino acid declines as the intake is decreased[101] (Figure 8).

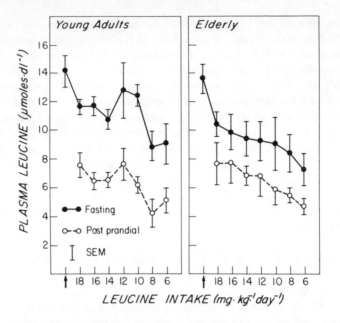

FIGURE 8.   Changes in plasma (drawn after an overnight fast and in the postprandial state) leucine concentrations in young adult and elderly men given amino acid diets providing graded levels of leucine. Intake of all other amino acids remained constant. Unpublished data of Perera, W. D. and Young, V. R.

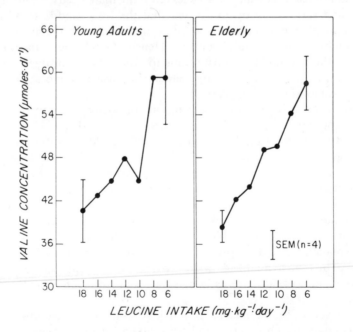

FIGURE 9.   Change in concentration of plasma valine with altered intakes of leucine in young adult and elderly men. Unpublished data of Perera, W. D. and Young, V. R.

In contrast, plasma valine levels rise with reduced intakes of leucine (Figure 9), possibly due to an effect of leucine on the uptake and metabolism of valine in muscle.[102] This pattern of change in plasma leucine and valine concentrations to reduced leucine intake is also observed in healthy elderly subjects (Figures 8 and 9). In other studies, we have found that the pattern and magnitude of reduction in plasma tryptophan to reduced tryptophan intakes is similar in both age groups,[103,104] and this also applies to the response of plasma valine to altered intakes of this amino acid.[105]

From these limited studies it appears that plasma amino acid levels are subject to the same regulation in both young and older subjects; that available data have not uncovered any major differences between these age groups. Again it is prudent to emphasize the limited extent of the published data and there is need to explore the response of plasma amino acids to a variety of nutritional and hormonal conditions in young and older subjects before a definitive statement is possible. For example, exogenous glucose influences the disposition of plasma amino acids[99] and this is brought about, at least in part, through the action of insulin. Altered insulin sensitivity in peripheral tissues has been demonstrated (e.g., Reference 106). For this reason it would be important to know whether changes in plasma amino acids in response to insulin or glucose administration are similar in young adults and elderly subjects.

B. Dynamic Status of Amino Acid Metabolism

Determinations of plasma amino acid concentrations do not furnish data about the rate of flow of the amino acids in this compartment, and as yet there is little published information about dynamic aspects of plasma amino acid metabolism. Thus, we have begun to investigate this problem with initial emphasis on the metabolism of some of the nonessential amino acids. These amino acids play a major role in tissue protein synthesis and participate in many reactions of intermediary metabolism and in the formation of physiologically active nitrogen-containing compounds. Among the nonessential amino acids, glycine has an important role in methyl group metabolism and in the formation of conjugates (e.g., glycocholic acid, hippuric acid), purines, creatine, and glutathione, in addition to being a substrate for protein synthesis. Through conversion to serine, glycine also participates in the formation of phosopholipids. Thus, the contribution of glycine to whole body amino acid metabolism would be expected to be of quantitative significance.

Using a procedure of continuous administration of ^{15}N-labeled glycine,[107] it is possible to estimate the amount of glycine entering the free glycine pool from the diet, from endogenous synthesis, or via release from body proteins due to their turnover, and the removal of glycine from the pool for protein synthesis and synthesis of other compounds requiring nitrogen and for urea formation. The model of glycine metabolism is shown in Figure 10, and measurement of glycine flux provides an estimate of the amount of glycine entering the pool from glycine synthesis in the tissues as well as from dietary sources and from glycine released by breakdown of body protein. Under steady state conditions, this is equal to the amount of glycine removed by incorporation into body protein and by metabolism through other pathways including synthesis of nonessential amino acids and eventual oxidation with conversion of nitrogen to urea.

Lapidot and co-workers[34,35,108] used a single-dose technique to estimate glycine flux from ^{15}N data in rabbits and human subjects, but their studies were of short duration (1 hour) and possibly measure only that portion of whole body glycine metabolism accounted for within the liver. The flux of glycine in adult human subjects was found to be 280 to 430 μmole kg^{-1}/hr^{-1} in the postabsorptive state, but in an earlier study by Watts and Crawhill[109] the flux of glycine was reported to be 590 μmoles kg^{-1} hr^{-1}, based on measurements over a longer period after glycine-^{15}N administration.

In our studies,[107] the magnitude of the glycine flux per kg body weight was found to be similar in young and old subjects; when expressed per kg body cell mass (BCM) elderly subjects tended to reveal a higher flux rate (Figure 11). This may occur because

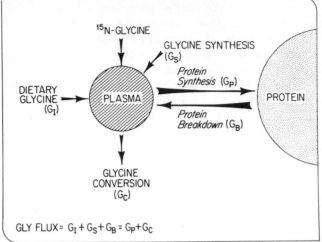

FIGURE 10.   Simplified model of whole body glycine metabolism studied with a continuous administration of ^{15}N-glycine. Glycine flux or flow of glycine through the free glycine pool. Under steady state conditions entry of glycine into the pool via diet (G_I), *de novo* synthesis (G_S), and from protein breakdown (G_B) is balanced by the removal of glycine via protein synthesis (G_p) and conversion to other products (G_C).

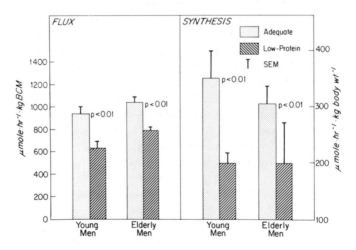

FIGURE 11.   Changes in glycine flux and in *de novo* glycine synthesis in young adult and elderly men following transfer from an adequate protein to a low-protein diet. (From Gersovitz, M., Bier, D., Matthews, D., Udall, J., Munro, H. N., and Young, V. R., *Metabolism*, in press, 1980.)

glycine flux is related to metabolism in visceral organs and the process of aging results in a selective loss of muscle, with consequent shift of metabolic emphasis to the viscera, as discussed above.

Glycine flux was found to be much reduced in response to a decrease in dietary protein intake in both young adults and elderly subjects (Figure 11). This is consistent with the general decrease in whole body nitrogen flux in response to inadequate protein diets[24] and to a reduction in the activity of liver enzymes associated with the synthesis of nonessential amino acids.[110] Little of the whole body glycine flux could be attributed to dietary glycine or glycine released by breakdown of body protein. Instead, *de novo* production of glycine was found to account for about 75% of the whole body glycine flux during adequate protein feeding and almost as large a percentage during the period of low protein intake.

These observations show that total synthesis of glycine by the body is extensive and is related closely to dietary protein intake. Since endogenous glycine synthesis is a major component of glycine flux, it can be concluded that formation of glycine provides a significant pathway for nitrogen derived from other amino acids. Support for an active metabolic glycine pool is provided by data on interorgan transport of glycine. Studies in fed sheep[111] show a net uptake by the liver of 3.9 mmol glycine and 1.2 mmol serine per hour from portal blood, most of it provided by release of these amino acids into the plasma by the gut and the kidneys. Combined net glycine and serine uptake from plasma by the liver of the sheep (5 mmol/hr, or 100 μmol kg^{-1}hr^{-1} body weight) would thus represent a significant interorgan flux in comparison with whole body glycine flux of 457 μmol kg^{-1}hr^{-1} that we have estimated in man. It should also be pointed out that the recent identification of an extensive interorgan translocation of glutathione (γ-glutamylcysteinyl-glycine) may reflect an additional significant route for glycine metabolism.[112]

Serine and glycine are interconvertible through the glycine cleavage system and via serine hydroxymethylase.[113,114] Thus, ^{15}N-glycine will donate its label to serine and this is reflected in the relatively constant ratio of 0.5 for the enrichment of ^{15}N in plasma serine to that in glycine that we observed in both age groups.[107] Furthermore, Fern and Garlick[115] found that in rat liver, an important site of serine synthesis from its precursor glycine, the specific radioactivity of free serine following a 6-hour infusion of [U-^{14}C] glycine equalled or exceeded that of free glycine. On the other hand, the ratio of the specific radioactivity of serine to glycine in plasma was about 0.3 and in other tissues the ratio was lower than in the liver. Thus, our results for the relative levels of enrichment of ^{15}N in the plasma serine and glycine pools presumably reflect the lower ^{15}N enrichment achieved in the precursor glycine pool in liver compared with that for plasma glycine as well as formation of serine from nitrogen sources that are poorly enriched with [15]N. Finally, the reduction in the rate of serine entry into the plasma compartment via diet and from body protein breakdown with the restricted protein intake would be in the same proportion as for changes found for glycine. Therefore we have concluded that serine biosynthesis in both young men and elderly individuals is also markedly reduced in response to the reduced protein intake.[107]

An important observation from this study of glycine metabolism, with ^{15}N-glycine as tracer, is the fact that there is a significant and extensive transfer of N among amino acids within the amino acid pools and this aspect of amino acid metabolism should be explored further. Studies with other nonessential amino acids, labeled with ^{13}C and ^{15}N, such as alanine, aspartic, and glutamic acids, would improve on understanding of the quantitative interrelationships among the nonessential amino acids and their importance in the maintenance of body nitrogen homeostasis during progression of the adult years.

V. PROTEIN AND AMINO ACID REQUIREMENTS

An objective of studies on the integrative aspects of body protein and amino acid metabolism, such as those discussed above, is to provide a basis for measurement of nutritional requirements and of the quantitative influence of factors that affect them. However, because many of the specific aspects of protein and amino acid metabolism cannot yet be related to the more practical issues of protein and amino acid requirements, the latter have been explored in a limited number of ways.

Much of the published data concerned with protein and amino acid requirements have been compiled in monograph form by Irwin and Hegsted,[116,117] which supplements several detailed reviews on the protein and amino acid requirements in the elderly.[118-120] Also, we have reviewed this area with particular reference to human aging.[8-10] Hence, a summary of the major issues and problems will be given here, with emphasis on a number of recent studies.

A. Requirements for Essential Amino Acids

The dietary requirement for total protein consists of a need for essential (indispensable) amino acids together with a source of nonspecific nitrogen used for synthesis of the nonessential (dispensable) amino acids and other physiologically important N-containing compounds.

Nitrogen balance has been used as the principal technique to determine the minimal requirements for the essential amino acids in human adults, and the available studies reveal a wide variability in the needs for individual essential amino acids among subjects of similar age and body weight.[16,116] The variation encountered is presumably due both to biological variation among individuals and to experimental and analytical error. Furthermore, it is also worth noting that the nitrogen balance data have been interpreted in different ways and this adds to the difficulties in comparing results among the various laboratories and in relation to the effects of advancing adult age. Thus, Rose[121] considered that the minimum requirement was met by the lowest level of intake of the amino acid which would maintain a "distinctly positive" N balance. On the other hand, Leverton and co-workers[122] chose the "equilibrium zone", defined as being within 5% of N equilibrium, as the end point in their assessment of the minimum essential amino acid needs in adult women.

Compared with studies of amino acid requirements in young adults, there have been few definitive studies of the essential amino acid requirements in the elderly (see Table 7 for summary). Tuttle, Swendseid, and colleagues conducted a series of studies of the essential amino acid requirements of "elderly" men. In the first study,[123] with five men aged 52 to 68 years, it was concluded that elderly subjects may have a higher requirement for one or more of the essential amino acids than younger persons. A second study by these investigators,[124] in subjects over 50 years of age, suggested that the requirements of one or more essential amino acids may also increase as the total dietary nitrogen intake rises. Seven subjects maintained nitrogen equilibrium on a diet providing 7 g total nitrogen daily and an intake of essential amino acids equivalent to that furnished by 39 g egg protein. Increasing the total nitrogen intake to 15 g per day by addition of glycine and diammonium citrate to the diet precipitated a negative nitrogen balance in seven of eight subjects. In further studies[125] the source of the dietary "nonspecific nitrogen" was found to be important in maintaining adequate protein nutrition in elderly subjects because nitrogen retention was higher when a mixture of nonessential amino acids was used in comparison with glycine as the source of supplemental nitrogen.

Two differing conclusions have been drawn for the minimal methionine requirements of the elderly. Tuttle et al.[126] gave a synthetic L-amino acid mixture, patterned as in egg protein, to six males, 58 to 73 years of age. Total nitrogen intake was 7 g per day. Four subjects receiving no cystine required 2.4, 2.7, 3.0, and 3.0 g, respectively, to achieve nitrogen equilibrium. Two other subjects receiving only small amounts of cystine (less than 50 mg) required greater than 2.1 g daily. These values for the S-amino acid needs of the elderly are considerably higher than published estimates for the young adult (Table 7). Tuttle et al.[126] also suggest that the requirement for lysine

Table 7
SOME PUBLISHED ESTIMATES OF
THE REQUIREMENTS FOR
INDIVIDUAL ESSENTIAL AMINO
ACIDS IN YOUNG ADULT AND
ELDERLY SUBJECTS

Amino acid	Age (year)	Estimated requirement (mg kg^{-1}day^{-1})	Ref.
Young adult			
S-amino acid		13	138
Lysine		12	138
Tryptophan		3	103
Threonine		7	137
Elderly			
S-amino acid (methionine)[a]	64	46	126
Lysine[a]	59	30	126
Tryptophan	73	2	104
Threonine	72	7	137

[a] The high values for methionine and lysine requirements suggested by Tuttle and co-workers have not
been confirmed and probably significantly overestimate actual requirements.[126]

is higher for the elderly. However, in contrast with these findings, six black men, 65 to 84 years, studied by Watts et al.[127] required lower intakes of the sulfur-containing amino acids to achieve N balance, compared with the needs in younger subjects.

The apparently contradictory findings in these various studies may be due to wide individual variation among subjects, to experimental errors in the use of the nitrogen balance technique and/or to differences in composition of the basal diets and amino acid mixtures used. It is also uncertain whether a higher requirement for methionine in elderly men, as reported by Tuttle et al.,[126] is due to an increased need for this amino acid or whether, and if true, it is related to a reduced efficiency of conversion of methionine to cystine in older individuals. The experimental diet used by Tuttle et al.[126] did not contain significant amounts of cystine and it may be pertinent that Gaull et al.[128] suggest that the newborn infant has a lower capacity to convert methionine to cystine compared with young adults. It would be worthwhile to explore whether aging influences the efficiency of conversion of methionine to cystine and, in consequence, the requirement for sulfur amino acids.

An alternative approach to the N balance technique that we have explored is based on measurement of the concentration of free amino acids in blood plasma. The relationships between the concentration of free amino acids in blood plasma; dietary amino acid intake has been the subject of a number of reviews.[98,99,129,130] It is quite clear that a reduced concentration of an essential amino acid in plasma indicates risk of a deficient level of the amino acid in the diet. Furthermore, the pattern of amino acids and concentration of a specific essential amino acid in plasma have been found to correlate with the ability of the dietary protein to support growth in experimental animals. Hence, various studies have demonstrated that, under well-defined conditions, a predictable relationship exists between the plasma concentration of the test amino acid and the intake of the amino acid in relation to the minimum requirement.[131-136]

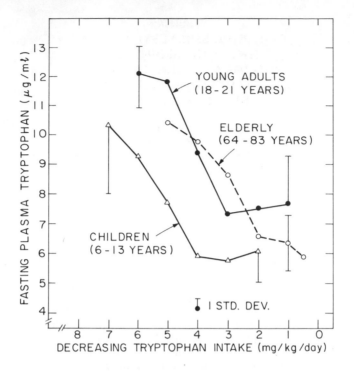

FIGURE 12.   Change in plasma tryptophan with altered tryptophan intake in groups of children, young adult men, and elderly subjects. Results combine data of separate experiments carried out in our laboratories. (From Young, V. R., Uauy, R., Winterer, J. C., and Scrimshaw, N. S., *Nutrition, Longevity, and Aging,* Rockstein, M. and Sussman, M. L., Eds., Academic Press, New York, 1976, 67. With permission.)

We have explored this approach for assessing the minimum requirements for tryptophan,[103] valine,[105] and threonine[137] in young adults. These studies have been extended to older subjects and in the first of this series,[105] involving 14 elderly subjects, 73 ± 5 years old, the relationships between plasma tryptophan concentration, tryptophan intake, and tryptophan requirement were examined. The experimental diet was based on an L-amino acid mixture, patterned as in egg protein, and provided N equivalent to about 0.5 g protein/kg body weight/day. Plasma tryptophan concentration decreased as tryptophan intake was reduced to the 2 mg/kg/day level (Figure 12). Thereafter, it remained relatively constant as the intake level was reduced further, indicating a tryptophan requirement in healthy, elderly subjects of approximately 2 mg/kg body weight per day. This is slightly lower than the values of 3 and 4 mg/kg as determined for young men and children, respectively, by the same plasma amino acid procedure.

This approach was also used to determine the threonine requirement in elderly subjects.[137] Plasma threonine levels decreased with graded reductions in threonine intake until the latter reached a level close to 7 mg/kg/day. A statistical evaluation of the plasma amino acid data suggested that the daily threonine requirement in elderly women, when expressed per unit of body weight, is the same as for young men. However, this probably means that the threonine requirement per unit of total body protein increases with age because lean body mass is less in proportion to total body weight in the older subject, as compared with young adults. This conclusion also applies to the valine requirement, based again on an interpretation of the plasma valine response curve.[105]

Table 8
SOME COMPARATIVE
ESTIMATIONS OF MEAN
OBLIGATORY, URINARY N
LOSSES, EXPRESSED PER KG
BODY WEIGHT AND PER G
CREATININE EXCRETION IN
YOUNG ADULT AND ELDERLY
SUBJECTS

| Group | Obligatory nitrogen excretion | | Ref. |
	(mgN /kg/day)	(mg/g creatinine)	
Young adult			
Women	25.2	1.5	139
Men	37	1.6	142
Men	38	1.7	143
Elderly			
Women	24.4	2.1	144
Men	34.5	2.2	145
Men	27.3	1.6	141

Note: A more extensive compilation of the available data has been presented by Bodwell et al.[160]

From the foregoing it is evident that information about requirements for individual essential amino acids in the aging human is still fragmentary and often contradictory. This is an unsatisfactory state of affairs particularly because estimations of the requirements for essential amino acids form the basis on which to design the "protein" component of both normal and therapeutic diets for use in the elderly and to assess the significance of dietary protein quality in this age group.

B. Requirement for Total Nitrogen (Protein)

The minimum physiological needs for total protein in adult humans have been determined using one of two N balance methods. These are (1) the factorial approach and (2) the N balance response curve method to directly determine the intake required to just maintain body N balance. In the former approach the losses of "obligatory" N via urine and feces are measured and summated together with additional corrections for N losses via the integument and other minor routes.[138] The aim of this method is to determine the total nitrogen loss occurring from the body when the subject receives, for a brief period, a protein-free but otherwise adequate diet. The minimum dietary protein requirement is then computed to be that amount of high quality protein necessary to balance endogenous N losses.

The major route of obligatory N loss in adult man is via the urine. For comparative purposes, Table 8 summarizes results obtained in our laboratories for young adult men and elderly males and females. As can be seen, obligatory urinary N excretion in healthy elderly women is comparable to that for young women, the latter determined by Bricker and Smith[139] and Hawley et al.[140] obtained with young women. Hence, for the same body weight, total daily obligatory urinary N loss appears to be similar in young and old women. Also, based on our findings, the obligatory urinary nitrogen output per unit of body weight in elderly men is essentially the same as that in young

Table 9
SOME COMPARATIVE
ESTIMATIONS OF
OBLIGATORY FECAL N
LOSSES IN YOUNG ADULTS
AND ELDERLY SUBJECTS

Group	Obligatory fecal N (mg kg^{-1}day^{-1})	Ref.
Young adult		
Women	8.4	139
Men	8.8	142
Men	14	143
Elderly		
Women	9.8	144
Men	12.2	145
Men	9.5	141

Table 10
SOME REPORTED VALUES FOR TOTAL
OBLIGATORY N LOSSES IN YOUNG
ADULTS AND ELDERLY SUBJECTS

Group	Sum of urine and fecal (mg N/kg/day)	Total losses[a] (mg N/kg/day)	Ref.
Young adult			
Women	33.1	38.1	139
Men	45.6	50.6	142
Men	52	57	143
Elderly			
Women	34.2	39.2	144
Men	46.7	51.7	145
Men	36.8	41.8	141

[a]   Assuming an additional N loss of 5 mg N/kg/day via skin and other miscellaneous routes (e.g., see Reference 138).

men. When expressed per unit of creatinine excretion, or per unit body cell mass, obligatory urinary nitrogen losses were higher in elderly than in young. These differences tend to parallel those discussed earlier for whole body protein turnover. However, other studies[141] have not confirmed these relationships and this may be due to differences in the characteristics of the small numbers of elderly subjects comprising the cross-sectional studies.

Similar comparisons may also be made for obligatory fecal N output and these estimates are given in Table 9. The reported values for adult males range from 9 to 23 mg N/kg body weight and the 1973 FAO/WHO Expert Group on Protein and Energy Requirements[138] chose a value of 12 mg N/kg as being a weighted mean for adults. The value of 8.7 mg N/kg for obligatory fecal N loss in young women reported by Bricker and Smith[139] closely compares with a mean value of 9.8 mg N/kg/day for the elderly women. Thus on the basis of these limited data for healthy elderly subjects the obligatory fecal N loss apparently is similar to that for young adults.

Total obligatory N losses for young adults have also been computed, as shown in Table 10, and compared with the values obtained with the elderly. From this compar-

Table 11
1973 FAO/WHO APPROACH TO THE FACTORIAL ESTIMATION OF
PROTEIN REQUIREMENTS AND ALLOWANCES FOR ADULT HUMANS

1. Total obligatory nitrogen losses (O_N) = Obligatory urinary nitrogen + obligatory fecal nitrogen + skin nitrogen and miscellaneous nitrogen.
2. Nitrogen requirement for maintenance (R_N) adjusted for efficiency of nitrogen utilization = O_N × 1.3.
3. Safe practical allowance (for milk or egg protein) adjusted for individual variability (SPA) = R_N × 1.3.
4. SPA predicted to be sufficient to cover needs of 97.5% of the population.

From *Energy and Protein Requirements,* World Health Organization Tech. Rep. Ser. 522, Food and Agriculture Organization, World Health Organization, Geneva, 1973.

ison, the total obligatory nitrogen loss in elderly men and women is similar to or somewhat lower than that for younger individuals. However, our estimate for elderly women is somewhat lower than the mean value of 49 mg N/kg for total obligatory N loss assumed for young women by the 1973 FAO/WHO Expert Group.[138]

From these values a prediction can now be made of the minimum needs for high quality protein in adult subjects, using the factorial calculation shown in Table 11. Thus our data on endogenous N losses in elderly people suggest that 0.42g protein (N × 6.25)/kg/day would be a *safe practical allowance* for healthy elderly women[144] and 0.52g for elderly men.[145] These compare with the 1973 FAO/WHO[138] values of 0.57g and 0.52g protein/kg/day for healthy adult men and women, respectively. However, as discussed below, these predictions underestimate the intake level that we consider minimally adequate for the older age group.

In addition to the factorial approach, the minimum physiological needs for dietary protein may be directly determined from the N balance response to graded protein intakes. Watkin[118] has carefully reviewed this topic and has discussed the factors which may account for the lack of agreement among the various studies, of which there are many, but few studies allow definitive conclusions to be drawn concerning the minimum protein needs of older people. Table 11 summarizes some of the N balance studies and conclusions drawn from them. Some investigators concluded that the need for protein was higher in the elderly than in young adults whereas others considered that there were no substantial differences between the requirements for protein in young and old adults. However, a number of the studies referred to in this table, as well as others reviewed by Watkin[118] and Irwin and Hegsted,[117] were not based on precise N balance determinations, and furthermore conclusions were made in reference to the then prevailing views on the estimated protein needs of younger adults. Also, the level(s) of protein intake tested in some of the studies did not necessarily evaluate the minimum intake which could maintain N equilibrium.

Several recent investigations in the elderly have made an attempt to standardize correlates of nitrogen balance in order to arrive at a reliable estimate of the protein requirement for this age group. Thus we[65] measured nitrogen balances in response to graded levels of egg protein intake by elderly men and women. Similarly, Cheng et al.[151] examined the nitrogen balance response to graded levels of dietary protein from a wheat-soy-milk mixture in young adults and elderly males. Since the relevance of both these studies to the elderly population at large may be limited because of their short duration (10 to 11 days at each protein level), nitrogen balance studies of longer duration seem desirable in order to assess whether there is adaptation to a given level of dietary protein intake that may complicate interpretation of results obtained in relatively brief diet periods. Therefore, we (Gersovitz, Motil, Munro, Scrimshaw, and Young — in preparation) have conducted a study to evaluate the current recommended

Table 12
SOME STUDIES ON N BALANCE AND PROTEIN NEEDS IN THE ELDERLY

Estimate and conclusion	Remarks	Ref.
N equilibrium in 7 of 8 women at 0.7 and 1.0 g protein/kg; dietary standards adequate	Healthy women, 52—74 years	146
Good nutritional state maintained at 54 ± 5 g protein	N balance assessed from diet records 20 women, 68—88 years	147
Protein needs not different from young adults	Review of studies with older men and women in a mental hospital	148
No evidence of qualitative or quantitative changes with age	Balance studies in healthy old men	118
Elderly require 0.7 g protein/kg/day	4 men, 69—76 years, poorly nourished subjects	149
Protein requirement for elderly women may be 20—30% less than for young women	9 women, 66—94 years old; maintained health at self-chosen intakes	150

daily protein allowance, as proposed by the Dietary Allowances Committee of the U.S. Food and Nutrition Board,[152] for older men and women by exploring the response of body protein metabolism to this level of dietary protein during a 30-day metabolic study period. An additional purpose of this investigation concerned the age-ranges of the present U.S. dietary protein allowances for older adults which are presently proposed for those aged 51 years and older without specific allowances for groups within this broad category.

The unpublished results for N balance obtained in this recent study are summarized in Table 12 and they indicate that 0.8 g egg protein/kg/day does not support an adequate body N balance in many elderly females, even after a 30-day adaptation period. Among elderly males, 0.8 g of egg protein/kg/day was insufficient to achieve N balance in any subject during the initial 10 days of feeding protein at this level. Since the mean nitrogen balance of the elderly males approached equilibrium by the end of the 30-day study, an adaptive response occurred in these subjects. Nevertheless, body nitrogen equilibrium was still not obtained by this time in three of the seven male subjects.

These findings differ from two other recent studies in elderly human subjects.[141,151] The degree of negative nitrogen balance observed in our elderly males during the initial 10 days of dietary protein intake was more marked than that observed on elderly male prisoners by Cheng et al.[151] who used, as in our unpublished study, a protein level of 0.8 g per kg/day for 11 days. However, these investigators provided their elderly subjects, as well as a control group of young adults, with any energy intake of 40 kcal/kg/day. This was probably in excess of their actual energy requirements under confinement and undoubtedly would have enhanced N retention beyond that which would have been achieved with an energy intake that more closely met requirements.[153-156] Although Zanni et al.[141] found N equilibrium in elderly males to be achieved at an intake of 0.6 gm protein·kg body weight, their subjects received a protein-free diet for 17 days immediately prior to the test period. It is well recognized that such an initial period of dietary protein deprivation will influence N balance response when protein is subsequently reincorporated into the diet. Thus the N retention observed by Zanni et al.[141] was probably more favorable than would have occurred in initially well-nourished subjects. For these various reasons it is likely that the protein requirements in elderly subjects were underestimated in these two recently published studies. A summary of these studies and our own is presented in Table 13.

Although the negative nitrogen balances observed in our elderly subjects were not marked at the 0.8 g protein/kg intake (Table 12), it should be emphasized that the nitrogen balance technique yields a conservative estimate of the protein requirement

Table 13
NITROGEN BALANCES IN ELDERLY MEN AND WOMEN GIVEN 0.8 g EGG PROTEIN /kg/day FOR 30 DAYS

	Elderly men	Elderly women
Number	7	8
Age (year)	72—82	74—99
Wt. (kg)	51—89	48—69
Energy intake (kcal/kg)[a]	32 ± 3	29 ± 5
Nitrogen balance[b] (mgN/kg/day)		
Days: 6—10	−7.4 ± 3[a]	−0.8 ± 1.9
16—20	1.5 ± 3.8	−8 ± 1.7
26—30	0.4 ± 3.4(3)[c]	−2.3 ± 2.8(4)

[a] Mean ± SD.
[b] Mean ± SEM.
[c] Number in parenthesis indicates number of subjects showing persistent negative balance during last 15 of 30 days.

From Gersovitz, M., Munro, H. N., and Young, V. R., unpublished.

when test N intakes fall within the submaintenance to near maintenance range of intake. Furthermore, because our experimental diet was based on a high quality egg protein product, this reinforces the view that a protein intake necessary to promote nitrogen equilibrium from mixed sources typical of the U.S. diet should be greater than 0.8 g/kg/day. Thus our findings do not support the current NAS/NRC dietary allowance[152] of 0.8g protein kg/day of mixed quality protein as being sufficient to cover the protein needs of a majority of the elderly population.

While the elderly generally require a lowered energy intake,[157] the above suggests that the needs for dietary protein do not appear to be similarly reduced. Furthermore, it is also possible that a lower, although adequate, energy intake per se may bring about a change in the efficiency of dietary N retention,[158] and this could also contribute to differences in the protein requirement of young adult and elderly subjects. Finally, because we have observed previously that healthy young adult males, with relatively higher proportion of body cell mass than older subjects, achieve body nitrogen equilibrium and maintain protein nutritional status during the long-term consumption of 0.8 g/kg/day of a good quality soy protein isolate (Wayler, Scrimshaw, and Young — unpublished data), it may also be that the efficiency of dietary nitrogen rentention per unit of existing body cell mass is lower in healthy elderly subjects than in young adults. Whether this is causally related to the redistribution in body protein metabolism with increasing age cannot be established at present.

In view of the growing proportion of elderly persons in the U.S. population and in other technically advanced nations, it is sobering to realize the limited and uncertain state of the knowledge concerning protein and amino acid needs for this age group.

VI. EFFECTS OF INFECTION AND OTHER STRESSFUL STIMULI ON PROTEIN NEEDS

In assessing the practical and health significance of the estimates of the protein needs discussed above, it is important to emphasize that the results of our own studies and

Table 14

COMPARISON OF FOUR RECENT STUDIES TO ASSESS PROTEIN
REQUIREMENTS IN ELDERLY SUBJECTS

Study	Authors' conclusions	Comments	Ref.
Cheng et al.	NRC allowance of 0.8 g/kg considered adequate	7 men; 61—72 years; 62 kg; 11-day periods; Energy intake: 40 kcal/kg; balance in 4/7 subjects	151
Zanni et al.	FAO/WHO 1973 safe level of 0.57 g egg protein/kg considered adequate	6 men; 63—77 years; 83 kg; *test protein followed 17-day protein-free period;* 15-day balance; energy intake: 31 kcal/kg.	141
Uauy et al.	Mean requirement 0.8 g/kg, women allowance >0.57<0.8 g/kg	7 women; 71—78 years; 69 kg; energy intake: 28 kcal/kg; 7 males; 68—74 years; 74 kg; energy intake: 32 kcal/kg	65
Gersovitz et al.	0.8 g egg protein/kg not adequate for long-term balance	7 women; 71—99 years; 62 kg; 7 men; 70—82 years; 71 kg; energy intake: 30 kcal/kg	unpublished

the estimations for protein allowances in the elderly are intended to apply to healthy individuals. However, superimposed infection, altered gastrointestinal function, and metabolic changes which often accompany chronic disease states would all be expected to reduce the efficiency of dietary N utilization. The net result would be to increase the amount of protein needed to maintain protein nutritional status. Because elderly people are more commonly affected by these factors, it is important to recognize their adverse effects on protein metabolism and nutrition. Furthermore, Watkin[118] has stated: "Socioeconomic factors and presence of disease have far more practical influence than age per se in determining the status of protein nutrition in the aged."

The qualitative effects of acute infection on dietary protein utilization and requirements have been well described[159] for some infections in a limited number of individuals. Unfortunately the available data are of little value for quantifying the effects of infection on nutrient needs in the elderly. However, it is known that any infection and other stressful stimuli of physical and psychological origin produce a tendency to negative nitrogen balance through the cumulative effect of several different mechanisms. Thus in spite of the potential for disease states to increase protein and amino acid needs in a majority of elderly people there are no studies which help to assess their quantitative influence on nutrient utilization and dietary requirements. Although this is a complex problem, there is an urgent need to explore the nutritional and dietary significance of disease states that are common to so many members of the elderly population.

VII. SUMMARY AND CONCLUSIONS

In this review an update of various aspects of whole body protein and amino acid metabolism during aging in human subjects has been given. The picture that emerges is one of a slow loss of total body protein with aging, due largely to a diminution in the size of the skeletal muscle mass. These changes are accompanied by a shift in the overall pattern of whole body protein synthesis and breakdown. With the use of ^{15}N-labeled amino acids to estimate the rate of whole body protein breakdown, and measurement of urinary N^r-methylhistidine excretion to determine the rate of muscle protein breakdown, muscle mass was estimated to account for about 30% of whole body protein turnover in the young adult, which declines to 20% or less in the elderly subject. Studies on albumin metabolism suggest that the regulation of albumin synthesis is altered with advancing old age in the human. Investigations have commenced on the influence of aging on the dynamic aspects of metabolism of specific amino acids, but they are limited and do not reveal any major differences between young adult and older individuals. Additional studies on this aspect of amino acid metabolism would be highly worthwhile in order to construct a comprehensive picture of the integrated metabolism of amino acids during human aging.

Recent studies concerned with determination of the requirements for individual essential amino acids and total protein are reviewed. However, the data are limited and often contradictory and some reasons for this are suggested. However, elderly individuals are more likely to be affected by various biological, environmental, and social factors that would tend to increase protein needs above those for younger adults. It is probable that, in practice, the protein needs in the elderly are higher than for the young. The reduction in energy intake, together with its possible consequences for dietary protein utilization, must also be considered in establishing safe and rational protein allowances. Until more data become available, we recommend that for food planning purposes, an appropriate allowance would be 12 to 14% of the total energy intake as dietary protein of nutritional quality comparable to that provided by North American and European type diets.

ACKNOWLEDGMENT

The authors' unpublished data referred to in this chapter have been obtained with the financial support of National Institute of Health (NIH) grants AM15856, AG01215, RR88, and a cooperative agreement with the USDA Human Nutrition Research Center on Aging at Tufts, Boston. The collaboration with Dr. Dennis Bier (HD10667) and Dr. John Burke (GM21700) has given us great opportunities and we are most grateful for this.

REFERENCES

1. **Forbes, G. B. and Reina, J. C.,** Adult lean body mass declines with age: some longitudinal observations, *Metabolism,* 19, 653, 1970.
2. **Rossman, I.,** Anatomic and body composition changes with aging, in *Handbook of the Biology of Aging,* Finch, C. E., and Hayflick, L., Eds., D Van Nostrand Reinhold, New York, 1977, 189.
3. **Korenchevsky, V.,** *Physiological and Pathological Aging,* Hafner, New York, 1961.
4. **Young, V. R., Winterer, J. C., Munro, H. N., and Scrimshaw, N. S.,** Muscle and whole body protein metabolism with special reference to man, in *Special Review of Experimental Aging Research,* Elias, M. F., Eleftheriou, B. E., and Elias, P. K., Eds., EAR, Bar Harbor, Maine.
5. **Hayflick, L.,** The cell biology of aging, *J. Invest. Dermatol.,* 73, 8, 1979.
6. **Adelman, R. C.,** Macromolecular metabolism during aging, in *Handbook on the Biology of Aging,* Finch, C. E. and Hayflick, L., Eds., D Van Nostrand Reinhold, New York, 1977, 63.
7. **Moldave, K., Harris, J., Sabo, W., and Sodnick, I.,** Protein synthesis and aging: studies with cell-free mammalian systems, *Fed. Proc.,* 38, 179, 1979.
8. **Young, V. R., Perera, W. D., Winterer, J. C., and Scrimshaw, N. S.,** Protein and amino acid requirements of the elderly, in *Nutrition and Aging,* Winick, M., Ed., John Wiley & Sons, New York, 1976, 77.
9. **Young, V. R., Uauy, R., Winterer, J. C., and Scrimshaw, N. S.,** Protein metabolism and needs in elderly people, in *Nutrition, Longevity and Aging,* Rockstein, M. and Sussman, M. L., Eds., Academic Press, New York, 1976, 67.
10. **Uauy, R., Scrimshaw, N. S., and Young, V. R.,** Human protein metabolism in relation to nutrient needs in the aged, in *Nutrition of the Aged,* Hawkins, W. W., Ed., Nutrition Society of Canada, Quebec, 1978, 53.
11. **Munro, H. N. and Young, V. R.,** Protein metabolism and requirements, in *Metabolic and Nutritional Disorders in the Elderly,* Exton-Smith, A. N. and Caird, F. I., Eds., John Wright and Sons, Bristol, U.K., 1980, 13.

12. **Schimke, R. T.,** Regulation of protein degradation in mammalian tissues, in *Mammalian Protein Metabolism,* Vol. IV, Munro, H. N., Ed., Academic Press, Inc., New York, 1970.

13. **Goldberg, A. L. and Dice, J. F.,** Intracellular protein degradation in mammalian and bacterial cells, *Ann. Rev. Biochem.,* 43, 835, 1974.

14. **Goldberg, A. L. and St. John, A. C.,** Intracellular protein degradation in mammalian and bacterial cells, Part II, *Ann. Rev. Biochem,* 45, 747, 1976.

15. **Ballard, F. J.,** Intracellular protein degradation, in *Essays in Biochemistry,* Campbell, P. N. and Aldridge, W. N., Eds., 13, Academic Press, New York, 1977.

16. **Young, V. R. and Scrimshaw, N. S.,** Nutritional evaluation of proteins and protein requirements, in *Protein Resources and Technology: Status and Research Needs,* Milner, M., Scrimshaw, N. S., and Wang, D. I. C., Eds., AVI Publishing, Westport, Conn., 1978, 136.

17. **Klein, P. D., Hatchey, D. L., Kreek, M., and Schoeller, D. A.,** Stable isotopes: essential tools in biological and medical research, in *Stable Isotopes: Application in Pharmacology, Toxicology and Clinical Research,* Baillie, T. A., Ed., University Park Press, Baltimore, 1978, 3.

18. **Schoenheimer, R.,** *The Dynamic State of Body Constituents,* Harvard University Press, Cambridge, Mass., 1942.

19. **Schoenheimer, R. and Rittenberg, D.,** The application of isotopes to the study of intermediary metabolism, *Science,* 87, 221, 1938.

20. **Schoenheimer, R. and Rittenberg, D.,** The study of intermediary metabolism of animals with the aid of isotopes, *Physiol. Rev.,* 20, 218, 1940.

21. **Sprinson, D. B. and Rittenberg, D.,** The rate of interaction of the amino acids of the diet with tissue proteins, *J. Biol. Chem.,* 180, 715, 1949.

22. **Sprinson, D. B. and Rittenberg, D.,** The rate of utilization of ammonia for protein synthesis, *J. Biol. Chem.,* 180, 707, 1949.

23. **San Pietro, A. and Rittenberg, D.** A study of the rate of protein synthesis in humans. II. Measurement of the metabolic pool and the rate of protein synthesis, *J. Biol . Chem.,* 201, 457, 1953.

24. **Waterlow, J. C., Garlick, P. J., and Millward, D. J.,** *Protein Turnover in Mammalian Tissues and in the Whole Body,* North-Holland, New York, 1978.

25. **Matwiyoff, N. A. and Ott, D. G.,** Stable isotope tracer in life sciences and medicine, *Science,* 181, 1125, 1973.

26. **Matthews, D. E., Ben-Galin, E., and Bier, D. M.,** Determination of stable isotope enrichment in individual amino acids by chemical ionization mass spectrometry, *Anal. Chem.,* 51, 80, 1979.

27. **Sweeley, C. C., Elliot, W. H., Fries J., and Ryhage, R.,** Mass spectrometric determination of unresolved components in gas chromatographic effluents, *Anal. Chem.,* 51, 1549, 1966.

28. **Matthews, D. E. and Hayes, J. M.,** Isotope-ratio-monitoring gas chromatography mass spectrometry, in *Stable Isotopes Proc. 3rd Int. Congr .,* Klein, E. R. and Klein, P. D., Eds., Academic Press, New York, 1979, 95.

29. **Waterlow, J. C.,** The assessment of protein nutrition and metabolism in the whole animal, with special reference to man, in *Mammalian Protein Metabolism,* Vol. 3, Munro, H. N., Ed., Academic Press, New York, 1969, 325.

30. **Waterlow, J. C., Golden, M. H. N., and Garlick, P. J.,** Protein turnover in man measured with ^{15}N: comparison of end products and dose regimes, *Am. J. Physiol.,* 235, E165, 1978.

31. **Garlick, P. J., Glugston, G. A., and Waterlow, J. C.,** Influence of low-energy diets on whole body protein turnover in obese subjects, *Am. J. Physiol.,* 238, E235, 1980.

32. **Irving, C. S., Nissim, R., and Lapidot, A.,** The determination of amino acid pool sizes and turnover rates by gas-chromatographic-mass spectrometric analysis, *Biomed. Mass. Spectrom.,* 5, 117, 1978.

33. **Nissim, I. and Lapidot, A.,** Plasma amino acid turnover rates and pools in rabbits: in vivo studies using stable isotopes, *Am. J. Physiol.,* 237, E418, 1979.

34. **Irving, C. S., Nissim, I., and Lapidot, A.,** Whole body amino acid pools and turnover rates determined by stable isotope gas-chromatographic-mass-spectrometric methodology, in *Monographs in Human Genetics,* Vol. 9, Sperling, O. and deVries, A., Eds., S. Karger, Basel, 1978, 50.

35. **Lapidot, A. and Nissim, I.,** Regulation of pool sizes and turnover rates of amino acids in humans: ^{15}N-glycine and ^{15}N-alanine single-dose experiments using gas chromatography-mass-spectrometry analysis, *Metabolism,* 29, 230, 1980.

36. **Picou, D. and Taylor-Roberts, T.,** The measurement of total protein synthesis and catabolism and nitrogen turnover in infants in different nutritional states and receiving different amounts of dietary protein, *Clin. Sci.,* 36, 283, 1969.

37. **Halliday, D. and McKeran, R. O.,** Measurement of muscle protein synthetic rate from several muscle biopsies and total protein turnover in man by continuous intravenous infusion of L-[α-15N]lysine, *Clin. Sci. Mol. Med.,* 49, 581, 1975.

38. **Halliday, D., Madigan, M., Ells, T., Richards, P., Bergstrom, J., and Furst, P.,** Metabolism of ^{13}C-α-ketoisovalerate and ^{13}C-phenylpyruvate in man, in *Stable Isotopes,* Proc. 3rd Int. Cong., Klein, E. R. and Klein, P. D., Eds., Academic Press, New York, 1979, 583.

39. James, W. P. T., Garlick, P. J., Sender, P. M., and Waterlow, J. C., Studies of amino acid and protein metabolism in normal man with L-[U-¹³C]tyrosine, *Clin. Sci. Mol. Med.*, 50, 525, 1976.

40. O'Keefe, S. J. D., Sender, P. M., and James, W. P. T., "Catabolic" loss of body nitrogen in response to surgery, *Lancet*, 2, 1035, 1974.

41. Waterlow, J. C., Lysine turnover in man measured by intravenous infusion of L-[U-14C]lysine, *Clin. Sci.*, 33, 507, 1967.

42. Matthews, D. E., Motil, K. J., Rohrbaugh, D. K., Burke, J. F., Young, V. R., and Bier, D. M., Measurement of leucine metabolism in man from a primed, continuous infusion of L-[1-¹³C] leucine, *Am. J. Physiol.*, 238, E473, 1980.

43. Bier, D. M. and Christopherson, H. L., Rapid micromethod for determination of ¹⁵N enrichment in plasma lysine: application to measurement of whole body protein turnover, *Anal. Biochem.*, 94, 242, 1979.

44. Golden, M. H. N. and Waterlow, J. C., Total protein synthesis in elderly people: a comparison of results with [¹⁵N-glycine and [¹⁴C] leucine, *Clin. Sci. Molec. Med.*, 53, 227, 1977.

45. Aub, M. B. and Waterlow, J. C., Analysis of a five-compartment system with continuous infusion and its application to the study of amino acid turnover, *J. Theor. Biol.*, 26, 243, 1970.

46. Conway, J. M., Bier, D. M., Motil, K. J., Burke, J. F., and Young, V. R., Whole body lysine flux in young adult men: effects of reduced total protein and of lysine intake, *Am. J. Physiol.*, 239, E192, 1980.

47. Soltesz, G. Y., Joyce, J., and Young, M., Protein synthesis rate in the newborn lamb, *Biol. Neonate*, 23, 139, 1973.

48. Millward, D. J., Garlick, P. J., Stewart, R. J. C., Nnanyelugo, D. O., and Waterlow, J. C., Skeletal muscle growth and protein turnover, *Biochem. J.*, 150, 235, 1975.

49. Nicholson, J. F., Rate of protein synthesis in premature infants, *Pediatr. Res.*, 4, 389, 1970.

50. Pencharz, P. B., Steffe, W. P., Cochran, W., Scrimshaw, N. S., Rand, W. M., and Young, V. R., Protein metabolism in human neonates: nitrogen-balance studies, estimated obligatory losses of nitrogen and whole body turnover of nitrogen, *Clin. Sci. Mol. Med.*, 52, 485, 1977.

51. Golden, M. H. N., Waterlow, J. C., and Picou, D., Protein turnover, synthesis and breakdown before and after recovery from protein energy malnutrition, *Clin. Sci. Mol. Med.*, 53, 473, 1977.

52. Golden, M. H. N., Waterlow, J. C., and Picou, D., The relationship between dietary intake, weight changes, nitrogen balance and protein turnover in man, *Am. J. Clin. Nutr.*, 30, 1345, 1977.

53. Kein, C. L., Rohrbaugh, D. K., Burke, J. F., and Young, V. R., Whole body protein synthesis in relation to basal energy expenditure in healthy children and in children recovering from burn injury, *Pediatr. Res.*, 12, 211, 1978.

54. Pencharz, P. B., Motil, K. J., Parsons, H. G., and Duffy, B. J., The effect of an energy-restricted diet on the protein metabolism of obese adolescents: nitrogen balance and whole body nitrogen turnover, *Clin. Sci.*, 59, 13, 1980.

55. Steffee, W. P., Goldsmith, R. S., Pencharz, P. B., Scrimshaw, N. S., and Young, V. R., Dietary protein intake and dynamic aspects of whole body nitrogen metabolism in adult humans, *Metabolism*, 25, 281, 1976.

56. Sharp, C. S., Lassen, S., Shonkman, S., Hazlet, J. W., and Kednis, M. S., Studies of protein retention and turnover using nitrogen-15 as a tag, *J. Nutr.*, 63, 155, 1957.

57. Winterer, J., Steffee, W. P., Perera, W. D. A., Uauy, R., Scrimshaw, N. S., and Young, V. R., Whole body protein turnover in aging man, *Exp. Gerontol.*, 11, 79, 1976.

58. Uauy, R., Winterer, J. C., Bilmazes, C., Haverberg, L. N., Scrimshaw, N. S., Munro, H. N., and Young, V. R., The changing pattern of whole body protein metabolism in aging humans, *J. Gerontol.*, 33, 663, 1978.

59. Rowe, J. W., Andres, R., Robin, J. D., Norris, A. H., and Shock, N. W., The effect of age on creatinine clearance in men: a cross-sectional and longitudinal study, *J. Gerontol.*, 31, 155, 1976.

60. Young, V. R. and Munro, H. N., Nᵀ-methylhistidine (3-methylhistidine) and muscle protein turnover: an overview, *Fed. Proc.*, 37, 2291, 1978.

61. Bilmazes, C., Uauy, R., Haverberg, L. N., Munro, H. N., and Young, V. R., Muscle protein breakdown in humans based on Nᵀ-methylhistidine (3-methylhistidine) content of mixed proteins in skeletal muscle and urinary output of Nᵀ-methylhistidine, *Metabolism*, 27, 525, 1978.

62. Lundholm, K. and Schersten, R., Leucine incorporation into proteins and cathepsin -D activity in human skeletal muscles. The influence of the age of the subject, *Exp. Gerontol.*, 10, 155, 1975.

63. Munro, H. N., Evolution of protein metabolism in mammals, in *Mammalian Protein Metabolism*, Munro, H. N., Ed., Academic Press, New York, 1969, 133.

64. Gan, J. C. and Jeffay, H., Origins and metabolism of the intracellular amino acid pools in rat liver and muscle, *Biochim. Biophys. Acta*, 148, 448, 1967.

65. Uauy, R., Scrimshaw, N. S., and Young, V. R., Human protein requirements: nitrogen balance response to graded levels of egg protein in elderly men and women, *Am. J. Clin. Nutr.*, 31, 779, 1978.

66. **Cahill, G. F., Jr.,** Starvation in man, *N. Engl. J. Med.,* 282, 668, 1970.
67. **Young, V. R.,** The role of skeletal and cardiac muscle in the regulation of protein metabolism, in *Mammalian Protein Metabolism,* Munro, H. N., Ed., Academic Press, New York, 1970, 585.
68. **Chinn, K. S. K.,** Prediction of muscle and remaining tissue protein in man, *J. Appl. Physiol.,* 23, 713, 1967.
69. **Rowe, J. W.,** Clinical research on aging. Strategies and directions, *N. Engl. J. Med.,* 297, 1332, 1977.
70. **Millward, D. J., Bates, P. C., Grimble, G. K., Brown, J. G., Nathan, M., and Rennie, M. J.,** Quantitative importance of non-muscle of N^r-methylhistidine in urine, *Biochem. J.,* 190, 225, 1980.
71. **Ove, P., Obenrader, M., and Lansing, A.,** Synthesis and degradation of liver proteins in young and old rats, *Biochem. Biophys. Acta,* 277, 211, 1972.
72. **Obenrader, M. F., Lansing, A. I., and Ove, P.,** Evidence relating to the amount of albumin mRNA to the increased albumin synthetic activity in old rats, *Adv. Exp. Med. Biol.,* 61, 289, 1975.
73. **Chen, J. C., Ove, P., and Lansing, A. I.,** In vitro synthesis of microsomal protein and albumin in young and old rats, *Biochem. Biophys. Acta,* 312, 589, 1973.
74. **Barrows, C. H.,** *The Effect of Age on Protein Synthesis,* Proc. 8th Int. Cong. Gerontol. Washington, D.C., Vol. 1, 179, 1969.
75. **Van Bezooijen, C. F. A., Grell, R., and Knook, D. L.,** Albumin synthesis by liver parenchymal cells from young and old rats, *Biochem. Biophys. Res. Comm.,* 71, 513, 1976.
76. **Van Bezooijen, C. F. A., Grell, R., and Knook, D. L.,** The effect of age on protein synthesis by isolated liver parenchymal cells, *Mech. Ageing Dev.,* 6, 293, 1977.
77. **Beatow, D. E. and Gandhi, P. S.,** Decreased protein synthesis by microsomes isolated from senescent rat livers, *Exp. Gerontol.,* 8, 243, 1973.
78. **Mainwaring, W. I. P.,** The effect of age on protein synthesis in mouse liver, *Biochem. J.* 113, 869, 1969.
79. **Comolli, R., Schubert, A., and Riboni, L.,** Changes in the activity and distribution of the ribosomal dissociation factor of rat liver during growth, *Mech. Ageing Dev.,* 11, 199, 1979.
80. **Yan, S. H. and Franks, J. J.,** Albumin metabolism in elderly men and women, *J. Lab. Clin. Med.,* 72, 449, 1968.
81. **Misra, D. P., Loudon, J. M., and Staddon, G. E.,** Albumin metabolism in elderly patients, *J. Gerontol.,* 30, 304, 1975.
82. **McFarlane, A. S.,** Measurement of synthesis rates of liver produced plasma proteins, *Biochem. J.,* 89, 277, 1963.
83. **Reeve, E. B., Pearson, J. R., and Martz, D. C.,** Plasma protein synthesis in the liver: method for measurement of albumin formation in vivo, *Science,* 139, 914, 1963.
84. **Gersovitz, M., Munro, H. N., Udall, J., and Young, V. R.,** Albumin synthesis in young and elderly subjects using a new stable isotope methodology: response to level of protein intake, *Metabolism,* 29, 1075, 1980.
85. **Peters, T.,** Serum albumin, in *the Plasma Proteins, Structure, Function and Genetic Control,* Vol. 1, Putnam, F. W., Ed., Academic Press, New York, 1975, 133.
86. **Rothschild, M. A., Oratz, M., and Schreiber, S. S.,** Albumin synthesis, in *Albumin, Structure, Function and Uses,* Rosenoer, V. M., Oratz, M., and Rothschild, M. A., Eds., Pergamon Press, New York, 1977, 227.
87. **Schreiber, G. and Urban, J.,** The synthesis and secretion of albumin, *Rev. Physiol. Biochem. Pharmacol.,* 82, 27, 1978.
88. **James, W. P. T. and Hay, A. M.,** Albumin metabolism: effect of the nutritional state and the dietary protein intake, *J. Clin. Invest.,* 47, 1958, 1968.
89. **Cohen, S. and Hansen, J. D. L.,** Metabolism of albumin and γ-globulin tracer studies in protein depletion states, *Clin. Sci.,* 23, 351, 1962.
90. **Munro, H. N., Hubert, C., and Baliga, B. S.,** Regulation of protein synthesis in relation to amino acid supply, in *Alcohol and Abnormal Protein Synthesis,* Rothschild, M. A., Oratz, M., and Schreiber, S., Eds., Pergamon Press, New York, 1975, 33.
91. **Pion R.,** The relationship between the levels of free amino acids in blood and muscle and the nutritive value of proteins, in *Proteins in Human Nutrition,* Porter, J. W. G. and Rolls, B. A., Eds., Academic Press, New York, 1973, 329.
92. **Elwyn, D. H.,** The role of liver in regulation of amino acid and protein metabolism, in *Mammalian Protein Metabolism,* Vol. 4, Munro, H. N., Ed., Academic Press, New York, 1970, 523.
93. **Peraino, C. and Harper, A. E.,** Observations on protein digestion in vivo. V. Free amino acids in blood plasma of rats force-fed zein, casein or their respective hydrolysates, *J. Nutr.,* 80, 270, 1963.
94. **Wehr, R. F. and Lewis, G. T.,** Amino acids in blood plasma of young and aged adults, *Proc. Soc. Exp. Biol. Med.,* 121, 349, 1966.
95. **Armstrong, M. D. and Stave, U.,** A study of plasma free amino acid levels. III. Variations during growth and aging, *Metabolism,* 22, 571, 1973.

96. Möller, P., Bergstrom, J., Erickson, S., Fürst, P. and Hellström, K., Effect of aging on free amino acids and electrolytes in leg muscle, *Clin. Sci.*, 56, 427, 1979.

97. Ackerman, P. G. and Kheim, T., Plasma amino acids in young and older adult human subjects, *Clin. Chem.*, 10, 32, 1964.

98. Young, V. R. and Scrimshaw, N. S., The nutritional significance of plasma and urinary amino acids, in *Protein and Amino Acid Functions*, Bigwood, E. J., Ed., Pergamon Press, Oxford, 1972, 541.

99. Munro, H. N., Free amino acid pools and their role in regulation, in *Mammalian Protein Metabolism*, Vol. 4, Munro, H. N., Ed., Academic Press, New York, 1970, 339.

100. McLaughlan, J. M., Nutritional significance of alterations in plasma amino acids and serum proteins, in *Improvement in Protein Nutrition*, Harper, A. E. and Hegsted, D. M., Eds., National Academy of Sciences, National Research Council, Washington, D. C., 1974, 89.

101. Ozalp, I., Young, V. R., Nagchaudhuri, J., Tontisirin, K., and Scrimshaw, N. S., Plasma amino acid response in young men given diets devoid of single amino acids, *J. Nutr.*, 102, 1147, 1972.

102. Hambraeus, L., Bilmazes, C., Dippel, C., Scrimshaw, N. S., and Young, V. R., Regulatory role of dietary leucine on plasma branched chain amino acid levels in young men, *J. Nutr.*, 106, 230, 1976.

103. Young, V. R., Hussein, M. A., Murray, E., and Scrimshaw, N. S., Plasma tryptophan response curve in relation to tryptophan requirements in young men, *J. Nutr.*, 101, 45, 1971.

104. Tontisirin, K., Young, V. R., Miller, M., and Scrimshaw, N. S., Plasma tryptophan response curve and trypophan requirements of elderly people, *J. Nutr.*, 103, 1220, 1973.

105. Young, V. R., Tontisirin, K., Ozalp, I., Lakshamana, F., and Scrimshaw, N. S., Plasma amino acid response curve and amino acid requirements in young men: valine and lysine, *J. Nutr.*, 102, 1159, 1972.

106. DeFronzo, R. A., Glucose intolerance and aging. Evidence for tissue insensitivity to insulin, *Diabetes*, 28, 1095, 1979.

107. Gersovitz, M., Bier, D., Matthews, D., Udall, J., Munro, H. N., and Young, V. R., Dynamic aspects of whole body glycine metabolism: influence of protein intake in young adult and elderly males, *Metabolism*, 29, 1087, 1980.

108. Lapidot, A., Nissim, I., and Irving, C. S., The diurnal rhythms in plasma amino acid pool sizes and turnover rates measured by gas chromatographic-mass spectrometric analysis of stable tracer ^{15}N-glycine, *Israel J. Chem.*, 77, 209, 1978.

109. Watts, R. W. E. and Crawhall, J. C., The first glycine metabolic pool in man, *Biochem. J.*, 73, 277, 1959.

110. Harper, A. E., Diet and plasma amino acids, *Am. J. Clin. Nutr.*, 21, 358, 1968.

111. Bergman, E. N. and Heitmann, R. N., Metabolism of amino acids by the gut, liver, kidneys, and peripheral tissues, *Fed. Proc.*, 37, 1228, 1978.

112. Griffith, O. W. and Meister, A., Glutathione: interorgan translocation, turnover, and metabolism, *Proc. Natl. Acad. Sci.*, 76, 5606, 1979.

113. Kikuchi, G., The glycine cleavage system: composition, reaction, mechanisms, and physiological significance, *Mol. Cell Biochem.*, 1, 169, 1973.

114. Yoshida, T. and Kikuchi, G., Major pathways of serine and glycine catabolism in various organs of the rat and cock, *J. Biochem.*, 73, 1013, 1973.

115. Fern, E. B. and Garlick, P. J., The specific radioactivity of the tissue free amino acid pool as a basis for measuring the rate of protein synthesis in the rat in vivo, *Biochem. J.*, 142, 413, 1974.

116. Irwin, M. I. and Hegsted, D. M., A conspectus of research or amino acid requirements of man, *J. Nutr.*, 101, 539, 1971.

117. Irwin, M. I. and Hegsted, D. M., A conspectus of research on protein requirements of man, *J. Nutr.*, 101, 385, 1971.

118. Watkin, D. M., The assessment of protein nutrition in the aged, *Ann. N. Y. Acad. Sci.*, 69, 902, 1957 to 1958.

119. Watkin, D. M., Protein metabolism and requirements in the elderly, in *Mammalian Protein Metabolism*, Vol. 2, Munro, H. N. and Allison, J. B., Eds., Academic Press, New York, 1964, 247.

120. Watkin, D. M., Nutrition for the aging and aged, in *Modern Nutrition in Health and Disease*, Goodhart, R. S. and Shil, M. E., Eds., Lea & Febiger, Philadelphia, 1980, 781.

121. Rose, W. C., The amino acid requirements of adult man, *Nutr. Abstr. Rev.*, 27, 631, 1957.

122. Leverton, R. M., Gram, M. R., Chaloupka, M., Bradovsky, E., and Mitchell, A., The quantitative amino acid requirements of young women. I. Threonine, *J. Nutr.*, 58, 59, 1956.

123. Tuttle, S. G., Swendseid, M. E., Mulcare, D., Griffith, W. H., and Bassett, S. H., Study of the essential amino acid requirements of men over fifty, *Metabolism*, 6, 564, 1957.

124. Tuttle, S. G., Swendseid, M. E., Mulcare, D., Griffith, W. H., and Bassett, S. H., Essential amino acid requirements of older men in relation to nitrogen intake, *Metabolism*, 8, 61, 1959.

125. Tuttle, S. G., Basset, S. H., Griffith, W. H., Mulcare, D. B., and Swendseid, M. E., Further observations on the amino acid requirements of older men. I. Effects of nonessential nitrogen supplements fed with different amounts of essential amino acids, *Am. J. Clin. Nutr.*, 16, 225, 1965.

126. **Tuttle, S. G., Basset, S. H., Griffith, W. H., Mulcare, D. B., and Swendseid, M. E.,** Further observations on the amino acid requirements of older men. II. Methionine and lysine, *Am. J. Clin. Nutr.,* 16, 229, 1965.

127. **Watts, J. H., Mann, A. N., Bradley, L., and Thompson, D. J.,** Nitrogen balances of men over 65 fed the FAO and milk patterns of essential amino acids, *J. Gerontol.,* 19, 370, 1964.

128. **Gaull, G., Rassin, D. K., Raiha, N. C. R., and Heinonen, K.,** Milk protein quantity and quality in low-birth weight infants. III. Effects on sulfur amino acids in plasma and urine, *J. Pediat.,* 90, 348, 1977.

129. **McLaughlan, J. M. and Morrison, A. B.,** Dietary factors affecting plasma amino acid concentrations in *Protein Nutrition and Free Amino Acid Patterns,* Leathem, J. H., Ed., Rutgers University Press, New Brunswick, 1968, 3.

130. **Ljungqvist, B. G.,** Plasma amino acid response to single test meals in humans. I. A background review, *Res. Exp. Med.,* 174, 1, 1978.

131. **Kang-Lee, Y. A. and Harper, A. E.,** Threonine metabolism in vivo: effect of threonine intake and prior indication of threonine dehydratase in rats, *J. Nutr.,* 108, 163, 1978.

132. **Brookes, I. M., Owens, F. N., and Garrigus, U. S.,** Influence of amino acid level in the diet upon amino acid oxidation by the rat, *J. Nutr.,* 102, 27, 1972.

133. **McLaughlan, J. M. and Illman, W. I.,** Use of free amino acid requirements of the growing rat, *J. Nutr.,* 93, 21, 1969.

134. **Mitchell, J. R., Becker, D. E., Jensen, A. H., Harman, B. G., and Norton, H. W.,** Determination of amino acid needs of the young pig by nitrogen balance and plasma free amino acids, *J. Anim. Sci.,* 27, 1327, 1968.

135. **Young, V. R. and Munro, H. N.,** Plasma and tissue tryptophan levels in relation to tryptophan requirements of weanling and adult rats, *J. Nutr.,* 103, 1756—1973.

136. **Kang-Lee, A. Y. and Harper, A. E.,** Effect of histidine activity on the metabolism of histidine in vivo, *J. Nutr.,* 107, 1427, 1977.

137. **Tontisirin, K., Young, V. R., Rand, W. M., and Scrimshaw, N. S.,** Plasma threonine response curve and threonine requirements of young men and elderly women, *J. Nutr.,* 104, 495, 1974.

138. Energy and Protein Requirements, World Health Organization Tech. Rep. Ser. 522, Food and Agriculture Organization, World Health Organization, Geneva, 1973.

139. **Bricker, M. L. and Smith, J. M.,** A study of the endogenous nitrogen output of college women with particular reference to the use of creatinine output in the calculation of the biological values of the protein of egg and sunflower seed flour, *J. Nutr.,* 44, 5530, 1951.

140. **Hawley, E. E., Merlin, J. R. Nassett, E. S., and Szymanski, T. A.,** Biological values of six partially-purified proteins, *J. Nutr.,* 36, 153, 1946.

141. **Zanni, E., Calloway, D. H., and Zezulka, A. Y.,** Protein requirements of elderly men, *J. Nutr.,* 109, 513, 1979.

142. **Scrimshaw, N. S., Hussein, M. A., Murray, E., Rand, W. M., and Young, V. R.,** Protein requirements of man, *J. Nutr.,* 102, 1595, 1972.

143. **Calloway, D. H. and Margen, S.,** Variation in endogenous nitrogen excretion and dietary nitrogen utilization as determinants of human protein requirement, *J. Nutr.,* 101, 205 1971.

144. **Scrimshaw, N. S., Perera, W. D. A., and Young, V. R.,** Protein requirements of man: obligatory urinary and fecal nitrogen losses in elderly women, *J. Nutr.,* 106, 665, 1976.

145. **Uauy, R., Scrimshaw, N. S., Rand, W. M., and Young, V. R.,** Human protein requirements: obligatory urinary and fecal nitrogen losses and the factorial estimation of protein needs in elderly men, *J. Nutr.,* 108, 97, 1978.

146. **Roberts, P. H., Kerr, C. H., and Ohlson, M. A.,** Nutritional status of older women. Nitrogen calcium, phosphorus retentions of nine women, *J. Am. Diet. Assoc.,* 24, 292, 1948.

147. **Albanese, A. A., Higgens, R. A., Orto, L. A., and Zwattoro, D. N.,** Protein and amino needs in the aged in health and convalescence, *Geriatrics,* 12, 443, 1957.

148. **Horwitt, M. K.,** Dietary requirements of the aged, *J. Am. Diet. Assoc.,* 29, 443, 1953.

149. **Kountz, W. B., Hofstatter, L., and Ackerman, P. G.,** Nitrogen balance studies in four elderly men, *J. Gerontol.,* 6, 20, 1951.

150. **Albanese, A. A., Higgens, R. A., Vestal, B., Stephanson, L., and Malsch, M.,** Protein requirements of old age, *Geriatrics,* 7, 109, 1952.

151. **Cheng, A. H. R., Gomez, A., Bergan, J. G., Lee, T-C., Monckeberg, F., and Chichester, C. O.,** Comparative nitrogen balance study between young and aged adults using three levels of protein intake from a combination of wheat-soy-milk mixture, *Am. J. Clin. Nutr.,* 31, 12, 1978.

152. Food and Nutrition Board, *Recommended Dietary Allowances,* 9th Revised Edition, National Research Council/National Academy of Sciences, Washington, D.C., 1980.

153. **Garza, C., Scrimshaw, N. S., and Young, V. R.,** Human protein requirements: effect of variations in energy intake within the maintenance range, *Am. J. Clin. Nutr.,* 29, 280, 1976.

154. **Garza, C., Scrimshaw, N. S., and Young, V. R.,** Human protein requirements: a long-term metabolic balance study in young men to evaluate the 1973 FAO/WHO safe level of protein intake, *J. Nutr.,* 107, 335, 1977.

155. **Inoue, G., Fujita, Y., and Niiyama, Y.,** Studies on protein requirements of young men fed egg protein and rice protein with excess and maintenance energy intakes, *J. Nutr.,* 103, 1673, 1973.

156. **Calloway, D. H.,** Nitrogen balance of men with marginal intakes of protein and energy, *J. Nutr.,* 105, 914, 1975.

157. **Shock, N. W.,** Energy metabolism, caloric intake and physical activity of the aging in *Nutrition in Old Age,* Carlson, L. A., Ed., Almquist and Wiksell, Uppsala, Sweden, 1972, 12.

158. **Butterfield-Hodgon, G. and Calloway, D. H.,** Protein utilization in man under two conditions of energy balance and work, *Fed. Proc.,* 36 (Abstr.), 1166, 1977.

159. **Beisel, W. R.,** Infectious diseases, in *Nutritional Support of Medical Practical,* Schneider, H. L., Anderson, C. E., and Coursin, D. B., Eds., Harper & Row, New York, 1977, 350.

160. **Bodwell, C. E., Schuster, E. M., Hyle, E., Brooks, B., Womack, M., Steele, P., and Ahrens, R.,** Obligatory urinary and fecal nitrogen losses in young women, older men and young men and the factorial estimation of adult human protein requirements, *Am. J. Clin. Nutr.,* 32, 2450, 1979.

Chapter 5

THE VITAMIN STATUS AND REQUIREMENTS OF THE ELDERLY

Barbara B. Fleming

TABLE OF CONTENTS

I. INTRODUCTION

Epidemiological research on the nutritional status of the older segment of the U.S. population is rather limited while research designed to determine the effect of age, per se, on vitamin requirements is essentially nonexistent. Good nutrition throughout life is an effective means of sustaining good health and minimizing degenerative changes in the elderly.[1] Knowledge of the vitamin status and vitamin requirements of this group is important in establishing nutrition guidelines for maintenance of optimal health.

Research designed to examine nutritional status and requirements of the elderly is becoming increasingly important since the number of individuals over the age of 65 is increasing proportionally more rapidly than any other age group.[2] Currently, the U.S. Bureau of the Census projects that at least 17% of the population will be over 65 years of age by 2030.

Individuals over 65 are the population group with the highest risk of illness and disability.[3] An estimated 85% of this group has some form of chronic disease[4,5] which may be related to inadequate nutrition or over-nutrition.[4] Diseases such as coronary heart disease,[6,7] hypertension,[8] osteoporosis,[9] and diabetes[7] are suspected of being nutritionally related to some degree and may possibly be modified by nutritional intervention. So in addition to the relationship between aging and nutrition, the interrelationships of aging, nutrition, and disease must be more fully explored. In 1976, the 10.5% of the population over the age of 65 accounted for 54% of all federal health expenditures.[1] Therefore, a significant potential benefit to be derived from greater knowledge of nutritional status and requirements of the elderly is health cost containment.

The objective of this paper is to examine the vitamin status and requirements of the elderly. The types of studies conducted in an effort to assess vitamin status of the elderly will be discussed, and findings from these studies will be reported for each of the vitamins. Approaches used in determining vitamin requirements of the elderly and findings with regard to requirements of each of the vitamins will be reviewed in the second section of this paper.

II. VITAMIN STATUS OF THE ELDERLY

The vitamin status of the U.S. elderly has been assessed by (1) dietary intake surveys, (2) measurement of vitamin levels in tissues or measurement of a biochemical function for which a specific vitamin is required, and (3) surveys of clinical signs of vitamin deficiency. Each of these three methods attempts to detect a stage of vitamin deficiency as outlined in Figure 1. Dietary intake data are compared to prevailing dietary standards in order to detect primary vitamin deficiency. Assessment of subclinical nutritional deficiency is based on detection of depleted blood, urine, or tissue stores of a nutrient, altered biochemical function, and/or altered metabolite levels. If the vitamin deficiency remains untreated, clinical symptoms appear and eventually death ensues.

A. Measurement of Dietary Intake as a Method of Assessment of Nutritional Status
1. Methods
Determination of dietary intake by each of the three major methods: (1) food rec-

Stage 1

Primary deficiency due to inadequate dietary intake

Secondary deficiency due to poor absorption, decreased reutilization, increased excretion or destruction, increased requirement

Stage 2

Depletion of tissue stores
Detected by blood, urine and tissue analysis

Stage 3

Biochemical abnormalities consisting of altered biological function followed by deterioration in the capacity of cells to function normally
Detected primarily by measurement of a biochemical system in which the vitamin functions, such as enzyme activity, and measurement of altered metabolite levels

Stage 4

Physiological symptoms such as general malaise, appetite loss, irritability, loss of body weight
Detected by clinical signs such as skin lesions, anemias, etc.

Stage 5

Mortality - if avitaminosis pathology progresses and is not corrected
Detected by vital statistics

FIGURE 1.   Stages in the development of vitamin deficiency.   Adapted from Krehl, W. A., *Geriatrics, 29,* 65, 1974 and from Brin, M., Dibble, M. V., Peal A., McMullen, E., Bourquin, A., and Chen, N., *Am. J. Clin. Nutr.,* 17, 240, 1965.

ords or diaries, (2) recall, or (3) dietary histories involves specific difficulties.[11,12] Food records or food diaries consist of determinations of present food intake generally by use of household measures or by weighing. This method is time-consuming, is not as suitable for meals eaten away from home, and may actually influence nutrient intake of subjects.

Dietary recall methods are also highly dependent on the cooperation and accuracy of the subjects in recalling foods eaten at some preceding period of time and, therefore, are subject to errors in estimation of kind and amounts of food eaten, particularly in the elderly. The frequently used 24-hr recall is considered an adequate method of intake assessment when used with large groups of subjects,[13-15] preferably groups of 50 or more.[14] However, the 24-hr recall tends to underestimate calories[13-17] and, like other short-term assessments, may not accurately reflect typical long-term patterns of food intake.[12-17]

Dietary histories based on food frequencies include information about general food patterns and habits for a period of time, up to a year. This method eliminates some of the seasonal variation in short-term reporting of intake and may more accurately reflect long-term patterns of intake. However, diet histories require much time and effort on the part of trained personnel and tend to overestimate protein consumption.[11] This method is also highly dependent on the subjects' accuracy in recalling food patterns.[13]

There is little research on the best dietary methods to be used with older subjects. The reliability of the 24-hr recall was not as great in elderly subjects as in younger subjects studied by Campbell and Dodds.[17] MacLeod[13] compared 24-hr recalls, 7-day dietary histories, and 7-day weighed food records of 200 normal, elderly individuals living at home. In this group, dietary histories overestimated protein intake and the 24-hr recall underestimated caloric intake. The 24-hr recall and the 7-day weighed record were well correlated and identified suboptimal nutrition in more cases than did the 7-day diet history.

After dietary data are obtained by food records, diet recall, or diet history, two major potential sources of error in analyzing and interpreting the data remain. First, food table values of nutrient content used in calculating diet composition are averages for a particular food, are dependent on methods of analysis used, and may not accurately reflect geographical and seasonal variation in nutrient content.[18] Secondly, the RDAs* generally used to evaluate intake are estimates based on extrapolation from a very limited number of studies, particularly in the case of RDAs for people over 51 years of age.[19]

B. Dietary Intake Standards

The RDAs are the most commonly used standards for the evaluation of intake. Two large national surveys, the TSNS[20] and the HANES,[21] developed their own standards for evaluation of dietary intake. These standards are given in Table 1 for comparison and for use in discussion of individual studies.

The RDAs were first formulated in 1941 and have been revised and updated nine times.[19,22-29] The RDAs are recommendations for the average daily amount of nutrients that healthy populations should consume over a period of time as determined by the Committee on Dietary Allowances of the Food and Nutrition Board of the National Research Council. Nutrient requirements are assumed to be normally distributed in healthy populations of adults. The mean requirement plus two standard deviations above the mean is the theoretical basis for estimating RDAs and is designed to be sufficient to cover 97.5% of the population.[30] The data on which the RDAs are based are limited; therefore, in many cases determination of a mean requirement is impossible. In addition, the criteria for determination of the requirement for each of the nutrients are varied. Although the term "required for optimal health" is used quite frequently, the definition of optimal health is completely arbitrary. It is very important to note that the nutrient requirements of the age group 51 years and older, in the words of the National Research Council itself, are "essentially an extrapolation from the nutrient needs of younger adults." The Committee on Dietary Allowances, after reviewing studies available to them in composing the 1980 requirements, concluded that studies of the nutrient needs of the elderly were inadequate for formulation of specific RDAs for the 51 year and older group.

A mean nutrient intake below the RDA for a particular group suggests that some individuals within the group are at nutritional risk. However, intake of a nutrient below the RDA is not conclusive evidence of nutritional inadequacy since the RDAs are designed to include a wide margin of safety. Inadequate nutrient intake accompanied by clinical and/or biochemical evidence of deficiency is more indicative of nutrient deficiency.

C. Dietary Intake Survey Findings

Three national surveys examined dietary intake of older individuals in the U.S. population (Table 2). The HFCS[31] was based on 24-hr food recalls of 14,000 individuals. Nine hundred and fifty-two of these subjects were older than 65 years. The TSNS[20] was heavily weighted toward people living in low income areas. Approximately 40,000

---

*   Recommended Dietary Allowances, formulated by the Food and Nutrition Board of the National Research Council.

subjects were given clinical examinations including wrist X-rays and hemoglobin and hematocrit determinations. A subgroup of 2128 persons over 60 years of age participated in a 24-hr dietary recall and additional biochemical evaluations. The HANES[21] collected data similar to the TSNS[20] dietary and clinical measurements on a total of 20,749 individuals between the ages of 1 and 74 years. A total of 3479 of these individuals were between 65 and 74 years.

Numerous studies on more geographically isolated segments of the elderly population have also been conducted. Intake data obtained by weighed food records, dietary recall, and less frequently by dietary histories were reported as the mean nutrient intake for the groups or as the percent of individual diets meeting a specified percentage of the current RDAs. Since the RDAs are designed to be two standard deviations higher than the average mean requirement, many investigators consider two thirds of the RDA an appropriate standard for evaluating intake. The mean nutrient intake is a good general indicator of the nutritional status of a population as a whole. However, the use of means alone can mask the fact that a substantial number of individuals within a group may have intakes below the RDA. Therefore, the percent of individual diets meeting a specified percentage of the RDA is a very important index in characterizing the nutritional status of a population. In most studies, the intake of vitamin A, ascorbic acid, thiamin, niacin, and riboflavin was determined and reported. Studies that examined dietary intake of older people are summarized in Table 2 and will be discussed in terms of individual nutrients. The mean nutrient intake of each population group will be compared to two thirds of the 1980 RDA in the following discussion. The values for percent of individual intakes below two thirds of the RDA were taken from each paper and are, therefore, based on current RDAs when the study was conducted as indicated in Table 2. Findings with regard to dietary intake of younger age groups are included in the tables for comparison.

1. Vitamin A

Mean intakes of vitamin A in the older population in two of the large national surveys (HANES,[21] HFCS[31]) were greater than two thirds of the 1980 RDA. All ethnic and age groups in the TSNS[20] except for certain Spanish-American groups had mean vitamin A intake above two thirds of the RDA. Most, but not all[39,44] other studies also reported mean intake of vitamin A above two thirds of the RDA. Therefore, vitamin A intake seems to be adequate in most population groups in terms of mean intake.

However, the number of individuals with low vitamin A intake suggests that the problem of low vitamin A intake is a serious one. The HANES,[21] TSNS,[20] and HFCS[31] reported that over half of the older individuals sampled had vitamin A intakes below two thirds of the RDA. Guthrie,[39] Pao,[50] Todhunter[52] and colleagues observed vitamin A intake below two thirds of the RDA in 66, 54, and 44% of their subjects, respectively. In the remainder of the studies, the percent of subjects at risk due to intakes less than two thirds of the RDA ranged from lows of 4%,[48] 7%,[47] and 9%,[36] and 12%[34] to more intermediate levels of 20 to 30%.[41,45,51]

2. Thiamin

Mean thiamin intake of older subjects in the TSNS,[20] HFCS,[31] and in almost all of the smaller groups (except for Brown,[32] Harrill,[41] and their co-workers) was greater than two thirds of the 1980 RDA. Twenty percent of the older men and women, 45% of the older women in the HFCS,[31] and 40% of the older subjects in the TSNS[20] consumed less than two thirds of the RDA. Thus a significant percent of these large population groups appeared to be at a risk of thiamin deficiency and other smaller studies confirmed this trend. Twenty to 40% of the subjects in the studies of Guthrie et al.,[39] Harrill and Cervone,[41] Lyons and Trulson,[48] Pao and Hill,[50] and Todhunter and Darby[52] consumed less than two thirds of the RDA.

Table 1
DIETARY INTAKE STANDARDS FOR OLDER ADULTS

Recommended Dietary Allowances

	1941	1943	1948	1953	1958
Reference	M^a 70 kg F^a 56 kg	M 70 kg, moderately active F 56 kg, moderately active	M 70 kg, physically active F 56 kg, moderately active	M age 65, 65 kg, 170 cm F age 65, 55 kg, 170 cm	M 65 years, 70 kg, 175 cm F 65 years, 65 kg, 163 cm
Calories	M 2500 F 2100	M 3000 F 2500	M 3000 F 2400	M 2600 F 1800	M 2550 F 1800
Thiamin (mg)	M 1.5 F 1.2	M 1.8 F 1.5	M 1.5 F 1.2	M 1.3 F 1.0	M 1.3 F 1.0
Riboflavin (mg)	M 2.2 F 1.8	M 2.7 F 2.2	M 1.8 F 1.5	M 1.6 F 1.4	M 1.8 F 1.5
Niacin (mg)	M 15 F 12	M 18 F 15	M 15 F 12	M 13 F 10	M 18 F 17
Ascorbic acid (mg)	M 75 F 70	M 75 F 70	M 75 F 70	M 75 F 70	M 75 F 70
Vitamin A (IU)	M 5000 F 5000	M 5000 F 5000	M 5000 F 5000	M 5000 F 5000	M 5000 F 5000

	1963	1968	1974	1980
Reference	M 55—75 years, 70 kg, 175 cm F 55—75 years, 58 kg, 163 cm	M 55—75+ years, 70 kg, 171 cm F 55—75+ years, 58 kg, 157 cm	M 51+ years, 70 kg, 172 cm F 51+ years, 58 kg, 162 cm	M 51+ years, 70 kg, 178 cm F 51+ years, 55 kg, 163 cm
Calories	M 2200 F 1600	M 2400 F 1700	M 2400 F 1800	M — F —
Thiamin (mg)	M 0.9 F 0.8	M 1.2 F 1.0	M 1.2 F 1.0	M 1.2 F 1.0
Riboflavin (mg)	M 1.3 F 1.2	M 1.7 F 1.5	M 1.5 F 1.1	M 1.4 F 1.2
Niacin (mg)	M 15 F 13	M 14 F 13	M 16 F 12	M 16 F 13

Ascorbic acid (mg)	M 70 / F 70	M 45 / F 60	M 60 / F 60
Vitamin A (IU)	M 5000 / F 5000	M 1000 RE[b] / F 800 RE	M 1000 RE / F 800 RE
Vitamin E (IU)	M 5000 / F 5000	M 15 / F 12	M 10 TE[c] / F 5 TE
Vitamin D (µg)	M 30 / F 25		M 5 / F 5
Folacin (mg)	M 0.4 / F 0.4	M 0.4 / F 0.4	M 0.4 / F 0.4
B_6 (mg)	M 2.0 / F 2.0	M 2.0 / F 2.0	M 2.2 / F 2.0
B_{12} (µg)	M 6 / F 6	M 3.0 / F 3.0	M 3.0 / F 3.0

	Standards used in TSNS[d]	Standards used in Hanes survey[e]
Reference M/F > 60	M 70 kg / F 55 kg	
Calories	M 2380 / F 1595	
Thiamin (mg)	M 1.0 / F 0.6	
Riboflavin (mg)	M 1.3 / F 0.9	
Niacin (mg)	M 15 / F 11	
Ascorbic acid (mg)	30	M and F 55
Vitamin A (IU)	3500	M and F 3500

[a] M = male, F = female.

[b] RE = Retinol equivalents. 1 retinol equivalent = 1 µg retinol or 6 µg β carotene.

[c] TE = α - tocopherol equivalents. 1 mg d-α tocopherol = 1 α TE.

[d] TSNS = Ten State Nutrition Survey.[20]

[e] HANES = Health and Nutrition Examination Survey.[21]

From Recommended Dietary Allowances, 1st to 9th eds., Food and Nutrition Board, National Research Council, National Academy of Sciencies, Washington, D.C., 1941 to 1980.

Table 2

DIETARY INTAKE STUDIES

Ref.	Location, year of study	Description of population	Methods	Findings
21	National—34 states and District of Columbia 1971—1972	Total group n = 10,126[a] 1—74 years,[b] M + F[c]; Older group n = 1,938 > 59 years, M + F	24-hr recall	*see Findings Table 21 below*
20	National 1968—1970	n = 3023, M + F, > 59 years, Mainly low income	24-hr recall, and food frequency chart	*see Findings Table 20 below*
31	National, 1965	n = 1,938, M + F > 60 years	24-hr recall	*see Findings Table 31 below*

Findings (Ref. 21) — Mean intake

Age	Ascorbic acid (mg)		Vitamin A (IU)
18—44	M	98	5186
	F	79	4018
45—59	M + F	90	5542
60+	M + F	96	6507
Total group (all ages)	Individual intake 38% < 30 mg		56% < 3000 IU

Findings (Ref. 20) — Mean Intake

Age	Thiamin (mg)	Riboflavin (mg)	Niacin (mg)	Ascorbic acid (mg)	Vitamin A (IU)
>59 M	1.14	1.76	19.06	59	4979
F	0.86	1.40	14.72	67	5172

Percent below the Ten State Standards

	Thiamin	Riboflavin	Niacin	Ascorbic acid	Vitamin A
Low income	45	27	35	45	57
High income	43	19	23	35	50

Findings (Ref. 31)

	Thiamin (mg)	Riboflavin (mg)	Niacin (mg)	Ascorbic acid (mg)	Vitamin A (IU)
M	1.17	1.70		66	5800
F	0.84	1.25			4976

			% Below 67% of 1964 RDA			
		Thiamin	Riboflavin	Niacin	Ascorbic acid (mg)	Vitamin A (IU)
Age	M					
65—74		20	26		43	41
75+		21	41		52	51
	F					
65—74		45	42		51	60
75+		45	49		54	60

Mean intake

	Thiamin (mg)	Riboflavin (mg)	Niacin (mg)	Ascorbic acid (mg)	Vitamin A (IU)
F					
Home	0.96	1.28	12.2	122	5439
instit.	0.69	1.20	8.2	58	3252
M					
Home	1.22	1.45	15.5	161	6249
instit.	0.78	1.22	9.8	67	3591

Percent below 50% of 1968 RDA

Riboflavin	Niacin	Ascorbic acid	Vitamin A
5	12	4	6

Percent individual values

	Thiamin <1.0mg	Riboflavin <2.0mg	Niacin <10mg	Ascorbic acid <50mg	Vitamin A <4000 IU
NS[e]	40	67	25	27	12
NS and S[e]	21	37	11	16	7

	Location	Method	Population
32	Rhode Island, 1977	7-day weighed intake	Nursing home residents, n = 20, M + F, x̄ age = 85, 1/2 ambulatory, 1/2 sedentary,
		10-day diet records	n = 23, M + F, independent, rural elderly, x̄ age = 77, healthy, middle income
33	Near Manhattan, Kan., (1975)[a]	Food frequency questionnaire, trained interviews	Nursing home residents, n = 102 F, > 70 years independent housing residents, n = 102 F, > 70 yr
34	Boston, Mass., 1962	1-week recall and 7-day recorded intake	n = 104 healthy M + F, 2/3 > 70 yr, (51—99 years), own homes and apartments

Table 2 (Continued)
DIETARY INTAKE STUDIES

Ref.	Location, year of study	Description of population	Methods
35	Syracuse, N.Y. 1963—65	n = 214, M + F, x̄ age = 71, housing unit residents	6-day food record
36	Lincoln, Neb., 1963	n = 32, F, x̄ age = 75 years, healthy, own homes	6 weighed intakes, 7-day recorded intake
37	San Mateo, Calif., 1948—49	n = 514, M + F > 50 years	7-day diet record
38	Location not given, 1978	n = 40, M + F, x̄ age = 72 years	3-day food record

Findings

Ref. 35 — Mean Intake

	Thiamin (mg)	Riboflavin (mg)	Ascorbic acid (mg)	Vitamin A (IU)
M	0.98	1.33	50	5348
F	0.88	1.31	54	5719

Percent less than 67% 1958 RDA

M	9	18	51	36
F	6	16	44	33

Ref. 36 — Mean intake

Thiamin (mg)	Riboflavin (mg)	Niacin (mg)	Ascorbic acid (mg)	Vitamin A (IU)
1.1	1.7	21	102	4885

Percent individual values < 67% of 1958 RDA

0	6	0	3	9

Ref. 37 — Mean intake

	Carotene (IU)	Preformed A (IU)	Total (IU)
M	5570	5070	10,640
F	4640	3810	8450

Ref. 38 — Mean intake

	Thiamin (mg)	Riboflavin (mg)	Niacin (mg)	Ascorbic acid (mg)	Vitamin A (IU)
M	1.34	1.78	16.2	110	5043
F	0.96	1.43	11.9	76	4712

39	Rural Pa., 1972	24-hr recall	n = 109, M + F, > 60 years, own homes and apartments, 1/2 low income

Mean intake

	Thiamin	Riboflavin	Ascorbic acid	Vitamin A
M	1.0	1.3	51	2999
F	0.9	1.2	64	2999

Percent less than 2/3 1968 RDA

Total group	42	45	45	66

40	Milwaukee, Wis., 1958	3-day food record, 1 week inventory	n = 65, M + F, 40—75 years, nursing home residents

Percent meeting 1958 RDA

Age		Vitamin A	Ascorbic acid
55—74	M	8	3
	F	10	5
75 +	M	7	3
	F	23	14

41	Fort Collins, Colo., 1977	3 consecutive days weighed intake	Nursing home residents, n = 46, private home residents, n = 24, x̄ age = 80, low/medium income

Mean intake

Thiamin (mg)	Riboflavin (mg)	Niacin (mg)	Ascorbic acid (mg)	Vitamin A (IU)
0.72	1.19	9.3	83	4338

Percent less than 2/3 1974 RDA

47	9	43	13	21

42	Cincinnati, Ohio, 1970	24-hr recall	n = 185, M + F, 45—90 years, own homes or apartments, low income

Mean intake

	Thiamin (mg)	Riboflavin (mg)	Niacin (mg)	Ascorbic acid (mg)	Vitamin A (IU)
Participants in meal program					
F	0.90	1.40	14	55	10,232
M	1.80	1.85	16	62	6,658
Subjects not provided with 1 meal per day					
F	0.82	1.11	10	52	5414
M	0.73	1.15	10	44	4429

Table 2 (Continued)
DIETARY INTAKE STUDIES

Ref.	Location, year of study	Description of population	Methods	Findings					
				Mean intake					
					Thiamin (mg)	Riboflavin (mg)	Niacin (mg)	Ascorbic acid (mg)	Vitamin A (IU)
43	West Lafayette, Ind., 1974	n = 44, M + F, age 63—93, nursing home (chronic illness prevalent)	5 or 6 nonconsecutive days of food intake	Age					
				63—84 years	1.0	1.5	10.3	102	7101
				85—93 years	0.9	1.4	9.7	108	6973
				Percent less than 80% 1948 RDA					
					Thiamin (mg)	Riboflavin (mg)	Niacin (mg)	Ascorbic acid (mg)	Vitamin A (IU)
44	New York City, 1955	n = 53, M + F, > 60 years, 68% on public aid	1-day diet record	M	70	55	59	67	63
				F	77	54	50	30	63
				Percent less than 80% 1953 RDA					
					Thiamin (mg)	Riboflavin (mg)	Niacin (mg)	Ascorbic acid (mg)	Vitamin A (IU)
45	Michigan, 1955	n = 117, F, 47—92 years	Diet recall diet history	White	70	70	70	55	70
				Black	70	70	70	55	80
				Mean intake as percent of 1974 RDA					
					Thiamin	Riboflavin	Niacin	Ascorbic acid	Vitamin A
46	Central Miss., 1978	n = 466, M + F, 59—96 years, Noninstitutionalized	1-day food records	Meal program partic- ipants	102	130	105	168	118
				Nonpartici- pants	102	115	95	166	119

			Percent of households less than 2/3 1963 RDA		
	Thiamin	Riboflavin	Ascorbic acid	Vitamin A	
	3	2	15	7	

47 Rochester, N.Y., 1965 n = 283 households, 456 M + F, x̄ age = 73, low income 7-day food recall

48 Boston, Mass., 1956 n = 100 M + F, >65 years, low to middle income Diet history

	Mean intake				
	Thiamin (mg)	Riboflavin (mg)	Niacin (mg)	Ascorbic acid (mg)	Vitamin A (IU)
M	1.29	2.00	15.69	105	10,973
F	0.94	1.58	11.60	95	8,571
	Percent below 2/3 1953 RDA				
M	32	26	10	17	10
F	20	17	2	26	4

49 Baltimore, Md., and D.C., 1966 n = 252 M, 20—99 years, 137 M > 55 years, middle to high income 7-day record

	Mean intake				
	Thiamin (mg)	Riboflavin (mg)	Niacin (mg)	Ascorbic acid (mg)	Vitamin A (IU)
20—34 years	1.67	2.70	23.1	106	11,900
35—44 years	1.38	2.21	20.1	107	7800
45—54 years	1.28	1.91	20.0	106	7800
55—64 years	1.20	1.83	18.5	115	7900
65—74 years	1.35	1.98	18.0	142	8900
75—99 years	1.20	1.87	15.0	119	8100

50 North Central and Southern U.S., 1965 n = 952 M + F, >65 years, subsample of 1965 USDA Survey non-farm 1-day diet recall

	Percent less than 2/3 1968 RDA				
	Thiamin	Riboflavin	Niacin	Ascorbic acid	Vitamin A
	34	39		49	54

Table 2 (Continued)
DIETARY INTAKE STUDIES

Ref.	Location, year of study	Description of population	Methods	Findings				
				Mean intake				
51	San Mateo, Calif., 1962	n = 141 M + F, x̄ age = 76, healthy	1-day diet record	M				
				50—54 years	1.1	1.7	15	88	7136
				60—64 years	1.0	2.0	15	74	10,058
				65—69 years	1.0	1.6	12	86	7300
				70—74 years	0.9	1.4	11	66	8983
				>75 years	1.1	1.7	11	85	9058
				F				
				50—54 years	1.0	1.6	14	86	7929
				60—64 years	0.9	1.4	12	98	8251
				65—69 years	0.9	1.4	12	86	7291
				70—74 years	0.9	1.5	10	77	7990
				>75 years	0.8	0.9	9	69	5170
				Percent less than 2/3 1964 RDA				
				M (x̄ age = 68 yr)	12	7	66	25	24
				F (x̄ age = 73 yr)	4	10	62	19	27

Ref.	Location, year of study	Description of population	Methods	Findings				
				Percent less than 66% 1974 RDA				
52	Tenn., 1973	n = 529, M + F, x̄ age = 74 years	24-hr recall	Thiamin	Riboflavin	Niacin	Ascorbic acid	Vitamin A
				43	37		67	44

				Percent less than 74% 1953 RDA				
				4	2	8	5	3
53	R.I., 1958	n = 48, M + F, 71% were > 60 years, ambulatory residents of public institute for the aged	14-day weighed food intake					

a n = Number of subjects.
b Age; $\bar{x}$ age = 70 indicates mean age of the population.
c M = male, F = female.
d When the year of study was not given, the year of the publication is given in parentheses.
e NS = not supplemented with vitamin capsules; S = supplemented with vitamin capsules.
f Approximation from bar graph.

3. Riboflavin

The mean intake of riboflavin was greater than two thirds of the 1980 RDA in every study. The percent of older individuals with values below approximately two thirds of the RDA ranged from a low of 2% in LeBovit's subjects[47] to a high of approximately 70% in Kelley's subjects.[45] The large national surveys (TSNS,[20] HFCS[31]) reported that from 19 to 49% of the older population consumed less than two thirds of the RDA.

4. Niacin

The mean niacin intake of older individuals was above two thirds of the 1980 RDA in all studies except that of Harrill and Cervone.[41] The TSNS[20] reported individual levels of intake below two thirds of the RDA in 35% of the low income group and in 23% of the high income group over 59 years of age. Some populations appeared to be at very low risk of deficiency with fewer than 10% of the individuals consuming less than two thirds of the RDA[36,48,53] while others reported that over 40% of the individuals consumed less than two thirds of the RDA.[41,51]

5. Ascorbic Acid

The mean intake of ascorbic acid exceeded the 1980 RDA in all studies. Only when individual intakes were examined did there appear to be any risk of ascorbic acid deficiency. The TSNS[20] reported that 45 and 35% of the high and low income subjects older than 59 years consumed less than two thirds of the RDA for ascorbic acid. The HANES[21] found that 28% of their population group consumed less than 30 mg ascorbic acid. Approximately 45% of the men and 52% of the women over 60 years of age in the HFCS[31] consumed less than two thirds of the RDA. Six other investigators reported ascorbic acid intake less than two thirds of the RDA in fewer than 30% of their subjects[34,36,41,47,48,53] while six reported that over 45% of their population groups consumed less than two thirds of the RDA.[35,39,40,50,52] A significant percent of the older population appeared to be at risk of ascorbic acid deficiency based on these studies.

6. Conclusions

The mean intakes of thiamin, riboflavin, niacin, ascorbic acid, and vitamin A were greater than two thirds of the RDA in almost all studies reported (Table 2). Mean niacin intake and mean thiamin intake were below two thirds of the RDA in 2 of 11 studies while mean vitamin A intake was below two thirds of the RDA in only 1 of 16 studies. Mean riboflavin and ascorbic acid intakes were adequate in all studies.

However, examination of the vitamin status of the populations in terms of individual intakes suggested the possibility of primary vitamin deficiencies. Thiamin intake was below two thirds of the RDA in 25% or more of the subjects in 6 of 11 studies. Riboflavin intake was below two thirds of the RDA in 25% or more of the subjects in 5 of 11 studies. Six of 11 studies reported ascorbic acid intake below two thirds of the RDA in more than 25% of the subjects with 3 of the 6 studies reporting intakes less than two thirds of the RDA in over half the subjects. Intake of vitamin A was below two thirds of the RDA in over 25% of the subjects examined in 7 of 11 studies (3 of the 7 reported intake less than two thirds of the RDA in over half of the subjects). Niacin intake was below two thirds of the RDA in more than 25% of the subjects in two studies and in more than half of the subjects in a third study out of a total of five studies reported. Thus ascorbic acid, vitamin A, and niacin intakes were less than two thirds of the RDA for each of the nutrients in over one fourth of the subjects in over one half of the studies. While these dietary deficiencies are not proof of biologically significant nutritional deficiencies, they do indicate that a significant proportion of the elderly population may be at risk of developing vitamin deficiencies.

Table 3
ICNND CRITERIA FOR VITAMIN ADEQUACY[a]

Nutrient	Metabolite or effect measured	Unit of measurement	Tissue in which measured	Level observed "Deficient"	Level observed "Low"
Thiamin	(a) Thiamin	μg/g creatinine		<27	27—65
	(b) TPP effect[b]	mg/24 hr	Urine	<0.04	0.041—0.096
		percent	Erythrocyte	>15	10—15
Riboflavin	Riboflavin	μg/g creatinine	Urine	<27	27—79
		mg/24 hr	Urine	<0.04	0.041—0.116
Niacin	N-methyl nicotinamide	mg/24 hr	Urine	<0.8	0.81—2.4
Vitamin B₆	Xanthurenic acid	mg/24 hr	Urine	>100	50—99
Ascorbic acid	Ascorbic acid	mg/dl	Plasma	<0.10	0.10—0.19
Vitamin A		μg/dl	Plasma	<10	10—19
Carotene		μ/dl	Plasma	<10	20—39

[a] Interdepartmental Committee for National Defense Manual for Nutrition Surveys, U.S. Government Printing Office, Washington, D.C., 1957.

[b] Brin, M., Erythrocyte as a biopsy tissue for functional evaluation of thiamin adequacy, *JAMA,* 187, 762, 1964.

D. Measurement of Tissue Levels and Biochemical Functions as Assessment of Vitamin Status

1. Methodology and Standards

Measurement of tissue levels of a nutrient and/or its metabolites or of a biochemical function involving the nutrient appears to be a more objective and accurate assessment of nutritional status. Low vitamin intake alone is not conclusive evidence of a deficiency state. However, as in the case of dietary intake, the significance of criteria used in biochemical assessment is not always known. The tissue levels of a nutrient required for optimal function of systems in which the nutrient is involved have not been determined for some vitamins nor, in fact, are the biological functions of all the vitamins known. In addition, correlations between dietary intake and tissue levels or excretion of the vitamin are not always high. Finally, the commonly used ICNND standards[54] by which biochemical parameters are evaluated are based on values in 25-year-old, physically active males, and thus, may not be valid for assessment of older populations.[35] The ICNND criteria are given in Table 3.

2. Vitamin A

Mean plasma vitamin A levels of older populations met or exceeded the ICNND level of adequacy of greater than 39 μg % vitamin A in serum in all studies (Table 4). Fewer than 1% of the individuals over 5 years old in the HANES[21] had low serum vitamin A values. In the TSNS[20], individual levels were adequate except in segments of the Spanish-American population. Fewer than 6% of the subjects studied by Gillum,[37] Dibble,[35] Brin,[10] Fisher[59] and their co-workers had inadequate serum vitamin A levels. Low or deficient serum vitamin A levels occurred in 17% of the group examined by Harrill and Cervone.[41] Serum levels of carotene reflect recent dietary intake more closely than serum levels of vitamin A since serum vitamin A content also reflects liver tissue stores.[66] Inadequate serum carotene was observed in less than 5% of the subjects examined by Dibble and co-workers[35] and by Harrill and Cervone.[41] The low vitamin A intake in the HANES, TSNS, and in several other studies was generally not reflected in inadequate serum levels of vitamin A and carotene.

Table 4
VITAMIN STATUS DETERMINED BY MEASUREMENT OF TISSUE LEVELS AND BIOCHEMICAL FUNCTION

Ref.	Location, year of study	Description of population	Findings
21	National (34 states and D.C.), 1971—1972	Total group: n = 10,126 M + F[b]; elderly group: n = 1,938 M + F, 59—74 years	See mean value and percent low or deficient tables below
20	National (10 states), 1972	n = 895 M, 1,233 F, > 59 years, mainly low income	See percent low or deficient tables below
55	Miami, Florida (1979)[c]	n = 193, M + F, > 60 years, mainly black, low income, urban, noninstitutionalized	See means below

Ref. 21 — Findings

Mean value — Vitamin A (serum, μg/dl)

Age	
1—5	37.2
18—44	60.5
45—59	64.5
>60	65.1

Percent low or deficient[a] — Vitamin A (serum)

Age	
1—5	3.45
18—44	0.04
45—59	0.10
	0.14

Ref. 20 — Findings: Percent low or deficient

Vitamin A and carotene (serum)

Age		White	Black	Span. Am.
17—44	M	3.7	5.9	24.1
	F	1.7	7.1	17.2
>59	M	2.6	2.9	14.8
	F	1.2	1.4	11.1

Ascorbic acid (serum)

Age		White	Black	Span. Am.
17—44	M	15.0	17.0	8.3
	F	8.8	12.9	9.0
>59	M	13.6	18.3	15.5
	F	7.0	9.2	2.6

Thiamin (urine)

Age	White	Black	Span. Am.
17—34	3.6	7.9	4.2
35—59	3.8	8.9	4.2
>59	4.8	8.0	9.6

Riboflavin (urine) — Low income states

Age	White	Black	Span. Am.
17—34	11.8	17.9	5.9
>59	5.8	14.7	11.3

High income states

Age	White	Black	Span. Am.
17—34	7.1	9.8	5.9
>59	5.5	12.9	1.9

Ref. 55 — Findings: Means

Folacin (red blood cell, ng/ml)

M 119
F 165

Folacin (serum, ng/ml)

M 7.59
F 12.2

Means

56 Michigan 1954

n = 143, M + F, residents of county institution, most with one or more diseases

Males

Age	Ascorbic acid (serum mg/dl)	Vitamin A (serum µg/dl)	Carotene (serum µg/dl)
40—49	0.60	42.5	102.5
60—69	0.38	41.4	90.9
70—79	0.55	41.2	84.0
80—89	0.55	55.6	90.8
>90	0.32	32.7	41.6

Females

Age	Ascorbic acid (serum mg/dl)	Vitamin A (serum µg/dl)	Carotene (serum µg/dl)
40—49	1.15	35.0	102.5
60—69	0.61	43.6	84.6
70—79	0.67	48.9	112.4
80—89	0.54	35.4	75.1
>90	1.27	24.4	74.1

10 New York (1965)

n = 234, M + F, $\bar{x}$ age = 71 years, community homes, public housing, veterans hospital

Means

Thiamin (urine, µg/g creatinine)	Riboflavin (urine, µg/g creatinine)	Ascorbic acid (plasma, mg/dl)	Vitamin A (plasma, µg/dl)	Carotene (plasma, µg/dl)
174	599	0.68	54.4	133.7
Rbc-transketo-lase 90/mg/10 ml/hr hexose formed TPP effect 6.7%				

Percent deficient

TPP effect	
urine	1
plasma	18

57 New York (1964)

n = 10 M, 62—96 years, community home

Thiamin (urine, mg/24 hr)	Riboflavin (urine, mg/24 hr)	N-methyl-nico-tinamide (urine, mg/24 hr)	Ascorbic acid (plasma, mg/dl)	Carotene (plasma, µg/dl)
urine 0.042 TPP effect— 15%	1.26	3.08	1.56	11.3

TPP

Table 4 (Continued)
VITAMIN STATUS DETERMINED BY MEASUREMENT OF TISSUE LEVELS AND BIOCHEMICAL FUNCTION

Ref.	Location, year of study	Description of population	Findings					
			Means					
			Thiamin (urine, μg/g creatinine)	Riboflavin (urine, μg/g creatinine)	Ascorbic acid (plasma, μg/dl)	Vitamin A (plasma, μg/dl)	B_{12} (plasma, mg/dl)	Carotene (plasma, μg/100 ml)
58	Indianapolis, Ind. (1957)	n = 201, M + F, 31—100 years, county home residents, ill or low SE	Age					
			41—50 142	707	0.88	49	0.54	115
			61—70 200	634	0.88	52	0.48	129
			71—80 151	504	0.84	59	0.45	105
			81—90 180	536	0.73	57	0.44	113
35	Syracuse, N.Y., 1963—1965	n = 214, M + F, > 50 years, housing unit, dwellers	TPP effect (percent)					
			Age					
			51—60 9.8					
			61—70 8.2					
			71—80 7.5					
			>80 8.6					
			Percent low or deficient					
			Urine or plasma values 41	17	7	1		3
			TPP effect 12					
			Means					
			Thiamin (urine, μg/g creatinine)	Riboflavin (urine, μg/g creatinine)		Vitamin A (plasma, μg/dl)		Carotene (plasma, μg/dl)
59	Utah (1978)	n = 187, M + F, x̄ age = 69, 5 rural, low income, communities						

				M	951	1396	50	330
				F	1781	2661	48	358

	Percent deficient or low			
M	2	1	0	0
F	2	1	0	0

B₁₂ values — percent incidence

	Age	
	20—49	50—94	80—89
<100 µg/ml	0.83	18.2	33.2
<150 µg/ml	7.02	45.4	
<200 µg/ml	23.2	74.0	

Means

	Vitamin A (plasma, µg/dℓ)	Carotene (plasma, µg/dℓ)
M	56	118
F	54	120

Age	Thiamin (urine µg/g creatinine)	Riboflavin (urine µg/g creatinine)	Niacin N-methyl nicotinamide (urine µg/g creatinine)	Ascorbic acid (plasma mg/dℓ)	Vitamin A (plasma µg/dℓ)	Carotene (plasma µg/dℓ)
62—75	258	139	7.2	1.2	53	155
76—85	120	148	6.2	1.2	53	129
86—99	78	95	4.2	1.4	53	125
TSNS Standards of Adequacy	>66		>1.6	>0.2	>30	>4

Ref	Study	Description
60	Baltimore, Md., 1956	Young subjects n = 248, 31—44 years; Healthy, older subjects, n = 89, x̄ age = 71; Nursing home residents n = 126, x̄ age = 74
37	San Mateo, Calif., 1948—1949	n = 215 M, n = 269 F, > 50 years, all healthy, 30 men in home for aged
41	Fort Collins, Colo. 1977	n = 46 (nursing homes) 24 (private homes), F, x̄ age = 80

Table 4 (Continued)

VITAMIN STATUS DETERMINED BY MEASUREMENT OF TISSUE LEVELS AND BIOCHEMICAL FUNCTION

Ref.	Location, year of study	Description of population	Findings
43	Midwest (1974)	n = 12 M, 32 F, age 63—93, diseases prevalent	Percent below TSNS standards (low or deficient) 17 15 1 14 1 Means Ascorbic acid (serum, mg/dℓ) Folic acid (plasma, mg/dℓ) Age 63—84 1.0 14.9 85—93 1.1 11.7
44	New York, N.Y., 1955	n = 49 M + F, > 60 years	Percent below stated value Ascorbic acid (plasma) < 0.4 µg/dℓ 31 Vitamin A (plasma) < 30 µg/dℓ 10 Carotene (plasma) < 50 µg/dℓ 12
61	St. Louis, Mo., 1947—1948	n = 220 inmates and patients (40—120 years) n = 29 younger M + F	Means Thiamin (plasma, µg/dℓ) Age 16—39 3.8 40—59 3.3 60—69 3.7 70—79 3.2 80 + 3.1
62	St. Louis, Mo., (1953)	n = 142 inmates, M + F, institutionalized	Means B$_6$ in blood (mg/dℓ) Mean for all ages 1.1

63 — San Mateo, Calif., 1948—1949 — n = 569, M + F, > 50 years, healthy

Ascorbic acid (plasma, mg/dℓ)

Age	Male	Female
16—39	0.82	1.02
40—59	0.59	0.48
60—69	0.42	0.42
70—74	0.41	0.43
75—79	0.35	0.41
80—103	0.33	0.40
Means		

64 — Baltimore, Md., (1960) — n = 60, $\bar{x}$ age = 25 n = 60 old, $\bar{x}$ age = 76

Ascorbic acid (plasma, mg/dℓ)

Age	Male	Female
50—54	0.73	1.10
55—59	0.75	1.13
60—64	0.94	1.21
65—69	0.91	0.99
70—79	0.76	0.99
>79	0.92	0.95
Means		

29% less than 0.4 mg/dℓ

Glutamate oxaloacetate transminase (serum-content units)

	Young	Old	M + F
M	16.5	13.0	
F	18.8	13.3	
Means			

Xanthurenic acid excretion (mg/24 hr urine)

Young	Old
6.5	32.6

65 — Baltimore, Md., 1971, 1973 — n = 617 M, 18—90 years, healthy community dwellers, middle to high socioeconomic status

B_6, (plasma ng/mℓ)

Age	
18—29	25.4
30—39	19.6
Means	

Glutamate oxaloacetate transminase (erythrocytes IU)

Age	
18—39	28

Table 4 (Continued)
VITAMIN STATUS DETERMINED BY MEASUREMENT OF TISSUE LEVELS AND BIOCHEMICAL FUNCTION

Ref.	Location, year of study	Description of population	Findings				
				Means			
			40—49	20.3	40—59	27.8	
			50—59	24.6			
			60—69	20.8	60—79	27.6	
			70—79	18.0	80—90	26.3	
			80—89	13.3			

a   Percent low or deficient values are assessed by ICNND Standards (Table 3).

b   M = male, F = female.

c   When the year of the study was not given, the year of publication is given in parentheses.

3. Thiamin

Mean urinary thiamin values for the older groups surveyed (except for Brin's study of nursing home patients)[57] were above the 0.096 mg/24 hr or 66 μg thiamin per gram of creatinine considered acceptable by ICNND standards. Mean thiamin excretion ranged from a low of 78 μg/g of creatinine in 86- to 99-year-olds[41] to a high of 1781 ug/g of creatinine in females over 69 years of age.[59] The TSNS[20] reported inadequate urinary thiamin excretion in only 5% of the whites, 8% of the blacks, and 10% of the Spanish-Americans studied. Low or deficient levels of thiamin were found in the urine of 90, 41, 18, 29, and 2% of the elderly individuals examined in other studies.[10,35,41,55,57,59]

Decreased erythrocyte transketolase activity is correlated with severity of thiamin deficiency.[67-69] The addition of thiamin pyrophosphate (TPP) to deficient cells restores transketolase enzyme activity (TPP effect). The TPP effect is sensitive to and specific for thiamin deficiency and probably a more valid indicator of nutritional status than urinary thiamin.[10] The use of the TPP effect for assessing thiamin nutriture usually results in classification of fewer individuals as thiamin deficient than does use of urinary thiamin. Using the TPP effect as a criterion of adequacy, 40, 12, and 15% of the populations examined by Brin et al.,[57] Dibble,[35] and Brin et al.[10] were thiamin deficient.

4. Riboflavin

Urinary riboflavin excretion is a direct indicator of riboflavin status since riboflavin itself is its own principal urinary excretory product.[70] In adults, excretion of more than 0.116 mg of riboflavin in 24 hr or more than 80 μg of riboflavin per gram of creatinine is considered indicative of acceptable riboflavin nutriture (ICNND). Mean urinary riboflavin excretion was above the ICNND standards in all surveys. Individuals with urinary riboflavin excretion less than ICNND standards constituted 0, 1, 17, and 28% of the total number of subjects studied by Brin,[57] Fisher,[59] Dibble,[35] and Harrill and Cervone[41], respectively. Riboflavin deficiency does not seem to be a serious problem, at least among the populations studied.

5. Niacin

Excretion of one of the major metabolic products of niacin, n-methyl nicotinamide, (NMN), is used as an index of niacin status. Mean excretion of NMN in the studies of Brin et al.[57] and Harrill and Cervone[41] was above the ICNND acceptable level of 1.6 mg/g of creatinine or 2.4 mg/24 hr. Only 1% of the individuals examined by Harrill and Cervone could be considered niacin deficient. However, five of the ten nursing home residents in Brin's study excreted levels of NMN below the ICNND accepted levels.[57] This very limited number of studies suggests that niacin deficiency is not a serious problem in the healthy, noninstitutionalized elderly.

6. Ascorbic Acid

The plasma ascorbic acid concentration of a population is a rough index of its ascorbic acid intake. White blood cell ascorbic acid concentration is a better measure of tissue stores, but the method is technically difficult and thus not used for large screenings.[70,71]

The mean serum ascorbic acid levels in all groups were above the ICNND acceptable level of 0.19 mg/100 mℓ of serum. Individuals with low or deficient levels of serum ascorbic acid constituted 8, 7, and 0% of the older populations studied by Brin,[10] Dibble,[35] Harrill[41] and their colleagues and fewer than 10% of the group over 59 years old surveyed in the TSNS.[20] Thus ascorbic acid deficiency appears to occur at a very low frequency and is not a cause for serious concern in the older populations surveyed.

7. Folic Acid

Folic acid status is assessed by determination of folic acid in serum and blood with levels above 7 to 16 ng/mℓ of serum considered normal.[66] Bailey et al.[55] reported adequate mean levels of both serum folacin and red blood cell folacin in females in a primarily black population. Black males in the same population had inadequate mean red blood cell folacin and adequate serum folacin levels. Mean levels of serum folic acid were adequate in subjects examined by Justice et al.[43]

8. Vitamin B$_6$

Plasma pyridoxal phosphate (PLP) concentrations and erythrocyte and plasma glutamate oxaloacetate transaminase (GOT) concentrations are used to assess B$_6$ nutriture. Several investigators reported lower mean plasma PLP concentrations in old vs. young subjects.[65,72,73] The PLP values for subjects aged 20 to 35 averaged 18.5 ng/mℓ, 11.3 ng/m, and 15 ng/mℓ in the studies of Chabner,[72] Hamfelt,[73] and Rose,[65] and co-workers, respectively. The PLP levels of subjects over 60 years of age averaged 3.4 ng/mℓ and 12.5 ng/mℓ in the studies of Hamfelt[73] and Rose. Ranke et al.[64] observed lower serum GOT levels in older subjects which were correctable by B$_6$ administration. Rose and associates[65] did not find lower plasma or erythrocyte GOT levels in their older subjects.

9. Vitamin B$_{12}$

Normal serum B$_{12}$ levels range from 200 to 900 pg/mℓ with levels below 80 pg/mℓ representing unequivocal B$_{12}$ deficiency according to the World Health Organization (WHO) Scientific Group on Nutritional Anemias.[74] Serum B$_{12}$ levels below 100 pg/mℓ were reported in 33% of 80- to 89-year-olds, 18% of 50- to 94-year-olds, and only 1% of 20- to 49-year-olds in the study of Gaffney and coworkers.[60] Twenty-six percent of the geriatric patients examined by Dawson and Donald[75] had serum B$_{12}$ levels less than 160 pg/mℓ, a value the authors considered the lower limit of normal. The age-related decrease in serum B$_{12}$ levels reported by Gaffney et al.[60] was not observed by Droller,[76] Shilling,[77] Shulman,[78] Davis,[79] and their co-investigators. In addition, B$_{12}$ levels in liver[80] and vascular tissues[81] did not differ between young and old subjects. Although some studies[60,75] have shown the existence of B$_{12}$ deficiency states in a significant percentage of the older population, several others[76-79] have failed to confirm this finding.

10. Conclusions

When means for urinary thiamin, urinary riboflavin, urinary NMN, plasma ascorbic acid, and plasma vitamin A and carotene were determined for samples of the elderly U.S. population, only urinary thiamin excretion was below ICNND standards in any of the studies. Mean urinary thiamin levels were below ICNND standards in two of five reported studies (Table 4). Means for urinary excretion and serum or plasma levels of the other vitamins were adequate.

In contrast, when individual values were examined, a significant percentage of the older population appeared to be at risk of nutritional deficiency. Plasma vitamin A and carotene levels were the nutrient levels which were adequate in the greatest percentage of subjects. The extent of deficiencies of vitamin intake shown in Table 2 was not totally reflected as inadequate serum and urinary levels of the vitamins.

E. Clinical Symptoms as Assessment of Vitamin Status

Relating clinical symptoms to specific vitamin deficiencies with any certainty is very difficult.[18] This is due to the nonspecific nature of many clinical symptoms, such as loss of appetite, irritability, etc. and to the increased reporting of these symptoms in the elderly. Studies which have attempted to correlate clinical signs of vitamin deficiency with blood level of vitamins in New York City school children[83] and in hospital patients in New Jersey[82] have shown no correlation between the presence or absence of hypovitaminemia and clinical signs of vitamin deficiency. This lack of correlation between clinical signs and vitamin levels in blood or urine was also reported in a number of studies dealing with older subjects.[34,37,44,57,84]

Kaplan et al.[44] observed clinical signs of vitamin deficiency, such as glossitis and gingivitis, in 50 of 53 subjects, although dietary intake was not at all indicative of this level of deficiency. Chieffi and Kirk[84] examined 106 individuals and observed a greater frequency of hyperkeratosis of the skin follicles and of localized conjuctival thickening in those with low plasma vitamin A levels. However, they did not find any correlation between plasma vitamin A levels and any other signs of vitamin A deficiency. Gillum, Morgan, and Sailer[37] also observed no correlation between plasma levels of vitamin A and clinical signs of deficiency in their subjects. Similarly, Davidson et al.[34] and Brin et al.[57] were unable to correlate clinical signs of deficiency with urinary levels of riboflavin and thiamin respectively.

F. Vitamin Status and Longevity

Several studies have suggested that vitamin status of the elderly may be important not only with regard to maintenance of health, but may also be associated with longevity. Chope[85] obtained dietary information from 577 San Mateo County, California residents over 50 years of age in 1948 to 1949. A follow-up study of these same subjects in 1952 suggested a relationship between mortality and the intake of vitamins A, C, and niacin. A mortality rate of 13.9% was observed in subjects consuming less than 5000 IU of vitamin A. For subjects consuming more than 5000 IU per day, the mortality rate was 5.4%. It must be noted that the number of subjects in which these associations were observed was rather small, so the data remain suggestive rather than conclusive.

In the same San Mateo County residents, Chope[85] observed a mortality rate of 18.5% among subjects consuming less than 50 mg of ascorbic acid per day and a mortality rate of only 4.5% among subjects consuming more than 50 mg ascorbic acid. Schlenker[86] also observed an association between ascorbic acid intake and mortality. In a 4-year follow-up of 100 subjects, mean intake of ascorbic acid was 51 mg among those who died and 73 mg among survivors. However, Schlenker's study also involved few subjects. In addition, the ages of the survivors (mean age of 52.1) differed from the age of those who died (mean age of 67.4). Wilson and his associates[87,88] also demonstrated small but significant relationships between leukocyte ascorbic acid levels of less than 12 $\mu g/10^8$ white blood cells and mortality in two studies of geriatric patients.

A relationship between niacin intake and mortality was suggested by Chope's followup study of San Mateo County residents.[85] Mortality rates during a 5-year period were 10.4, 8.2, and 5.6% in subjects consuming less than 10 mg of niacin, 10 to 13 mg of niacin, and over 14 mg of niacin, respectively. Numbers of deaths among subjects were small so that the data were not conclusive.

Associations between vitamin intake and longevity observed by these authors may be merely coincidental rather than causal. However, the possible implications of these findings are certainly exciting and should be followed by controlled studies to examine the effect of varied levels of vitamin intake on longevity.

III. VITAMIN REQUIREMENTS

The first obstacle to determining the effect of age on vitamin requirements is determining the basis for the vitamin requirements. The requirement for a vitamin has been defined as the "minimum intake that will maintain normal function and health".[29]

Health has been defined by the World Health Organization as a "state of complete physical, mental, and social well-being and not merely the absence of disease or infirmity".[89] Clearly, there exists ample room for arbitrary decisions regarding vitamin requirements within the context of these definitions. As a result, there is not always agreement on the basis for determining when the requirement has been met.[90] Once the criteria for "normal function and health" are determined, then these criteria must be used in assessing vitamin requirements of representative healthy segments of each age group to determine if age, per se, affects vitamin requirements.

A. Methodology

Assessment of vitamin requirements is based on a number of techniques: (1) survey-type studies of nutrient intake of normal, disease-free populations, (2) epidemiological observations of clinical consequences of nutrient deficiencies correctable by dietary improvement, (3) measurements of adequacy of a molecular function in which a particular nutrient participates, (4) nutrient balance studies that measure nutritional status in relation to intake, and (5) studies in which depletion of a nutrient is followed by repletion.

There are difficulties inherent in the design and execution of both survey and laboratory type studies. The problems associated with dietary intake surveys have been discussed previously. Laboratory experiments with human subjects involve tremendous amounts of time and money along with a great deal of cooperation from the subjects who may have to consume monotonous diets and collect urine and feces. Laboratory studies, therefore, are usually of short duration and are based on few subjects. As a result of the difficulty of conducting large-scale surveys and controlled laboratory studies, requirements for some nutrients are based on estimates or extrapolation from animal studies.

In addition to problems of design and execution of dietary surveys and laboratory studies, there are some other very important difficulties in vitamin requirement assessment. Marks[91] stated that the main problem in assessment of dietary requirements is the determination of the significance of the criteria used for assessment. Determination of the level of vitamin intake which will prevent clinical signs of deficiency seems clear-cut, but the stage at which clinical evidence of deficiency appears is far advanced (Figure 1). In addition, clinical symptoms may be nonspecific and often do not correlate highly with dietary and subclinical evidence of deficiency as discussed previously. One of the first measurable effects of deficiency is a decrease in tissue stores of the vitamin followed by a decrease in biochemical function. The tissue levels associated with decreased biochemical function are not known for all nutrients nor are the biochemical functions of all vitamins known.[92] In the elderly, another complicating factor is that renal insufficiency may affect assessment of requirements based on urinary excretion of the vitamin or its metabolites.

B. Studies on Vitamin Requirements of the Elderly

There is a scarcity of data available on the effect of age on vitamin requirements. Possibly partly as a result of this deficiency, studies in which vitamin levels in blood or tissues were lower in old adults than in younger adults[60,61,93,94] have been used to suggest that vitamin requirements are increased in older individuals. Findings of lower tissue levels of vitamins in the elderly are not evidence of increased requirements and, in fact, may only reflect the observed decreased nutrient intake of the elderly. There are a number of factors which may result in decreased nutrient intake or may influence nutritional status of elderly subjects apart from an influence on dietary intake (Table 5).

Studies dealing with the effect of age on vitamin requirements will be discussed in the following section. It will be quite evident that very little is known about this topic.

Table 5

FACTORS THAT INFLUENCE NUTRITIONAL REQUIREMENTS AND NUTRITIONAL STATUS IN THE ELDERLY

I.   Intrinsic factors
    1.   Age, sex, and genetic factors
    2.   Physical and physiological changes with age
        a.   Oral changes — edentulousness, reduced perception of smell and taste
        b.   Decreased basal metabolic rate and decreased lean body mass
    3.   Pathological states
        a.   Acute conditions — such as trauma, infection, burns
        b.   Chronic conditions — such as diabetes, arthritis, and osteoporosis

II. Extrinsic factors
    1.   Diet
        a.   Level of nutrient intake
        b.   Chemical form of the nutrients and their interactions
        c.   Food processing and preparation methods
    2.   Economic factors
        a.   Low or reduced income
        b.   Lack of adequate facilities for food preparation and storage
    3.   Social and psychological factors
        a.   Isolation — frequently due to death of spouse, accompanied by loneliness and apathy
        b.   Cultural food habits and attitudes
        c.   Level of education
    4.   Decreased physical activity
    5.   Medications and/or surgery
    6.   Stress
    7.   Alcoholism

C. Water-Soluble Vitamins

1. Thiamin

Horwitt[95] measured thiamin levels under conditions of depletion and repletion in young (mean age of 34) and old (mean age of 70) subjects and observed no significant differences in initial serum levels or in rates of depletion or repletion between the two age groups. Horwitt's study, while scientifically sound, involved only six old and five young subjects and thus remains to be confirmed.

In a series of investigations with rats, Mills et al.[96,97] reported that the thiamin requirement per kilogram of diet increased with age, based on thiamin required for optimal weight gain of rats maintained in the cold (68°F) and the heat (90 to 91°F). However, since older rats consumed less food per unit of body weight, the thiamin requirement was actually less per unit of body weight in the older rats. Thus there certainly appears to be no increase in the thiamin requirement per unit of body weight as a function of age.

2. Riboflavin

Horwitt[95] measured urinary excretion of riboflavin in young (mean age of 34) and old (mean age of 70) subjects under conditions of depletion and repletion of riboflavin and found no differences between the two groups. In rats, the riboflavin requirement also does not increase with age based on determination of the dietary concentration of the vitamin required for optimal growth from weaning to 24.5 months.[97] Thus the riboflavin requirement does not appear to increase with age, although, once again, the available data are limited.

3. Niacin

There are no studies in humans specifically assessing the effect of age on niacin requirements. In rats, there does not appear to be any change in the niacin requirement with age from weaning to 24.5 months.[97]

4. Vitamin B₆

Ranke and co-workers[64] were among the first to suggest an effect of age on vitamin B₆ requirements as a result of observed differences in serum GOT and xanthurenic acid excretion following a trytophan load test in a group of young subjects (mean age of 25) compared to a group of nursing home residents (mean age of 76). However, the serum GOT levels and xanthurenic acid excretion could be brought to levels similar to those of young adults by administration of oral doses of 15 mg of vitamin B₆ per day for 3 weeks which suggests that older subjects consumed less of the vitamin initially. The decreased vitamin levels in plasma and the decreased serum GOT in older subjects have not been conclusively shown to be a function of age and not of diet or other extrinsic factors.[65,73,98] In a study designed to explore the effect of age on the vitamin B₆ requirement, Mills[97] reported no effect of age on the dietary concentration of B₆ required for growth of rats from weaning to 24.5 months.

5. Vitamin B₁₂

Gaffney and co-workers[60] suggested that vitamin B₁₂ requirements increase with age as a result of findings of a decrease of 35% in serum B₁₂ levels of males between the ages of 25 and 70. However, findings of a decrease in plasma levels are not evidence of altered requirements nor were age-related declines in blood[76-79] or in tissue[80,81] levels of B₁₂ observed by other investigators. Thus there are really no definitive data on the effect of age on B₁₂ requirements.

6. Other Water-Soluble Vitamins

The dietary concentration of choline and pantothenic acid required by rats for optimal growth did not increase between weaning and 24.5 months.[97]

7. Ascorbic Acid

There are no human studies designed to compare ascorbic acid requirements of the elderly to those of younger adults. However, Purinton and Schuck[99] determined the ascorbic acid requirements of groups of women aged 15 to 20, 20 to 25, and 25 to 50 by determining the quantity of ascorbic acid excreted in the 24 hr following administration of a saturation test dose. These authors reported that older women had lower ascorbic acid requirements than either group of younger women.

D. Fat-Soluble Vitamins

1. Vitamin E

Grinna[100] examined the effect of different levels of vitamin E in the diet on liver microsomes and nutrition of aging rats. Liver levels of tocopherol were similar in 11-, 42-, and 67-week-old rats. When vitamin E deficient diets were fed to 11-, 42-, and 67-week-old rats, signs of vitamin deficiency appeared after 7 weeks in 11-week-old rats, after 16 weeks in 42-week-old rats, and not at all in 67-week-old rats. These data indicate that the vitamin E requirement of rats decreases with age. Since there are no studies on the effect of age on the vitamin E requirements of humans, no basis exists for any change in the RDA of the elderly from that of younger adults.

2. Other Fat-Soluble Vitamins

There are not any studies either to suggest or to disprove that age alters the requirement for any of the other fat-soluble vitamins.

3. Conclusions

Much remains to be learned about vitamin requirements of all age groups before appropriate guidelines for vitamin requirements of the elderly can be established. Definitive studies on the effect of age on requirements of the vitamins are almost totally lacking. The limited data available suggest that there is no general increase in requirements for the vitamins as a function of age. The only vitamins for which a decrease in allowances with advancing age is suggested are those based on energy allowances, specifically thiamin, riboflavin, and niacin. However, the increasing frequency of disease and the increased use of medication in the elderly increase the risk of vitamin deficiency in this group. Other factors, such as lowered income, loneliness, and disinterest in food also affect vitamin status of this group (Table 5). Since a major change with age appears to be increased difficulty in maintaining homeostasis of various systems under conditions of stress,[101-103] it is important to examine vitamin requirements of the elderly under conditions of stress and disease.

IV. SUMMARY

The mean intakes of thiamin, riboflavin, niacin, ascorbic acid, and vitamin A were greater than two thirds of the RDA in almost all studies reported. However, the vitamin status of the elderly did not appear to be quite as good when individual intakes were examined. Ascorbic acid, vitamin A, and niacin intakes were less than two thirds of the RDA in over one fourth of the subjects in over one half of the studies reported. Nutrient intake of two thirds of the RDA is generally considered adequate since the RDAs represent the mean requirement for a nutrient plus approximately two standard deviations above the mean. The risk of primary vitamin deficiency increases the lower the mean nutrient intake of a population or the greater the number of individuals within a population consuming less than two thirds of the RDA for a nutrient.

Means for urinary riboflavin, urinary N-methyl nicotinamide, plasma ascorbic acid, plasma vitamin A, and plasma carotene were above ICNND standards in the elderly populations examined. Mean urinary thiamin levels were low in two of five studies. However, a percentage of each population examined appeared to be at risk of nutritional deficiency based on individual urinary and plasma levels of the vitamins.

These data suggest that a significant proportion of the elderly population may be at risk of developing nutritional deficiencies. However, the RDAs used for assessment of dietary intake are, in the words of the committee that devised them, "essentially an extrapolation from the nutrient needs of younger adults".[19] In addition, the ICNND standards used for assessment of biochemical findings are based on values found in 25-year-old healthy, physically active males.[35] Thus the standards used for evaluation of the vitamin status of the elderly may be totally inappropriate.

Information on the vitamin requirements of the aged is so limited that no definitive statement can be made. The limited data available suggest that there is no general increase in the requirement for the vitamins as a function of age. However, increased disease, apathy, loneliness, and a number of other social and economic factors place the elderly at potentially increased risk of vitamin deficiency. If nutrition is to be used as an important tool in sustaining optimal health, it is important that we increase our knowledge of vitamin requirements of all age groups. This knowledge is almost completely lacking in regard to the elderly population.

REFERENCES

1. Butler, R. N., Nutrition and Aging, Testimony before the Senate Select Committee on Nutrition and Human Needs, September 23, 1977.
2. Demographic Aspects of Aging and the Older Population in the United States, Bureau of the Census, U.S. Department of Commerce, Series P-23, 59, 1976.
3. Shank, R. E., Nutritional characteristics of the elderly — an overview, in *Nutrition, Longevity, and Aging,* Rockstein, M. and Sussman, M. L., Eds., Academic Press, New York, 1976, 9.
4. Watkin, D. M., Biochemical impact of nutrition on the aging process, in *Nutrition, Longevity, and Aging,* Rockstein, M. and Sussman, M., Eds., Academic Press, New York, 1976, 47.
5. Krehl, W. A., The influence of nutritional environment on age, *Geriatrics,* 29, 65, 1974.
6. Goodman, D. S. and Smith, F. R., "Hyperlipidemia, arteriosclerosis and ischemic heart disease", in *Nutrition and Aging,* Winick, M., Ed., John Wiley & Sons, New York, 1976, 177.
7. Bierman, E. L., Obesity, carbohydrate, and lipid interactions in the elderly, in *Nutrition and Aging,* Winick, M., Ed., John Wiley & Sons, New York, 1976, 171.
8. Kark, R. M. and Opama, J. H., Nutrition and cardiovascular-renal diseases, in *Modern Nutrition in Health and Disease,* 5th ed., Goodhart, R. S. and Shils, M. E. Eds., Lea & Febiger, Philadelphia, 1973, 852.
9. Jowsey, J., Prevention and treatment of osteoporosis, in *Nutrition and Aging,* Winick, M., Ed., John Wiley & Sons, New York, 1976, 131.
10. Brin, M., Dibble, M. V., Peel, A., McMullen, E., Bourquin, A., and Chen, N., Some preliminary findings on the nutritional status of the aged in Onondaga County, New York, *Am. J. Clin. Nutr.,* 17, 240, 1965.
11. Marr, J., Individual dietary surveys: purposes and methods, *World Rev. Nutr. Diet.,* 13, 105, 1971.
12. O'Hanlon, P. and Kohrs, M. B., Dietary studies of older Americans, *Am. J. Clin. Nutr.,* 31, 1257, 1978.
13. MacLeod, C. C., Methods of dietary assessment, in *Symposia of Swedish Nutrition Foundation — Nutrition in Old Age,* Carlson, L. A., Ed., Alomqvist and Wilfell, Uppsala, Sweden, 1972, 118.
14. Young, C. M., Hagan, G. C., Tucker, R. E., and Foster, W. D., A comparison of dietary study methods. II. Dietary history vs. seven-day record vs. 24-hour recall, *J. Am. Diet. Assoc.,* 28, 218, 1952.
15. Chalmers, F., Clayton, M., Gates, L., Tucker, R., Wertz, C., Young, C., and Foster, W., The dietary record — how many and which days?, *J. Am. Diet. Assoc.,* 28, 711, 1952.
16. Madden, J. P., Goodman, S. J., and Guthrie, H., Validity of the 24-hour recall, *J. Am. Diet. Assoc.,* 68, 143, 1976.
17. Campbell, V. A. and Dodds, M. L., Collecting dietary information from groups of older people, *J. Am. Diet. Assoc.,* 51, 29, 1967.
18. Kelsey, J. L., A compendium of nutritional status studies and dietary evaluation studies conducted in the United States, 1957 to 1967, *J. Nutr.,* 99, 119, 1969.
19. Food and Nutrition Board, *Recommended Dietary Allowance,* 9th ed., Food and Nutrition Board, National Research Council, National Academy of Sciences, Washington, D.C., 1980.
20. Ten State Nutrition Survey 1968 to 1970. I. Historical development. II. Demographic data. III. Clinical, anthropometry, dental. IV. Biochemical. V. Dietary and highlights, U.S. Department of Health, Education, and Welfare Publication No. (HSM) 72, 8130, 1972.
21. Preliminary findings of the first health and nutrition examination survey, United States, 1971 to 72. Dietary intake and biochemical findings, U.S. Department of Health, Education and Welfare Publication No. (HRA) 74, 1219, 1974.
22. Food and Nutrition Board, *Recommended Dietary Allowances,* 1st ed., Food and Nutrition Board, National Research Council, National Academy of Sciences, Washington, D.C., 1941.
23. Food and Nutrition Board, *Recommended Dietary Allowances,* 2nd ed., Food and Nutrition Board, National Research Council, National Academy of Sciences, Washington, D.C., 1943.
24. Food and Nutrition Board, *Recommended Dietary Allowances,* 3rd ed., Food and Nutrition Board, National Research Council, National Academy of Sciences, Washington, D. C., 1948.
25. Food and Nutrition Board, *Recommended Dietary Allowances,* 4th ed., Food and Nutrition Board, National Research Council, National Academy of Sciences, Washington, D.C., 1953.
26. Food and Nutrition Board, *Recommended Dietary Allowances,* 5th ed., Food and Nutrition Board, National Research Council, National Academy of Sciences, Washington, D.C., 1958.
27. Food and Nutrition Board, *Recommended Dietary Allowances,* 6th ed., Food and Nutrition Board, National Research Council, National Academy of Sciences, Washington, D. C., 1963.
28. Food and Nutrition Board, *Recommended Dietary Allowances,* 7th ed., Food and Nutrition Board, National Research Council, National Academy of Sciences, Washington, D.C., 1968.

29. Food and Nutrition Board, *Recommended Dietary Allowances,* 8th ed., Food and Nutrition Board, National Research Council, National Academy of Sciences, Washington, D.C., 1974.

30. Young, V. B., Diet and nutrient needs in old age, in *Biology of Aging,* Behnke, J. A., Finch, C. E., and Moment, G. B., Eds., Plenum Press, New York, 1978, 151.

31. Consumption of Households in the U.S., Spring, 1965, Household Food Consumption Survey, 1965 to 1966, Consumer and Food Economics Divisions, Agricultural Research Service, U.S. Department of Agriculture, Washington, D.C., 212, 1968.

32. Brown, P. T., Bergan, J. G., Parsons, E. P., and Krol, I., Dietary status of elderly people, *J. Am. Diet. Assoc.,* 71, 41, 1977.

33. Clarke, M. and Wakefield, L., Food choices of institutionalized vs. independent living elderly, *J. Am. Diet. Assoc.,* 66, 600, 1975.

34. Davidson, C. S., Livermore, J., Anderson, P., and Kaufman, S., The nutrition of a group of apparently healthy aging persons, *Am. J. Clin. Nutr.,* 10, 181, 1962.

35. Dibble, M. V., Brin, M., Thiele, V. F., Peel, A., Chen, N. and McMullen, E., Evaluation of the nutritional status of elderly subjects, with a comparison between fall and spring, *J. Am. Geriatr. Soc.,* 15, 1031, 1967.

36. Fry, C., Fox, P., Meltz, H., and Linkswiler, H., Nutrient intakes of healthy older women, *J. Am. Diet. Assoc.,* 42, 218, 1963.

37. Gillum, H. L., Morgan, A. F., and Sailer, F. S., Nutritional status of the aging. V. Vitamin A and carotene, *J. Nutr.,* 55, 655, 1955.

38. Grotkowski, M. L. and Sims, L. S., Nutritional knowledge, attitudes, and dietary practices of the elderly, *J. Am. Diet. Assoc.,* 72, 499, 1978.

39. Guthrie, H. A., Black, K., and Madden, J. P., Nutritional practices of elderly citizens in rural Pennsylvania, *Gerontology,* 12, 330, 1972.

40. Hankin, J. H. and Antonmattei, J. C., Survey of food service practices in nursing homes, *Am. J. Public Health Natl. Health,* 50, 1137, 1960.

41. Harrill, I. and Cervone, N., Vitamin status of older women, *Am. J. Clin. Nutr.,* 30, 431, 1977.

42. Joering, E., Nutrient contribution of a meals program for senior citizens, *J. Am. Diet. Assoc.,* 59, 129, 1971.

43. Justice, C., Howe, J., and Clark, H., Dietary intakes and nutritional status of elderly patients, *J. Am. Diet. Assoc.,* 65, 639, 1974.

44. Kaplan, L., Landes, J. H., and Pincus, J., The nutritional status of noninstitutionalized aged persons, *Geriatrics,* 10, 287, 1955.

45. Kelley, L., Ohlson, M. A., and Harper, L. J., Food selection and well-being of aging women, *J. Am. Diet. Assoc.,* 33, 466, 1957.

46. Kohrs, M. B., O'Hanlon, D. S., and Ekland, D., Contribution of the older Americans nutrition program to one day diet intake, *J. Am. Diet. Assoc.,* 72, 487, 1978.

47. LeBovit, C., The food of older persons living at home, *J. Am. Diet. Assoc.,* 46, 289, 1965.

48. Lyons, J. S. and Trulson, M. F., Food practices of older people living at home, *J. Gerontol.,* 11, 66, 1956.

49. McGandy, R. B., Barrows, C. H., Spanias, A., Meredith, A., Stone, J. L., and Norris, A. H., Nutrient intakes and energy expenditure in men of different ages, *J. Gerontol.,* 21, 587, 1966.

50. Pao, E. M. and Hill, M. M., Diets of the elderly — nutrition labeling and nutrition education, *J. Nutr. Educ.,* 6, 96, 1974.

51. Steinkamp, E. C., Cohen, N. L., and Walsh, H. E., Resurvey of an aging population — fourteen year follow-up, *J. Am. Diet. Assoc.,* 46, 103, 1965.

52. Todhunter, N. E. and Darby, W. J., Guidelines for maintaining adequate nutrition in old age, *Geriatrics,* 33, 49, 1978.

53. Tucker, R., Brin, C., and Wallace, M., Nutrient intake of older institutionalized persons, *J. Am. Diet. Assoc.,* 34, 819, 1958.

54. Manual for Nutrition Surveys, Interdepartmental Committee on National Defense, U.S. Government Printing Office, Washington, D.C., 1957.

55. Bailey, L. B., Wagner, P. A., Cristakis, G. J., Araiyo, P. E., Appledorf, H., Davis, C. G., Masteryann, J., and Dinning, J. S., Folacin and iron status and hematological findings in predominately black elderly persons from urban low-income households, *Am. J. Clin. Nutr.,* 32, 2346, 1979.

56. Brewer, W. D., Turnwall, M. E., Wagoner, E., Lee, J., Alsup, B., and Ohlson, M. A., Nutritional status of the aged in Michigan, *J. Am. Diet. Assoc.,* 32, 810, 1956.

57. Brin, M., Schwartzberg, S. H., and Davies, D. A., A vitamin evaluation program as applied to 10 elderly residents in a community home for the aged, *J. Am. Geriatr. Soc.,* 12, 493, 1964.

58. Chernish, S. M., Oscar, M. H., Touts, P. J., and Kohlstaidt, K. G., The effect of intrinsic factor on the absorption of vitamin B_{12} in older people, *Am. J. Clin. Nutr.,* 5, 651, 1957.

59. Fisher, S., Hendricks, D. G., and Mahoney, A. W., Nutritional assessment of senior rural Utahns by biochemical and physical measurement, *Am. J. Clin. Nutr.,* 31, 667, 1978.

60. **Gaffney, G. W., Hornick, A., Okuda, K., Meier, P., Chow, B. F., and Shock, N. W.,** Vitamin B_{12} serum concentrations in 528 apparently healthy human subjects of ages 12 to 94, *J. Gerontol.,* 12, 32, 1957.

61. **Kirk, E. and Chieffi, M.,** Vitamin studies in middle-aged and old individuals. III. Thiamine and pyruvic and blood concentrations, *J. Nutr.,* 38, 353, 1949.

62. **Kirk, J. E. and Chieffi, M.,** Vitamin studies in middle-aged and old individuals. XI. The concentration of total ascorbic acid in whole blood, *J. Gerontol.,* 8, 301, 1953.

63. **Morgan, A. F., Gillum, H. L., and Williams, R. I.,** Nutritional status of the aging. III. Serum ascorbic acid and intake, *J. Nutr.,* 55, 431, 1955.

64. **Ranke, E., Tauber, S. A., Horonick, A., Ranke, B., Goodhart, R., and Chow, B. F.,** Vitamin B_6 deficiency in the aged, *J. Gerontol.,* 15, 41, 1960.

65. **Rose, C. S., Gyorgy, P., Butler, M., Andres, R., Norris, A. H., Shock, N. W., Tobin, J., Brin, M., and Spiegel, H.,** Age differences in vitamin B_6 status of 617 men, *Am. J. Clin. Nutr.,* 29, 847, 1976.

66. **Goodhart, R. S. and Shils, M. E.,** *Modern Nutrition in Health and Disease,* 5th ed., Lea & Febiger, Philadelphia, 1973.

67. **Brin, M., Shoket, S. S., and Davidson, C. S.,** Effect of thiamine deficiency on glucose oxidative pathway of rat erythrocytes, *J. Biol. Chem.,* 230, 319, 1958.

68. **Brin, M., Tai, M., and Kalinsky, H.,** Effects of thiamine deficiency on erythrocyte hemolysate transketolase, *J. Nutr.,* 71, 273, 1960.

69. **Dreyfus, D. M.,** Clinical application of blood transketolase determination, *New Engl. J. Med.,* 267, 596, 1962.

70. **Standstead, H. H. and Pearson, W. N.,** Clinical evaluation of nutrition status, in *Modern Nutrition in Health and Disease,* 5th ed., Goodhart, R. S. and Shils, M. E., Eds., Lea & Febiger, Philadelphia, 1973, 572.

71. British Medical Council Special Report, No. 280, London, 1953.

72. **Chabner, B. A., DeVita, V. J., Livingston, D. M., and Oliverio, V. T.,** Abnormalities of tryptophan metabolism and plasma pyridoxal phosphate in Hodgkins disease, *N. Engl. J. Med.,* 282, 838, 1970.

73. **Hamfelt, A.,** Age variation of vitamin B_6 metabolism in man, *Clin. Chem. Acta,* 10, 48, 1964.

74. Scientific Group on Nutritional Anemias, World Health Organization, Technical Report Series, No. 405, World Health Organization, Geneva, 1968.

75. **Dawson, A. A. and Donald, D.,** The serum vitamin B_{12} in the elderly, *Gerontol. Clin.,* 8, 220, 1966.

76. **Droller, H. and Dossett, J. A.,** Vitamin B_{12} levels in senile dementia and confusional states, *Gerontol. Clin.,* 1, 96, 1959.

77. **Shilling, R. F.,** The absorption and utilization of vitamin B_{12}, *Am. J. Clin. Nutr.,* 3, 45, 1955.

78. **Shulman, R.,** A survey of vitamin B_{12} deficiency in an elderly psychiatric population, *Br. J. Psychiatr.,* 113, 241, 1967.

79. **Davis, T. R. A., Gershoff, S. N., and Gamble, D. F.,** Review of studies of vitamin and mineral nutrition in the United States, 1950 to 1968, *J. Nutr. Educ.,* 1, 41, 1969.

80. **Swendseid, M. E., Hvolboll, E., Shick, G., and Halsted, J.,** The vitamin B_{12} content of human liver tissue and its nutritional significance. A comparison study of various age groups, *Blood,* 12, 24, 1957.

81. **Hosodo, S. and Kirk, J. E.,** Vitamin B_{12} content of human vascular tissue in individuals of various ages, *J. Gerontol.,* 24, 298, 1969.

82. **Leevy, C. M., Cardi, L., Frank, O., Gillene, R., and Baker, H.,** Incidence and significance of hypovitaminemia in a randomly selected municipal hospital population, *Am. J. Clin. Nutr.,* 17, 259, 1965.

83. **Baker, H., Frank, O., Feingold, S., Christakis, G., and Liffer, H.,** Vitamins, total cholesterol, and triglycerides in 642 New York City school children, *Am. J. Clin. Nutr.,* 20, 850, 1967.

84. **Chieffi, M. and Kirk, E.,** Vitamin studies in middle-aged and old individuals. II. Correlation between vitamin A plasma content and certain clinical and laboratory findings, *J. Nutr.,* 37, 67, 1949.

85. **Chope, H. D.,** Relation of nutrition to health in aging persons. A four year follow-up of a study in San Mateo County, *Calif. State J. Med.,* 81, 5, 1954.

86. **Schlenker, E. D.,** The Nutritional Status of Older Women, Ph.D. thesis, Michigan State University, East Lansing, 1976.

87. **Wilson, T. S., Weeks, M. M., Mukherjie, S. K., Murrell, J. S., and Andrews, C. J.,** A study of vitamin C levels in the aged and subsequent mortality, *Gerontol. Clin.,* 14, 17, 1972.

88. **Wilson, T. S., Datta, S. B., Murrell, J. S., and Andrews, C. J.,** Relation of vitamin C levels to mortality in a geriatric hospital: a study of the effect of vitamin C administration, *Age and Ageing,* 2, 163, 1973.

89. **Anon.,** On a definition of health (editorial), *Calif. Med.,* 112, 63, 1973.

90. **Arroyave, G.,** Standards for the diagnosis of vitamin deficiency in man, in *Metabolic Adaptation and Nutrition,* PAHO/WHO Sci. Publ., No. 222, World Health Organization, Washington, D.C., 1971, 88.

91. **Marks, J.,** *The Vitamins in Health and Disease — A Modern Reappraisal,* Churchill Livingstone, London, 1968.
92. **Darke, S. J.,** Requirement for vitamins in old age, in *Symposia of the Swedish Nutrition Foundation — Nutrition in Old Age,* Carlson, L. A., Ed., Almqvist and Wilfsell, Uppsala, Sweden, 1972, 107.
93. **Andrews, J., Letcher, M., and Brook, M.,** Vitamin C supplementation in the elderly: a 17-month trial in an old persons home, *Br. Med. J.,* 2, 416, 1969.
94. **Brook, M. and Grimshaw, J. J.,** Vitamin C concentration of plasma and leukocytes as related to smoking habit, age, sex of humans, *Am. J. Clin. Nutr.,* 21, 1254, 1968.
95. **Horwitt, M. K.,** Dietary requirements of the aged, *J. Am. Diet. Assoc.,* 29, 443, 1958.
96. **Mills, C. A., Cottingham, E., and Taylor, E.,** The effect of advancing age on dietary thiamine requirements, *Arch. Biochem.,* 9, 221, 1946.
97. **Mills, C. A.,** B vitamin requirements with advancing age, *Am. J. Physiol.,* 153, 31, 1948.
98. **Lumeng, L. and Li, T. K.,** Vitamin B_6 metabolism in chronic alcohol abuse, *J. Clin. Invest.,* 53, 693, 1974.
99. **Purinton, H. J. and Schuck, C.,** A study of normal human requirements for ascorbic acid and certain of its metabolic relationships, *J. Nutr.,* 26, 509, 1943.
100. **Grinna, L. S.,** Effect of dietary α tocopherol on liver microsomes and mitochondria of aging rats, *J. Nutr.,* 106, 918, 1976.
101. **Adelman, R. C.,** Loss of adaptive mechanisms during aging, *Fed. Proc.,* 38, 1968, 1979.
102. **Kronenberg, R. S. and Drage, C. W.,** Attenuation of the ventilatory and heart rate responses to hypoxia and hypercapnia with aging in normal men, *J. Clin. Invest.,* 52, 1812, 1973.
103. **Shock, N. W.,** The science of gerontology, in *Proc. Seminars, 1959 to 61, Durham, N. C.: Council on Gerontology,* Jeffers, E. C., Ed., Dirke View Press, Durham, N. C., 1962, 123.

Chapter 6

TRACE ELEMENTS IN AGING RESEARCH: EMPHASIS ON ZINC, COPPER, CHROMIUM, AND SELENIUM

J. Cecil Smith, Jr., and Jeng M. Hsu

TABLE OF CONTENTS

I. INTRODUCTION

In the past, aging has been associated only with the elderly. In the broader concept, aging begins at conception and continues until death. The roles of the macronutrients for optimal health throughout the life span have long been recognized. Only recently however, have the roles of trace elements in health and disease been appreciated.

The metabolic roles of trace elements in aging have become of concern to nutritionists and were the subject of a symposium.[1] Many of the trace elements are specifically involved in enzyme activity and exhibit altered levels in a variety of diseases. The incidence of most of these diseases is positively correlated with age. It has been suggested that changes in quantity of a single trace element or alterations of trace element ratio may be important in the process of mammalian physiologic aging.[2] Based on the observation that the major steps of genetic information transfer are mediated by metal ions, Eichorn[3] speculated that it might be possible to ameliorate the aging process by controlling the metal ion environment.

The free radical theory of aging has recently been advanced.[4] This theory proposes that the aging process may be a sum of ever-present deleterious "free radical" reactions that are continuously in progress in the tissues. Thus longevity would reflect the ability to cope with and to minimize random free radical reactions. It has been speculated that formulation of human diets to limit free radical build-up might add 5 to 10 years of healthy, productive life.[4] Free radical reactions may be initiated and sustained by numerous trace element-containing metalloenzymes. The availability and concentration of certain trace elements in the diet and/or in a specific tissue might alter the production of the free radicals. For example, the seleno-metalloenzyme, glutathione peroxidase, catalyzes the breakdown of free radicals, such as hydrogen peroxide. Likewise, superoxide dismutase, a copper metalloenzyme, catalyzes the breakdown of a highly reactive form of oxygen that is also a free radical. The concentration of copper in a specific tissue may affect the activity of the enzyme. In turn, the copper concentration in the tissue might be altered by age.

A major limitation for trace element research has been the lack of longitudinal studies in which the subjects are followed for several decades.[5,6] Instead, most investigations have involved measurements of trace element nutriture in different age groups. Many differences among individuals of different ages result from variables other than aging.[7] Various age groups prefer different foods. The aged are subject to unidentifiable physiologic and structural changes which result from subclinical or overt disease. Thus a lower 24-hr urinary chromium excretion in an 80-year-old, compared with a 20-year-old, is not necessarily due to differences in age per se. Other factors that might contribute to changes in the metabolism of trace elements include decreased food (caloric) intake, decreased physical activity, changes in absorption and utilization of nutrients, and drug interaction. Decreased caloric intake in elderly people results in a decreased nutrient intake (including trace elements).[6]

Although it is usually assumed that impaired absorption of nutrients accompanies aging, the absorption of trace elements at various ages has not been definitively studied. According to Shock,[5] "present evidence indicates that older people do not show significant impairment in the ability to absorb a specific item from the diet". In contrast, Jacobs and Owen[8] reported that the absorption of iron was depressed in older age groups.

The dietary preferences of the elderly include foods that are high in refined sugars[9] and are poor sources of trace elements.[10] High-sugar products may be eaten in preference to better sources of the trace elements, such as seafoods or meats. In general, the foods that contain the highest concentration of trace elements are also the most expensive. Although oysters are an excellent source of zinc, their expense (and availability)

Table 1
PERCENTAGE OF U.S.
HOUSEHOLDS REPORTING
HEALTH PROBLEMS

Conditions	Households reporting health problems[a] (%)
Obesity	30
High blood pressure	22
Allergy	20
Heart disease	9
Kidney problems	8
Diabetes	7

[a] Based on approximately 1400 households.

From Jones, J. L., *National Food Situation,* 159, 27, 1977. With permission.

prevents them from being a significant source of dietary zinc for most Americans. Dental problems may prevent intake of foods, such as nuts or meats that are high in trace metals. Lastly, decreased intake of water and fluids by the elderly contributes to a lower total daily intake of trace elements.

An editorial recently asked, "What does a healthy control control?"[11] The authors stressed that in many studies the control fluids or tissues are from "normals" who are usually young and healthy persons, such as medical students. In addition, the normals may not be age-matched with the experimental subjects. Thus any differences between the control and experimental group that were associated with age would not be identified. Traditionally, subjects have been considered normal if they are ambulatory, can carry out routine daily activities, and are willing to donate a specimen for analysis. Few individuals, however, escape all health problems. A survey by the U.S. Department of Agriculture questioned approximately 1400 households from different regions and social levels.[12] In more than 60% of all households at least one person had health problems, either diagnosed by a physician or self-ascribed. Health problems with respect to a specific disease or condition are shown in Table 1. The most common problems were obesity, hypertension, and allergies which were reported in 30, 22, and 20% of the households, respectively. In about 40% of all households, someone had changed a dietary pattern to meet an existing health problem.

Knowledge of the "normal" ranges of trace elements for different age groups should include concentrations in "soft" and "hard" tissues as well as in body fluids such as blood and urine. Standard height and weight tables have been developed for different aged groups. Thus normal ranges of trace elements in tissues also should be developed for different aged groups. Recently a workshop sponsored by the National Science Foundation and the American Institute of Nutrition focused the need for data on the mineral composition of human tissues.[12a] Although data are available on the concentration of selected trace elements in many human tissues, the accuracy must be questioned due to complexities of analyses and the likelihood of contamination.

The most extensive compilation of mineral concentration in human tissue is the work of Iyengar et al.,[13] but the data were from tissues of adults whose ages were not reported. In definitive studies normal ranges should be developed for other trace elements for different age groups. At present the data for parameters of trace element metabolism for different age groups, such as each decade of life, are nearly nonexistent. In order to enhance trace element research concerning aging, a range of nor-

Table 2
PLASMA ZINC CONCENTRATIONS IN DIFFERENT AGE GROUPS

Age group	µg/dℓ
Premature infants	187 ± 20 (16)[a]
First week	164 ± 15 (12)
2nd week — 3 months	96 ± 14 (11)
4—11 months	127 ± 8 (15)
1—5 years	130 ± 10 (11)
6—11 years	113 ± 5 (12)
Adults	109 ± 2 (126)

[a]   Mean ± SEM, number of individuals in ( ).

From Berfenstam, R., *Acta Paediatr.*, 41, 33, 1952. With permission.

mal values for various tissues should be developed from a population of different ages and clinically verified to be in optimum health. Optimum health may be defined as freedom from disease and ideal function of the biochemical, physiological, and mental processes. Difficult decisions would include, for example, whether to accept the impaired glucose tolerance often associated with the aging process as normal as well as deciding what are "normal" blood pressure levels for different age groups in the U.S.

Longitudinal studies would be ideal, but might require nearly 100 years — which is certainly longer than one scientific lifetime. Since longitudinal studies involving trace elements are scarce, we will confine this discussion to studies in which the parameters of trace element metabolism were compared among different age groups. The discussion will be limited to studies of normal humans except where no such data are available. Reviews by Hsu[14], Smith[15], Mason[16], Mertz[17,18] and Burk[19] are recommended for general information about current knowledge on the metabolism of zinc, copper, chromium, and selenium.

II. ZINC METABOLISM AT DIFFERENT AGES

A. Plasma or Serum

The most complete report of plasma zinc concentration for different age groups from premature infants to adults was reported by Berfenstam in 1952.[20] The data (Table 2) indicate that plasma zinc was highest for premature infants (187 ± 20 µg/dℓ, mean ± SEM), lowest for infants between 2 weeks and 3 months (96 ± 14 µg/dℓ), and intermediate for the other age groups. The level for adults, 109 ± 2 µg/dℓ, was the lowest reported, except that for infants ages 2 weeks to 3 months. Our laboratory[20a] reported a plasma zinc concentration of 96 ± 12 µg/dℓ (mean ± SD) for normal adults compared with 89 ± 13 µg/dℓ, $P < 0.02$, for healthy children ages 3 to 13 years (Table 3). A more recent study examined the age-plasma zinc concentration relationship in 156 children from infancy to 18 years.[21] Infants and children to age 3 had slightly lower plasma zinc concentrations (67 ± 12 µg/dℓ) than their older counterparts (3 to 19 years, 73 ± 11 µg/dℓ) $P < 0.01$. Ohtake and Tamura[22] reported no significant differences among serum zinc levels of 156 healthy Japanese children between ages 6 and 12 years.

Most recent studies indicate that young children may have lower levels of plasma zinc (perhaps related to periods of rapid growth) than adults. However, most studies suggest that in adults, plasma zinc does not change significantly with age.[23-26] Never-

Table 3
PLASMA ZINC CONCENTRATIONS IN
ADULTS AND CHILDREN

Group	Mean ± SD (μg/100 dℓ)	Significance level
Adults (age 23—62 years)	96 ± 12 (89)[a]	P
Children (age 3—13 yrs)	89 ± 13 (26)	<0.02

[a]   Mean ± SD, number of subjects in ( ).

From Halsted, J. and Smith, J. C., Jr., *Lancet*, 1, 322, 1970. With permission.

theless, a few studies have suggested that plasma zinc does change with advancing age, especially after 40 or 50 years.[27,28] However, the results among the studies are not consistent and need clarification.

B. Erythrocytes

Berfenstam[20] reported a direct correlation between age and erythrocyte zinc concentration. Zinc level in cells was lowest in premature children (347 μg/dℓ) and highest in adults (1244 μg/dℓ).

C. Hair

Hair has been used as a convenient tissue for examination because it is readily available, accessible without special equipment, and may be sampled and stored without refrigeration. However, total hair zinc concentration may not accurately indicate current zinc status. In one study of prepubescent children, plasma zinc concentrations were low, whereas hair concentrations were normal.[29] Levels of zinc in plasma and hair were not significantly correlated. The use of hair as a diagnostic biopsy material for assessing trace element status was recently reviewed.[30,31]

It is generally agreed that zinc concentration decreases markedly during the first few months of life[32,33] (Figure 1). Erten et al.[34] studied 115 healthy subjects aged 0 to 15 years and reported that hair zinc increased with age. The authors suggested that hair zinc concentration was low during periods of most rapid growth. The data also suggested that the converse is true, i.e., hair zinc concentration may increase during periods of growth retardation. Data from our laboratory indicated that small-for-age children had significantly higher hair zinc concentrations than normal controls.[35]

D. Urine

Urinary zinc excretion in different age groups was recently reported by Elinder et al.[36] who studied 132 "normal" Swedes, including 50 pairs of identical twins. The data were presented as average milligrams of Zn per gram creatinine. Based on single urine specimens, 24-hr urinary zinc excretion was calculated for the various age groups. The accuracy of such a technique has not been established. The calculated values for 24-hr zinc excretion reported by Elinder et al.[36] apparently were not correlated with age.

E. Tissue

Liver zinc concentrations were nearly twice as high in infants younger than 3 months as in subjects older than 1 year.[37] In contrast, zinc levels in the kidney and spleen were similar for both age groups. In heart, brain, and lung, however, zinc concentration was lower for subjects older than 1 year than for subjects less than 3 months. Although

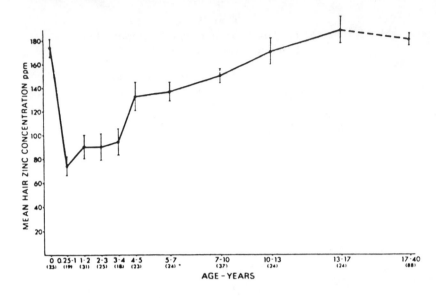

FIGURE 1.   Mean concentrations of zinc in hair of subjects from infancy to age 40. SEM indicated on graph; number of subjects in each age group is given in parentheses. (From Hambidge, K. M., Hambidge, C., Jacobs, M., and Baum, J. O.,, *Pediatr. Res.*, 6, 868, 1972. With permission.)

the study needs confirmation, the data suggest that the liver may serve as a zinc storage organ, especially for the young infants.

Schor et al.[38] reported that the zinc concentration of the bone (rib cartilage) was highest in infants but declined rapidly between 0.5 to 2.5 years of age. Inexplicably, the zinc level then increased between 25 and 90 years of age to a level similar to that in the infants. Although the subjects were considered "non-dwarfed" and thus normal, apparent cause of death was disease. There was no evidence, however, that any specific disease altered the bone zinc concentrations. One interpretation of the data is that bone zinc may accumulate throughout life. Such speculation needs verification.

F. Metabolic Balance

Metabolic balance is defined as the comparison of the intake of a nutrient with its total excretion, mainly via feces, urine, and sweat. In general young infants apparently are in negative zinc balance with excretion higher than intake; growing children are in positive balance (net retention of zinc); and adults are in equilibrium, assuming dietary zinc is adequate. Thus metabolic zinc balance is apparently age related. For example, Vorobieva[39] reported that zinc retention was 53% in 2-year-old children compared with 4% in 5- to 9-year-old children. The difference was reflected in the balances of these age groups. The estimated daily requirements for children range from 0.300 mg/kg for 3- to 6-year olds, to 6.2 mg (total) for 7- to 12-year olds.[40] Adult males maintained equilibrium on a zinc intake of 12.5 mg/day.[41]

G. Recommended Dietary Allowance

At present the RDA for zinc (15 mg) pertains to all groups older than 11 years, except pregnant and lactating females.[42] The actual zinc requirement, however, probably differs among individuals older than 11 years (Table 4). The RDAs should include specific recommendations for the elderly.

Table 4

RECOMMENDED DIETARY ALLOWANCES FOR ZINC, COPPER, CHROMIUM, AND SELENIUM ACCORDING TO AGE

Subjects	Age (years)	Zinc (mg)	Copper[a] (mg)	Chromium[a] (mg)	Selenium[a] (mg)
Infants	0.0—0.5	3	0.5—0.7	0.01—0.04	0.01—0.04
	0.5—1.0	5	0.7—1.0	0.02—0.06	0.02—0.06
Children	1—3	10	1.0—1.5	0.02—0.08	0.02—0.08
	4—6	10	1.5—2.0	0.03—0.12	0.03—0.12
	7—10	10	2.0—2.5	0.05—0.20	0.05—0.20
Adolescents and adults	11 +	15	2.0—3.0	0.05—0.20	0.05—0.20

[a] Estimated safe and adequate daily dietary intake.

From Recommended Dietary Allowances, 9th ed., Food and Nutrition Board, Nutrition Research Council, Academy of Sciences, Washington, D.C., 1980. With permission.

III. COPPER METABOLISM AT DIFFERENT AGES

A. Plasma or Serum

Studies of children have suggested that the plasma or serum copper concentration is highest for infants and decreases during adolescent years to a normal adult level. There is no general agreement about the serum copper concentration during the adult years. For example, Klevay[43] reported no consistent difference in the plasma copper levels that were associated with age after studying more than 200 Panamanians. In contrast, Harman[44] found a linear increase in serum concentration of copper between the ages of 20 and 60 years.

Studies involving normal plasma copper concentrations in females of child-bearing age may be complex because oral contraceptive use and pregnancy result in a marked increase in plasma copper concentration.[45] Thus women who are pregnant, as well as those receiving oral contraceptives, must be excluded from studies of "normals".

Cartwright and Wintrobe[46] reported a longitudinal study of serum copper levels in two physicians for periods of 8 and 12 years. The data, however, shed little light on the effect of age on serum copper because, although the trends were upward, both men had a low initial level of 68 μg/dℓ. Indeed, it was suggested that both individuals might have been heterozygous for Wilson's disease. This disease is characterized by an aberration in copper metabolism and is accompanied by low serum copper concentrations.

B. Hair

Klevay[43] reported the copper content of hair on a random sample of 431 Panamanians. He concluded that the concentration fell during the first decade of life and remained relatively constant thereafter with no significant correlation to age after 8 years. Likewise, studies by Eads and Lambdin[47] reported that age (from 9 to 60 years) did not affect copper concentration in the hair. In contrast, Petering et al.[48] studied 211 individuals of both sexes ranging in age from 1 to 80 years and concluded that hair copper was related to age (and sex).

C. Tissue

Several studies have reported that concentrations of copper in the liver were markedly higher in newborns than in adults.[37,49,50] During the first few months after birth the levels decreased rapidly to those found in adults. This rapid decrease suggests that

Table 5
SIGNS AND SYMPTOMS WHICH
MAY BE ASSOCIATED WITH
CHROMIUM DEFICIENCY

Impaired glucose tolerance
Elevated circulating insulin
Glycosuria
Fasting hyperglycemia
Elevated serum cholesterol and triglycerides
Mental confusion

From Anderson, R. A., *Sci. Total Environ.,*
17, 13, 1981. With permission.

the newborn liver serves as a store for copper and that dietary copper may be more critical after the decrease in stores occurs.

Schor et al.[38] reported a decrease in the copper concentration of the rib cartilage during the first 2.5 years of life with a steady increase for subjects up to 90 years.

D. Metabolic Balance

Balance studies suggest dietary requirements of 0.05 to 0.1 mg of Cu/kg/day for young children and preadolescents.[16] These levels are approximately twice the estimated requirement for growing infants. Studies carried out in recent years (since analytic methods have improved) indicate a daily requirement between 1 and 2 mg for adults.

E. Recommended Dietary Allowance and Actual Intake

Because the requirement has been estimated at between 1 and 2 mg for adults, the RDA has been established as 2.0 to 3.0 mg — a level considered "safe and adequate" for "adults", 11 years and older.[42] The range for infants less than 6 months is 0.5 to 0.7 mg.

Recently, reports have indicated that dietary copper intake appears to be considerably less than the RDA.[51,52] It was suggested that the increased consumption of processed foods has contributed to a lowered copper intake. Prolonged inadequate intake of dietary copper may have marked deleterious effects on overall health, especially in age groups, such as the elderly, that are at risk. A recent hypothesis stated that the ratio of zinc to copper in the diet may be responsible, in part, for cardiovascular problems.[53,54] Although this concept is speculative, there is evidence that a dietary deficiency of copper in animals results in impaired collagen and elastin formation leading to vascular complications.[55] Likewise, inadequate copper nutriture in animals has been produced not only by feeding a diet low in copper, but by the interference of other trace elements with copper-dependent biochemical processes. The antagonistic elements are cadmium, zinc, and molybdenum. Possibly some of those may accumulate with age and thus present greater problems for the elderly.

IV. CHROMIUM METABOLISM AT DIFFERENT AGES

Although chromium has recently been established as an essential element for humans,[42] few definitive data are available concerning the effect of age on parameters of chromium nutriture. Indeed, these parameters are just being established[56] (Table 5). Chromium analyses have presented numerous difficulties for several reasons including the following: low concentration in body fluids; lack of highly sensitive instrumen-

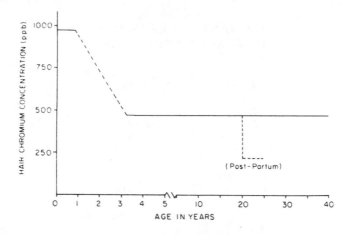

FIGURE 2. Hair chromium concentration in different age groups of U.S. subjects. (From Hambidge, K. M., *Newer Trace Elements in Nutrition*, Mertz, W. and Cornatzer, W. E., Eds., Marcel Dekker, New York, 1971, chap. 9. With permission.)

tation; and the contamination problems that are related to sample collection and preparation.

A. Plasma, Serum, and Whole Blood

The normal mean plasma or serum chromium concentrations reported have varied between 0.73 to 150 ng/mℓ.[57] Thus any attempt to determine the effect of age on serum concentrations must be accomplished by comparing various age groups within a single study with analysis by one method. A certified standard reference serum would help establish interlaboratory accuracy and allow comparison among laboratories.

Vir and Love[58] studied 196 subjects, who were 65 years or older. In general, plasma chromium concentrations showed no consistent relationship with age. Whole blood chromium also apparently was unrelated to age for males ranging from 22 to 47 years or older.

B. Hair

There is general agreement that hair chromium changes markedly with age. An initial high level at birth declines during the first 3 years and then appears to remain relatively constant to 40 years of age[32] (Figure 2).

To illustrate the effect of age on chromium concentration of hair in infants, Hambidge analyzed sections of hair from an infant 18 months of age who had its first haircut.[59] The hair was assumed to have grown at a rate of 1 cm/month since the child's hair was 18 cm long. The hair closest to the scalp (grown when the child was near 18 months) was much lower in chromium (144 ppb) than hair grown when the child was younger — 9 to 18 months (940 ppb). This technique offers promise for assessing the change in hair trace element concentration as related to age of infants.

C. Urine

Although urine is a useful parameter for assessing chromium nutriture, urinary chromium excretion is extremely low in normal adults (< 1.0 μg/24 hr).[60-62] Published values, however, often are tenfold of that level due to problems of methodology and instrumentation. A limited number of reports have compared the urinary chromium excretion in different age groups (Table 6). Gurson et al.[63] reported that daily 24-hr urinary chromium showed a stepwise increase until age 35. Hambidge[59] reported that

Table 6
URINARY EXCRETION IN DIFFERENT AGE GROUPS

Subject	Urinary excretion (ng/24 hr)
Children	
< 2 years	748 ± 422 (7)[a]
2—7 years	1692 ± 905 (12)
> 7 years	1808 ± 851 (12)
Adults	
20—35 years	3080 ± 1900 (5)
45—85 years[b]	2770 ± 1110 (19)

[a] Mean ± S.D., number of subjects in ( ).
[b] Institutionalized.

From Gurson, C. T., Sane, G., Mertz, W., Wolf, W. R., and Sokucii, S., *Nutr. Rep. Int.,* 12, 9, 1979. With permission.

young adults excreted more chromium daily than did younger children, suggesting a correlation of age with chromium excretion.

D. Tissue

Schroeder et al.[64] reported that the tissue concentration of chromium decreased with increasing age for U.S. subjects. The authors based their conclusion on human autopsy tissue that was analyzed for chromium by emission spectroscopy. In contrast, a recent study[65] concerning the concentration of chromium in autopsy tissue of diabetic and nondiabetic American Indians (Pima Tribe) showed no correlation between age and tissue level. Thus chromium tissue concentration should be clarified, since a lower chromium concentration in the elderly might suggest depletion, due to insufficient dietary intake.[17]

E. Metabolic Balance

It is doubtful whether conventional metabolic chromium balance can yield useful data since the absorption of chromium appears to be less than 2%.[66] Thus most of the chromium is excreted. However, it is possible that young, fast-growing subjects may be in more positive chromium balance than adults. No data related to this area are available.

F. Recommended Dietary Allowance

The recent RDA ranges for chromium are 0.01 to 0.04 mg/day for infants less than 6 months of age and 0.05 to 0.20 mg/day for children or adults 11 years or older[42] (Table 4).

V. SELENIUM METABOLISM AT DIFFERENT AGES

A. Plasma, Serum, Red Blood Cells, and Whole Blood

Several investigators have compared the concentrations of selenium in the whole blood, RBC, and plasma of elderly subjects with those of younger ones.[67-69] Using neutron activation analysis, Kasparek et al.[68] noted a gradual decrease in serum selen-

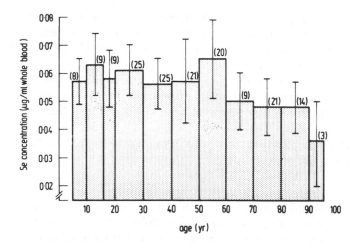

FIGURE 3. Whole blood selenium concentrations of different aged groups of New Zealanders. Standard deviation shown on bars and number of subjects in ( ). (From Robinson, M. F., Godfrey, P. J., Thompson, C. D., Rea, H. M., and van Rij, A. M., *Am. J. Clin. Nutr.*, 32, 1477, 1979. With permission.)

ium after age 34, whereas Robinson et al.,[69] using fluorescence analysis, reported no significant decline until after age 60 (Figure 3).

B. Hair
Schroeder et al.[70] measured hair selenium in eight individuals of ages 3.5 to 84 years. There was no apparent correlation of hair selenium level with age.

C. Tissue
In six subjects ranging in age from 9 months to 69 years, Schroeder et al.[70] reported no correlation between age and selenium concentration in various tissues. However, there were too few samples in this study to draw any conclusion. In addition, the tissues were obtained at autopsy; thus the cause of death may have affected the selenium levels. A recent study of normal and diseased human liver tissue showed no correlation between age and liver selenium concentration.[71,72]

D. Metabolic Balance
Although Schroeder et al.[70] estimated that 60 μg of selenium was necessary to maintain equilibrium for adults, studies from New Zealand indicated that less than 50 μg were adequate.[73]

E. Recommended Dietary Allowance
The recent RDA ranges for selenium are 0.01 to 0.04 mg/day for infants less than 6 months of age and 0.05 to 0.20 mg/day for children or adults 11 years or older[42] (Table 4).

VI. SUMMARY

A. Zinc
Most recent studies apparently support the belief that plasma (serum) zinc concentrations are lower in children than in adults, although the early extensive study of Berfenstam[20] reported that adults had lower levels than most other age groups. It is important to clarify whether plasma zinc decreases with age, since a decrease might

be an indication of depletion. At present, however, most reports suggest that adult age is not a factor. Two studies indicated that plasma zinc decreased with advancing age.[27,28] Hair zinc concentration apparently decreases markedly during the first few months of life, then tends to remain relatively constant.[32,33]

Hair and plasma zinc concentrations are not correlated.[29] Likewise, hair zinc is affected by the rate of growth and may be low during periods of rapid growth. Thus, hair zinc concentration can not be used as the sole criterion for assessment of zinc status.

Recent studies indicated that dietary zinc intakes are inadequate for several segments of our population, including the elderly.

B. Copper

The majority of studies indicate that the plasma (or serum) copper concentration is highest for infants and decreases during the adolescent years to a normal adult level. With respect to adults, most studies suggest a very slight and gradual increase in serum copper in older subjects, especially males. However, these studies need clarification since they are contradictory. We could find only one report suggesting differences in erythrocyte copper concentrations with age.[43]

Reports conflict concerning copper concentration in hair for various age groups. Perhaps of more importance is the question of the relevancy of hair copper concentration as a reflection of copper nutriture.

In regard to tissue concentration, it is rather well established that copper in the liver is much higher in newborns than of infants and children above 3 months. This suggests that the liver serves as a storage site for copper during the first few months of life; thereafter all copper required for metabolic purposes after infancy must be supplied from dietary sources.

C. Chromium

Some published data are available regarding normal serum or plasma chromium levels for subjects of different age groups. Their accuracy, however, must be questioned because of prior problems with analytic procedures and contamination. Nevertheless, there is general agreement that from a comparative viewpoint, hair concentration of the newborn is very high and decreases rapidly during the first few years of life, after which it remains constant.

No definitive conclusions can be drawn regarding urinary chromium excretion in different age groups due to the problems of analysis. Chromium concentration in tissue was reported to be lower in old than in young people. A more recent investigation, however, showed no correlation between age and tissue levels. Measurement of metabolic chromium balance is difficult because of the small retention rate. No studies have delineated the effect of age on chromium balance.

D. Selenium

There apparently is agreement that the concentrations of selenium in plasma, serum, RBC, and whole blood are lower in old than in young persons, especially after 60 years. In one report, no apparent relationship was found between selenium and age. Only two studies reported selenium concentrations in tissues. Again, no correlation with age was found. The question of metabolic balance remains unclear, although studies suggest that the 50 to 200 μg recently recommended as an RDA is adequate. To date, however, no definitive studies have reported metabolic balances for different age groups.

VII. AREAS FOR FUTURE RESEARCH

Longitudinal studies are needed for assessment of groups or populations over several years. These studies would allow a comparison of the individual subjects as each aged. Certified reference standards are needed also for the concentrations of various trace elements in serum and human tissues. Standards would permit the comparison of data from year to year and among laboratories. Data also are needed for the concentrations of trace elements in tissues from "normal" humans rather than from those who have died from disease-related causes. Another problem concerning tissue concentration of trace elements is the variability among methods of sample preparation and analysis.

Automated analytical methods for determining trace elements should be improved. Because of methodology problems, few data are available, for example, for the concentrations of chromium and selenium in human tissues. On the other hand, methodologies for zinc and copper in tissues are well established and many data are available for those elements.

Data for metabolic balances for different age groups were available for zinc, copper, and selenium but not for chromium possibly because of analytical problems. Apparently more balance studies are needed for selenium and chromium, although recommended daily ranges of intakes have already been established. Certainly, recommendations should be reassessed since they now do not consider the possibility that requirements change with age above 11 years.

ACKNOWLEDGMENT

It is a pleasure to thank Renato Ferretti for his assistance in the preparation of this manuscript.

REFERENCES

1. Hsu, J. M., Davis, R. L., and Neithamer, R. W., Eds., *The Biomedical Role of Trace Elements in Aging,* Eckerd College Gerontology Center, St. Petersburg, Fla., 1976.
2. Lawton, A. H., Trace Elements in Aging, in *The Biomedical Role of Trace Elements in Aging,* Hsu, J. M., Davis, R. L., and Neithamer, R. W., Eds., Eckerd College Gerontology Center, St. Petersburg, Fla., 1976, 1.
3. Eichorn, G. L., cited in meeting brief from Chicago, *Chem. Eng. News,* 50, 12, 1973.
4. Harman, D., Free radical theory of aging: nutritional implications, *Age,* 1, 145, 1978.
5. Shock, N. W., Physiologic aspects of aging, *J. Am. Diet. Assoc.,* 56, 491, 1970.
6. Smith, J. C., Jr., Golden ages and trace elements, in *The Biomedical Role of Trace Elements in Aging,* Hsu, J. M., Davis, R. L., and Neithamer, R. W., Eds., Eckerd College Gerontology Center, St. Petersburg, Fla., 1976, 7.
7. Exton-Smith, A. N., Physiological aspects of aging: relationship to nutrition, *Am. J. Clin. Nutr.,* 25, 853, 1972.
8. Jacobs, A. M. and Owen, G. M., The effect of age on iron absorption, *J. Gerontol.,* 24, 95, 1969.
9. Albanese, A. A., Nutrition and health of the elderly, *Nutr. News,* 39, 5, 1976.
10. Schroeder, H. A., *The Trace Elements and Man,* Devin-Adair, Old Greenwich, Conn., 1973.
11. Desforges J. F., Hollenberg, N. K., Ingelfinger, F. S., Molt, R. A., and Smith, A. L., What does a healthy control control? *N. Engl. J. Med.,* 296, 1165, 1977.
12. Jones, J. L., Are health concerns changing the American diet? in *National Food Situation,* Economic Research Service, U.S. Department of Agriculture, 159, 27, 1977.
12a. Smith, J. C., Jr., Anderson, R. A., Ferretti, R., Levander, O. A., Morris, E. R., Roginski, E. E., Veillon, C., Wolf, W. R., Anderson, J. J. B., and Mertz, W., Evaluation of published data pertaining to mineral components of human tissue, *Fed. Proc.,* 40, 2120, 1981.

13. **Iyengar, G. V., Kollmer, W. E., and Bowen, H. J. M.,** *The Elemental Composition of Human Tissues and Fluids,* Verlag Chemie, Weinheim, West Germany, 1978.

14. **Hsu, J. M.,** Current knowledge on zinc, copper, and chromium in aging, *World Rev. Nutr. Diet.,* 33, 42, 1979.

15. **Smith, J. C., Jr.,** Marginal nutritional states and conditioned deficiencies, in *Alcohol and Nutrition,* Li, T. K., Schenker, S., and Lumeng, L., Eds., Research Monogr. 2, National Institute on Alcohol Abuse and Alcoholism, Rockville, Md., 1979, 23.

16. **Mason, K. E.,** A conspectus of research on copper metabolism and requirements of man, *J. Nutr.,* 109, 1979, 1979.

17. **Mertz, W.,** Chromium occurrence and function in biological systems, *Physiol. Rev.,* 49, 163, 1969.

18. **Mertz, W.,** Chromium — an overview, in *Developments in Nutrition and Metabolism — Chromium in Nutrition and Metabolism,* Vol. 2, Shapcott, D. and Hubert, J., Eds., Elsevier/North-Holland Biomedical Press, New York, 1979, 1.

19. **Burk, R. F.,** Selenium in man, in *Trace Elements in Human Health and Disease, Essential and Toxic Elements,* Vol. 2, Prasad, A. S. and Oberleas, D., Eds., Academic Press, New York, 1976, chap. 30.

20. **Berfenstam, R.,** Studies on blood zinc, *Acta Paediatr.,* 41, 33, 1952.

20a. **Halsted, J. A. and Smith, J. C., Jr.,** Plasma-zinc in health and disease, *Lancet,* 1, 322, 1970.

21. **Butrimovitz, G. P.,** The Determination of Plasma Zinc by Atomic Absorption Spectrophotometry and Plasma Zinc Intervals Throughout Childhood, Ph.D. thesis, University of Maryland, College Park, 1977, 1.

22. **Ohtake, M. and Tamura, T.,** Serum zinc and copper levels in healthy Japanese children, *Tohoku, J. Exp. Med.,* 120, 99, 1976.

23. **Butt, E. M., Nusbaum, R. E., Gilmour, T. C., Didio, S. L., and Mariano, Sr.,** Trace metal levels in human serum and blood, *Arch. Environ. Health,* 8, 52, 1964.

24. **Chooi, M. K., Todd, J. K., and Boyd, N. D.,** Influence of age and sex on plasma zinc levels in normal and diabetic individuals, *Nutr. Metab.,* 20, 135, 1976.

25. **Davies, I. J. T., Musa, M., and Dormandy, T. L.,** Measurement of plasma zinc, *J. Clin. Pathol.,* 21, 359, 1968.

26. **Hansson, L., Huunan-Seppala, A., and Mattila, A.,** The content of calcium, magnesium, copper, zinc, lead, and chromium in the blood of patients with rheumatoid arthritis, *Scand. J. Rheumatol.,* 4, 33, 1975.

27. **Lindeman, R. D., Clark, M. L., and Colmore, J. P.,** Influence of age and sex on plasma and red-cell zinc concentrations, *J. Gerontol.,* 26, 358, 1971.

28. **Bjorksten, F., Aromaa, A., Knekt, P., and Malinen, L.,** Serum zinc concentrations in Finns, *Acta Med. Scand.,* 204, 67, 1978.

29. **McBean, L. D., Mahloudji, M., Reinhold, J. G., and Halsted, J. A.,** Correlation of zinc concentrations in human plasma and hair, *Am. J. Clin. Nutr.,* 24, 506, 1971.

30. **Katz, S. A.,** The use of hair as biopsy material for trace elements in the body, *Am. Lab.,* 11, 44, 1979.

31. **Maugh, T. H., II,** Hair: a diagnostic tool to complement blood serum and urine, *Science,* 202, 1271, 1978.

32. **Hambidge, K. M., Hambidge, C., Jacobs, M., and Baum, J. O.,** Low levels of zinc in hair, anorexia, poor growth, and hypogensia in children, *Pediatr. Res.,* 6, 868, 1972.

33. **Hambidge, K. M. and Walravens, P. A.,** Zinc deficiency in infants and preadolescent children, in *Trace Elements in Human Health and Disease, Zinc and Copper,* Vol 1, Prasad, A. S. and Oberleas, D., Eds., Academic Press, New York, 1976, 21.

34. **Erten, J., Arcasoy, A., Candor, A. O., and Cin, S.,** Hair zinc levels in healthy and malnourished children, *Am. J. Clin. Nutr.,* 31, 117, 1978.

35. **Krebs, N. F.,** Hair Zinc Concentrations in Small-for-Age and Normal-Sized Functionally Retarded Children, Master's thesis, University of Maryland, College Park, 1979, 1.

36. **Elinder, C. G., Kjellstrom, T., Linnman, L., and Pershagen, G.,** Urinary excretion of cadmium and zinc among persons from Sweden, *Environ. Res.,* 15, 473, 1978.

37. **Nusbaum, R. E., Alexander, G. V., Butt, E. M., Gilmour, T. C., and Didio, S. L.,** Some spectrographic studies of trace element storage in human tissues, *Soil Sci.,* 85, 95, 1958.

38. **Schor, R. A., Purssin, S. G., Jewett, D. L., Ludowieg, J. J., and Bhatnagar, R. S.,** Trace levels of manganese, copper, and zinc in rib cartilage as related to age in humans and animals, both normal and dwarfed, *Clin. Orthoped.,* 93, 346, 1973.

39. **Vorobieva, A. I.,** Copper and zinc balance in the organism of children aged 2, 6, and 8 to 10 years, *Vopr. Pitan.,* 26, 28, 1967.

40. **Halsted, J. A., Smith, J. C., Jr., and Irwin, M. I.,** A conspectus of research on zinc requirements of man, *J. Nutr.,* 104, 345, 1974.

41. Spencer, H., Osis, D., Kramer, L., and Norris, C., Intake, excretion, and retention of zinc in man, in *Trace Elements in Human Health and Disease, Zinc and Copper,* Vol. 1, Prasad, A. S. and Oberleas, D., Eds., Academic Press, New York, 1976, chap. 21.

42. Food and Nutrition Board, *Recommended Dietary Allowances,* 9th ed., Food and Nutrition Board, Nutrition Research Council, National Academy of Sciences, Washington, D.C., 1980.

43. Klevay, L. M., Hair as a biopsy material. II. Assessment of copper nutriture, *Am. J. Clin. Nutr.,* 23, 1194, 1970.

44. Harman, D., The free radical theory of aging. Effect of age on serum copper levels, *J. Gerontol.,* 20, 151, 1965.

45. Smith, J. C., Jr. and Brown, E. D., Effects of oral contraceptive agents on trace element metabolism: a review, in *Trace Elements and Human Disease,* Vol. 2, Prasad, A. S., Ed., Academic Press, New York, 1976, chap. 38.

46. Cartwright, G. E. and Wintrobe, M. M., Copper metabolism in normal subjects, *Am. J. Clin. Nutr.,* 14, 224, 1964.

47. Eads, E. A. and Lambdin, C. E., A survey of trace metals in human hair, *Environ. Res.,* 6, 247, 1973.

48. Petering, H. G., Yeager, D. W., and Witherup, S. O., Trace metal content of hair. I. Zinc and copper content of human hair in relation to age and sex, *Arch. Environ. Health,* 23, 202, 1971.

49. Bruckmann, G. and Zondek, S. G., Iron, copper, and manganese in human organs at various ages, *Biochem. J.,* 33, 1845, 1939.

50. Widdowson, E. M., McCance, R. A., and Spray, C. M., The chemical composition of the human body, *Clin. Sci.,* 10, 113, 1951.

51. Klevay, L. M., Reck, S. J., and Barcome, D. F., Evidence of dietary copper and zinc deficiencies, *JAMA,* 241, 1916, 1979.

52. Holden, J. M., Wolf, W. R., and Mertz, W., Zinc and copper in self-selected diets, *J. Am. Diet. Assoc.,* 75, 23, 1979.

53. Klevay, L. M., Coronary heart disease: the zinc/copper hypothesis, *Am. J. Clin. Nutr.,* 28, 764, 1975.

54. Klevay, L. M., The ratio of zinc to copper of diets in the United States, *Nutr. Rep. Int.,* 11, 237, 1975.

55. Underwood, E. J., *Trace Elements in Human and Animal Nutrition,* 4th ed., Academic Press, New York, 1977, chap. 3.

56. Anderson, R. A., Nutritional role of chromium, *Sci. Total Environ.,* 17, 13, 1981.

57. Versieck, J., De Rudder, J., Hoste, J., Barbier, F., Lemey, G., and Vanballenberghe, L., Determination of the serum chromium concentration in healthy individuals by neutron activation analyses, in *Developments in Nutrition and Metabolism, Chromium in Nutrition and Metabolism,* Vol. 2, Shapcott, E. and Hubert, J., Eds., Elsevier/North-Holland, New York, 1979, 59.

58. Vir, S. C. and Love, A. H. G., Chromium status of the aged, *Int. J. Vitam. Nutr. Res.,* 48, 402, 1978.

59. Hambidge, K. M., Chromium nutrition in the mother and the growing child, in *Newer Trace Elements in Nutrition,* Mertz, W. and Cornatzer, W. E., Eds., Marcel Dekker, New York, 1971, chap. 9.

60. Guthrie, B. E., Wolf, W. R., Veillon, C., and Mertz, W., Chromium in urine, in *Trace Substances in Environmental Health,* Vol. 12, A symposium, Hemphill, D. D., Ed., University of Missouri, Columbia, 1978, 490.

61. Guthrie, B. E., Wolf, W. R., and Veillon, C., Background correction and related problems in the determination of chromium in urine by graphite furnace atomic absorption spectrometry, *Anal. Chem.,* 50, 1900, 1978.

62. Veillon, C., Wolf, W. R., and Guthrie, B. E., Determination of chromium in biological materials by stable isotope dilution, *Anal. Chem.,* 51, 1022, 1979.

63. Gurson, C. T., Sane, G., Mertz, W., Wolf, W. R., and Sokucii, S., Nutritional significance of chromium in different chronological age groups and in populations differing in nutritional background, *Nutr. Rep. Int.,* 12, 9, 1979.

64. Schroeder, H. A., Balassa, J. J., and Tipton, I. H., Abnormal trace metals in man — chromium, *J. Chronic Dis.,* 15, 941, 1962.

65. Eatough, D. J., Hansen, L. O., Starr, S. E., Astin, M. S., Larsen, S. B., Izatt, R. M., and Christensen, J. J., Chromium in autopsy tissue of diabetic and non-diabetic American (Pima) Indians, in *Proc. 3rd Int. Symp. on Trace Element Metabolism in Man and Animals,* Kirchgessner, M., Ed., Institut für Ernahrungsphysiologie der Technischen Universität München, Freising-Weihenstphan, 1978, 204.

66. Doisy, R. J., Streeten, D. H. P., Freiberg, J. M., and Schneider, A. J., *Trace Elements in Human Health and Disease,* Prasad, A. S., Ed., Academic Press, New York, 1976, 79.

67. **Dickson, R. C. and Tomlinson, R. H.,** Selenium in blood and human tissues, *Clin. Chim. Acta,* 16, 311, 1967.
68. **Kasparek, K., Shicha, H., Siller, V., and Feinendegen, L. E.,** Normaluverte von Spurenelementen im menschlichen Serum und korrelation zum Lebensalter und zur Serum-Wiweiss-Konzentration, *Strahlentherapie,* 142, 468, 1972.
69. **Robinson, M. F., Godfrey, P. J., Thompson, C. D., Rea, H. M., and van Rij, A. M.,** Blood selenium and glutathione peroxidase activity in normal subjects and in surgical patients with and without cancer in New Zealand, *Am. J. Clin. Nutr.,* 32, 1477, 1979.
70. **Schroeder, H. A., Frost, D. V., and Balassa, J. H.,** Essential trace metals in man: selenium, *J. Chronic Dis.,* 23, 227, 1970.
71. **Ferretti, R. J.,** unpublished data, 1981.
72. **Levander, O. A.,** Selenium and chromium in human nutrition, *J. Am. Diet. Assoc.,* 66, 338, 1975.
73. **Robinson, M. F.,** The moonstone: more about selenium, *J. Hum. Nutr.,* 30, 79, 1976.

Chapter 7

DIETARY ANTIOXIDANTS AND AGING ON MEMBRANE FUNCTIONS

Albert Y. Sun and Grace Y. Sun

TABLE OF CONTENTS

I. INTRODUCTION

Many hypotheses are known to provide an explanation to the intriguing mechanism of cellular aging. They include the hypothesis on oxidative damage to cellular components, the theory on somatic mutation and genetically programmed cell death, the cybernetic theory, and aging due to hormonal imbalance, enzyme deterioration, altered autoimmune reactions, etc.[2,58] Among these, the ones related to oxidative damage to cellular membranes may be the most important in explaining the biochemical changes observed in the cellular aging process.[40,104,128]

Cell membranes are important as a permeability barrier for regulating the transport of substances across the boundaries of different cellular compartments. In the brain tissue, some membranes serve as a structural support for various types of metabolic functions while others are excitable upon stimulation. Phospholipids are structural components of all biological membranes, and these lipid molecules are comprised of fatty acids with different degrees of unsaturation. These double bonds within the fatty acid molecules are the primary target of lipid peroxidation processes. Therefore, questions are raised as to whether vitamin E and other dietary antioxidants can effectively retard organ damage due to lipid peroxidation. This article is an attempt to review the past studies concerning age-related changes in membrane structure and functions and to evaluate the effects of dietary vitamin E and other antioxidants on some cellular membrane processes. Several reviews concerning the subject of lipid peroxidation,[57,128] lipid changes in aging brain,[49] free radical reactions and aging,[41,55,63] nutrition and aging,[145] and the membrane hypothesis of aging[104] have been published recently and the readers can refer to these excellent reviews for more information.

II. LIPID PEROXIDATION AND ANTIOXIDANTS

In metabolically active membranes, a high degree of fatty acid unsaturation is necessary to maintain these membranes in a liquid crystalline state in order to facilitate the translocation of small molecules.[138] However, these unsaturated fatty acids are highly susceptible to attack by free radicals. The reactions regarding enzymic peroxidation of polyunsaturated fatty acids (PUFA) for prostaglandin biosynthesis have been reviewed[53,85] and will not be discussed here. In general, the PUFA which are esterified to membrane phospholipids may undergo spontaneous peroxidation initiated by enzymic or nonenzymic means.[73,88] Many environmental factors are known to give rise to free radical reactions. These include ionizing radiation,[5] excessive exposure to ultraviolet light and contacting air pollutants such as NO_2 and O_3.[13,44,64] Furthermore, lipid peroxides may be generated in the body organs due to intake of chemical initiators such as alcohols,[24,25] carbon tetrachloride, or chloroform.[74,93] In the presence of oxygen, the free radical reactions are self-propagating and may result in the formation of hydroperoxide and malonyldialdehyde (MDA) as shown in Figure 1. The hydroperoxides may undergo further peroxidation in the presence of Fe^{++} ions.[55,124] This interaction may result in complete destruction of the entire fatty acid molecule leading to structural and functional damage to the membranes.[63]

A number of enzymic systems are known to utilize and activate oxygen and are potentially active in generating free radicals which in turn can promote lipid peroxidation.[55] These reactions include ADP-activated lipid peroxidation coupled to the microsomal·NADPH oxidation system,[45] hydroxyl free radical production during metabolism of flavin enzyme,[31] the xanthine oxidase system, as well as other reactions in which superoxide anion radicals ($.O_2^-$) and singlet oxygen are produced.[31,52,55,124] The superoxide anion generated in the microsomes may react with H_2O_2, a product of

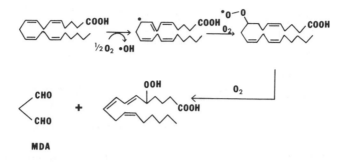

FIGURE 1.   Peroxidation reactions of arachidonic acid.

NADPH oxidation, and together with Fe^{3+} may form a hydroxy radical (.OH) through the reaction sequence[31] as indicated in Equations 1 to 3:

$$H_2O_2 + \cdot O_2^- \longrightarrow \cdot OH + O_2 + OH^- \qquad (1)$$

$$\cdot O_2^- + Fe^{3+} \longrightarrow O_2 + Fe^{2+} \qquad (2)$$

$$Fe^{2+} + H_2O_2 \longrightarrow \cdot OH + Fe^{3+} + OH^- \qquad (3)$$

Lipid peroxidation damage can be quenched by free radical scavengers or through some other biological protection systems. Peroxidation initiated by superoxide anion can be inhibited by the enzyme superoxide dismutase (SOD), which is known to catalyze the dismutation of $.O_2^-$ as shown in Equation 4.

$$2.O_2^- + 2H^+ \xrightarrow{\text{SOD}} H_2O_2 + O_2 \qquad (4)$$

Actually, the hydrogen peroxide formed is less toxic than the superoxide anion or the hydroxyl radicals because it can be "detoxified" by the action of catalase or glutathione peroxidase (GSH-Px). Reiss and Gershon[75] reported that the level of superoxide dismutase in rat liver was decreased threefold during aging. Glutathione peroxidase is known to contain selenium as an integral component of the enzyme.[78,79] Therefore, it is not surprising that the activity of glutathione peroxidase is dependent on the dietary content of selenium.[33,68] Its action on lipid peroxides (L-OOH) to form less harmful fatty acid alcohols has been suggested by Tappel[126] as shown in Equation 5:

$$L\text{--}OOH + 2GSH \xrightarrow{\text{GSH-Px}} L\text{--}OH + H_2O + GSSG \qquad (5)$$

On the other hand, McCay et al.[59] found no evidence for the formation of such alcohols (L-OH) in vitro due to the action of glutathione peroxidase, and they suggested that perhaps this enzyme merely exerts its protective effect by preventing free radical attack on the lipid molecules. Another possibility is that glutathione peroxidase only acts on free fatty acids and not those which are already esterified. An increase in lipid peroxidation activity in biomembranes was detected (by measuring the hydrocarbon evolved) from animals fed a selenium deficient diet.[26,37] The blood of elderly persons was found to have a lower level of selenium than the younger age group.[131] Thus despite the yet unknown mechanism of action of glutathione peroxidase, dietary selenium appears to be an important element in maintaining the active functioning of this enzyme which in turn can provide protection of the biomembranes against oxidative changes.[77]

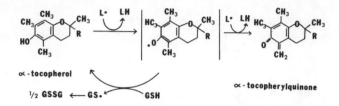

FIGURE 2.   Mechanism of α-tocopherol in quenching free radicals.

Ascorbic acid is considered to be a pro-oxidant when present at low concentration[89] and an antioxidant when present at high concentration.[87] In the brain tissue, the activity of catalase and glutathione peroxidase is much lower than in other nonneural tissues. Consequently, the high physiological level of ascorbic acid present in the brain cytoplasm may be an important factor for protecting the membranes against peroxidative damage.[87]

Free radical scavengers such as vitamin E or coenzyme Q may also protect biomembranes from peroxidative damage. Vitamin E is probably the most important antioxidant in the diet. It is lipid soluble, and after ingestion it appears to orient itself at some specific sites within the biomembranes. The protective effect of vitamin E on lipid peroxidation is due to its ability to quench free radicals and lipid peroxide radicals by converting the tocopherol to tocopheryl quinone as shown in the reactions indicated in Figure 2. The intermediate, a phenolic radical, is rather stable and can be reduced back to tocopherol by glutathione.

The susceptibility of tissue lipids to lipid peroxidation is not only dependent on the level of the membrane polyunsaturated fatty acids, but also on their vitamin E content. Cornwell et al.[19] showed that the rate of proliferation of smooth muscle cells in culture could be influenced by the unsaturated fatty acid as well as the presence of oxidants and antioxidants. Therefore, addition of antioxidants such as α-naphthol and vitamin E (either in the presence of trienoic and tetraenoic fatty acids) could give a stimulatory effect to the rate of cell proliferation. Vitamin E level in mammalian body organs seems to vary among tissues and membranes. On a per milligram protein basis, there is two- to threefold more tocopherol in the heart and lung tissue than in the liver and kidney.[130] Surprisingly, only a very low level of tocopherol was found in the red blood cell membranes (9ng/mg protein). Hatman and Kayden[42] reported that the vitamin E level in the white cells was approximately 30 times higher than that in the red cells. Hyperlipidemic individuals who take vitamin E supplement can achieve an unusually high level of the vitamin in all types of their blood cell membranes. These results are in favor of a protective role of dietary vitamin E on blood cell membranes, especially leukocytes which are important for the body defense mechanism Vitamin E deficiency was shown to give a greater accumulation of aging pigments[20,51,129] as well as other age-related changes.[103] Morphological examination also indicated obvious testicular degeneration in rats suffering from vitamin E and selenium deficiency (Sun, unpublished data). Thermally oxidized dietary lipids were shown to elicit a higher incidence of nutritional encephalopathy in the vitamin E deficient chick.[9] These deficiency symptoms imply that oxidative damage has occurred in the cellular and subcellular membranes due to a lack of protection by the antioxidant.[86] Although there is little information regarding whether Vitamin E level in body tissues may change as a function of age, indications such as an increase in oxidative products of lipids in serum with advancing age[125] do suggest that dietary supplement of the vitamin to the aged may be beneficial towards retarding some of the aging processes.

Other antioxidants such as butylated hydroxyanisole (BHA), butylated hydroxytoluene (BHT), diphenyl-*p*-phenylenediamine (DPPD) and ethoxyquin have been shown to prevent vitamin E deficiency.[18] these antioxidants may play a protective role against the free radical damage caused by prooxidants such as halomethanes, ethanol, ozone as well as other photoactivated carcinogens.[16,23,24,55,56] Some of these synthetic radical scavengers were also shown to prolong the average life span of mice[39] and reduce the accumulation of age pigments in body organs.[129] In fact, a number of these antioxidants, like α-mercaptoethylamine and ethoxyquin, have been tested as possible anti-aging agents.

III. EVIDENCE OF LIPID PEROXIDATION IN BIOLOGICAL SYSTEMS

The linear accumulation of chromolipids in body tissue with age has been one of the most striking subcellular modifications observed in aged animals.[83,94] Histological and biochemical examinations of the lipofuscin or age pigments indicate that they are comprised of conjugated polyunsaturated fatty acids.[72] These age pigments have the characteristic fluorescence spectra with a maximum at 470 nm when excited at 365 nm. The spectra of solvent extractable fluorescent age pigments from the aged animals are qualitatively similar to the chemical products formed when unsaturated fatty acids and γ-dicarbonyl substances are reacted with amino compounds such as ethanolamine.[129] Chio et al.[12] attempted to produce pigments similar to the lipofuscin observed in the natural process by subjecting subcellular membranes to peroxidation reactions. Casselman[10] also showed that the more unsaturated the lipids the greater chance these lipids would undergo in vitro oxidation to form the pigments. Tappel[128] showed that when mice were placed on a normal protein diet supplemented with a high level of antioxidants, there was a lower rate of lipid peroxidation as indicated by the decrease in fluorescent product formed.

The accumulation of lipofuscin pigments in nonreplaceable, fixed postmitotic cells is regarded as an age-related process.[8,84,95] Lipofuscin substances are found to accumulate with increasing age in some mammalian tissues, and these substances are believed to originate from in vivo lipid peroxidation reactions.[69,91,127,128] Lipofuscin formation could be induced by stress such as the state of chronic anoxia[96,97] and hyperoxia.[143] Sulkin and colleagues[96,97] observed the presence of lipofuscin pigments in nerve cells of young rats after prolonged treatments of acetanilide, vitamin E deficient diet, and chronic anoxia. Since tissue aging is a continuous process starting from conception until death, it is not surprising to find that lipid peroxidation and lipofuscin pigment formation are also part of this progressive process. However, whether lipofuscin is indeed the basic element underlying the aging process remains to be demonstrated.

Another evidence of lipid peroxidation in biological systems is the production of hydrocarbon gases, such as ethane and pentane,[21,22,26,27,37] which are produced during oxidative degradation of linoleic, linolenic, and arachidonic acid. The amount of gases evolved correlated well with the disappearance of these fatty acids and the formation of conjugated dienes.[27] Therefore, measurement of hydrocarbon gases has been a useful index for estimating the extent of lipid peroxidation during aging as well as in experimental conditions related to the effects of dietary antioxidants.

IV. EFFECTS OF AGING ON MEMBRANE LIPIDS AND FUNCTIONS

Membrane phospholipids are comprised of a glycerol backbone through which long chain hydrocarbons are linked in the form of ester or ether linkages. Not only do the phospholipid profiles vary widely among different body organs, but each phospholipid class within a specific type of subcellular membrane may be associated with a characteristic acyl group profile.[111,112] For example, the phospholipid acyl groups of grey matter in human brain are characterized by a high proportion of the (n-3) family such as 22:6(n-3), whereas the acyl groups of white matter are comprised largely of monoenes such as 18:1 and 20:1.[114] Unlike the brain, fatty acids in the adrenal gland are highly enriched in the (n-6) family but contain very little of the (n-3) family.[110,137] Within the brain tissue, the acyl group profile of phosphatidylcholines differs greatly from that of phosphatidylethanolamines, and acyl groups from the same phospholipid in synaptosomal membranes differ also in composition from those in the myelin.[121]

The physical properties of the hydrocarbon sidechains of phospholipids are of paramount importance to the membrane functions.[92] Many membrane-associated processes are dependent on the mode of packing and/or length of the hydrocarbon side chains. Due to the involvement of the acyl groups in membrane functions, many membrane-bound enzymes, antigens, and receptors are known to require specific phospholipids for expression of their activities.[102,136] Since membrane fatty acids are the primary target for lipid peroxidation, it is obvious that dietary deficiencies, drugs, and compounds which may exert oxidative or antioxidative effects on the membrane lipids may also affect the normal membrane functions.

Membrane phospholipids are undergoing constant turnover although the exact mechanism governing the turnover process is not well understood.[43] Different types of subcellular membranes are known to exhibit different rates of turnover of the phospholipid acyl groups.[109,113,119] In general, metabolic turnover of cellular phospholipids is more rapid in the endoplasmic reticulum as compared to other types of subcellular membranes. Thus although the endoplasmic reticulum is probably highly susceptible to changes due to dietary intervention, the components of this type of membrane may not be altered as a function of age due to its active metabolism. In this regard, the myelin is a better membrane model for correlating age-related changes because it can be isolated from brain in a relatively pure form, and this type of membrane is largely devoid of enzymes for active metabolism of its phospholipids. Rouser and Yamamoto[80,81] suggest that there is a decrease of myelin lipids during aging of human brain. The decrease in 2′,3′-cyclic nucleotide 3′-phosphodiesterase activity in human brain with age[7,134] also supports the age-related decrease in myelin since this enzyme is highly enriched in the myelin membrane and is used as a marker enzyme for assessing the myelin activity in brain. Wisniewski and Terry[142] gave morphologic evidence showing that myelin is lost from axons in aged brain. Berlet and Volk[4] further reported that the amount of myelin isolated from human brain homogenates decreased with age, and that the rate of decline was especially obvious around the fifth and sixth decades.[4] The decrease in brain myelin towards advancing age may be associated with the gradual decline in nerve conduction activity which is commonly observed in the aged. Furthermore, pathological symptoms associated with diseases involving demyelination may also exhibit parallel signs of premature aging.

We have studied the lipid changes in brain myelin during aging. Experiments were carried out with a number of brain species including tissues from the rodents,[115] the corpus callosum from rhesus monkey,[116] and the frontal cortex from human brain.[49,104] It is interesting to note that some obvious differences do exist with regard to the acyl group profile of the myelin phospholipids among various brain species (Table 1). For example, myelin isolated from human and monkey brain indicated a higher proportion of 22:4 but a lower proportion of 20:1 than those from the rodent brain. Although it is not clear whether the species-related differences in acyl group composition of myelin are in any way associated with the functional activities of the membrane, there are some differences regarding the age-related changes in myelin components from rodents and humans. For example, myelin deposition in the rodent brain is shown to be a continuous process throughout the entire life span,[47,115] whereas this same process is shown to reach a maximum level and then decline in the human.[4] Therefore, the phos-

Table 1
ACYL GROUP COMPOSITION (%, WT) OF
ETHANOLAMINE PHOSPHOGLYCERIDES OF
MYELIN ISOLATED FROM DIFFERENT
SPECIES OF THE MAMMALIAN BRAIN

Fatty acids	Human (61—67 years)	Rhesus monkey	Ox	Rat	Mouse
16:0	2.9	3.4	4.2	4.4	7.1
18:0	6.0	7.3	7.3	9.0	12.0
18:1	41.3	35.8	46.2	43.8	33.0
20:1	8.1	10.7	13.2	18.9	14.5
20:3	—	2.8	0.8	—	1.0
20:4	8.7	11.3	7.5	7.7	12.9
22:4	21.6	17.8	12.4	4.8	9.9
22:6	5.8	3.1	2.7	3.7	6.9
24:4	1.3	3.9	—	—	—

Note: Myelin was isolated from brain tissue according to the procedure described by Sun and Horrocks.[112] The ethanolamine phosphoglycerides were separated by two dimensional thin-layer chromatography as described in Horrocks and Sun.[48] Fatty acids of the phospholipids were converted to methylesters and were analyzed by gas-liquid chromatography.[112]

pholipid acyl groups in myelin isolated from human and primate brains indicated a more obvious change with age than those from the rodents. Myelin isolated from human frontal cortex also indicated a decrease in phosphatidylcholines and phosphatidylethanolamines and an increase in ethanolamine plasmalogens with advancing age (samples obtained between ages 15 and 90 years).[104] Among the phospholipids, there was a general increase in the monoenoic acyl groups and a decrease in the polyunsaturated acyl groups with advancing age.[49,104,116] The age-related decrease in polyunsaturated fatty acids in brain myelin is probably a process due to peroxidation induced by some naturally occurring free radicals. However, it is not known whether a dietary supplement of antioxidants may help to retard these changes.

The synaptic plasma membrane is probably more susceptible to peroxidative changes than the myelin due to its high content of polyunsaturated fatty acids.[121] Little is known about age-related changes in this type of neuronal brain membrane. The decrease in polyunsaturated fatty acid content in the frontal grey matter of aged human brain[6] suggests that the age-related changes in synaptosomal membranes are similar to those described in myelin. When the synaptosomal membranes were subjected to an in vitro lipid peroxidation process, a decrease in $(Na^+ + K^+)$-ATPase activity was observed.[98] There is no difference in the activity of this membrane-bound enzyme with respect to age (as determined from three different age groups).[101] However, when the enzyme preparations from these same age groups were tested for their response towards ethanol, there was a decrease in the resistance of the synaptosomal ATPase to inhibition by ethanol with advancing age.[101] This same phenomenon was observed in the membrane preparations from both human and rodent brain. Since ethanol may exert its effect by interacting with the hydrophobic sites of the membranes,[100,101] the decrease in response of the ATPase towards ethanol with age suggests that some physical properties of the membranes may have been altered as a consequence of advancing age.

There are also indications that an increasing level of endogenous lyso-phospholipids is formed in rat brain synaptosomes with advancing age.[104] The increase in lyso-phospholipids may be associated with a change in the membrane lipid metabolism such as an increase in phospholipid degradation activity and a decrease in the rate of reutilization.[54] This explanation is supported by the finding that synaptosomes isolated from 28-month-old rat brain were less active in reacylating the lyso-phosphatidylcholines with arachidonate as compared to synaptosomes isolated from young adults (Sun, unpublished data). Furthermore, the incorporation in vivo of labeled palmitate into brain glycerolipids was lower in the aged mice (28 months of age) than the young adults (10 months of age).[108] Lyso-phospholipids are products of phospholipase A action, and an accumulation of these compounds in membranes is not desirable on account of their detergent-like property.[139] Parce et al.[70] showed that the phospholipase A_2 activity in liver mitochondria was activated during in vitro aging. The acyl-CoA:lyso-phospholipid acyltransferase is an important enzyme for membrane acyl group turnover because it can couple with the phospholipase A to convert the lyso-compounds back to the membrane phospholipids.[54] This membrane-bound enzyme has been shown to respond to cell stimuli[29] and to drugs which may disturb the physical property of the membranes.[34,90,117,118] These results imply that modification of membrane acyl groups due to aging or dietary intervention can be attributed to a change in the enzymic systems responsible for metabolic turnover of the phospholipids.[120]

V. EFFECTS OF DIETARY ANTIOXIDANTS ON MEMBRANE LIPIDS AND FUNCTIONS

There is sufficient evidence to justify a serious consideration of the physiological importance of lipid peroxidation in the pathologic development of certain organ diseases such as atherosclerosis in the aorta and ceroid lipofuscinosis (Batten disease) in the nervous tissues. Excessive lipid peroxidation can cause extensive damage to the mitochondrial membranes leading to appearance of mitochondrial ghosts with obvious loss of matrix material.[62] Pfeifer and McCay[71] showed that excess peroxidation of liver mitochondria could give rise to a loss of the unsaturated mitochondrial lipids, decrease in oxidative phosphorylation, and electron transport activities. The $(Na^+ + K^+)$-ATPase activity of brain synaptic plasma membranes was inhibited by subjecting the membranes to in vitro lipid peroxidation.[98,102] Interactions between peroxidized lipids and proteins have been shown to result in a loss of membrane enzyme activity, polymerization and scissioning of polypeptide chains, accelerated formation of brown pigments, and destruction of labile amino acid residues such as histidine, lysine, cysteine, and methionine.[57]

Our laboratory has investigated the effects of dietary antioxidants on some age-related membrane processes.[1,32,103,105] The experiment involved feeding rats with various dietary regimens either deficient in vitamin E and selenium (Group I),[78] or supplemented with vitamin E (Group II), selenium (Group III), BHT (Group IV), and vitamin E plus selenium (Control). Rats reared on a basal diet which was deficient in vitamin E and selenium for 8 months achieved only half the body weight as compared to controls (Figure 3). The animals fed a basal diet supplemented with BHT were also poor in body growth. On the other hand, the groups given a basal diet supplemented with either vitamin E or selenium did not show obvious decrease in body weight. The mean life span of male rats in the vitamin E and selenium deficient group (I) was shortened by about 1 year, and all of them died before reaching 19 months of age. Animals fed a diet supplemented with vitamin E appeared to be more healthy in general, whereas severe deficiency symptoms were observed in experimental animals lacking the dietary vitamin E.

Since the brain membranes are more vulnerable to lipid peroxidation due to enrichment of polyunsaturated fatty acids in their phospholipids,[121] they were used to study

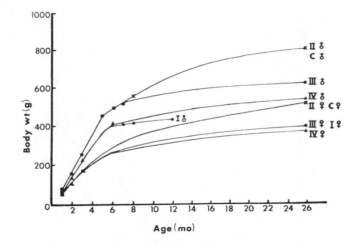

FIGURE 3. Effect of dietary vitamin E, selenium, and BHT on growth rate of male and female rats. Diets were initiated after weaning and were given *ad lib* together with tap water. At the beginning of the experiment, 20 male and female rats were placed in each group. **Group I:** Rats were fed a basal diet[78] deficient in vitamin E and selenium. **Group II:** Rats were fed a basal diet supplemented with vitamin E (50 IU of DL-α-tocopherol per kg of diet). **Group III:** Rats were fed with a basal diet supplemented with sodium selenite (0.5 ppm). **Group IV:** Rats were fed with a basal diet supplemented with butylated hydroxytoluene (BHT) (0.5%). **Group C:** Rats were fed with a basal diet supplemented with both vitamin E (50 IU/kg) and selenite (0.5 ppm). Each curve represents the average body weight at the time of measurement.

the vulnerability of membrane lipids to oxidative attack. As shown in Figure 4, malonyldialdehyde (MDA) formation was higher in the group fed a vitamin E and selenium deficient diet than the ones given a dietary supplement of either vitamin E or selenium. On the other hand, the group fed a basal diet supplemented with BHT was just as vulnerable to lipid peroxidation as the vitamin E and selenium deficient group. The increase in membrane peroxidation activity observed in the vitamin E and selenium deficient group seems to reflect a change in the structural components of the membranes, possibly due to perturbation of the membrane lipids. These results are in agreement with previous studies indicating that the susceptibility to lipid peroxidation can be influenced by the tissue level of vitamin E.[17,60,82] However, the exact relationship between membrane susceptibility to lipid peroxidation and the physicochemical properties of the membranes remains to be further investigated.

Although vitamin E deficiency has been shown to result in an altered microsomal protein synthesis[76] as well as some other enzyme activities,[35,66,144] it is not clear whether dietary selenium and BHT could prevent the membrane modifications due to vitamin E deficiency. In this experiment, the activities of two membrane-dependent transport processes were studied in an attempt to correlate these membrane processes with the effects of dietary antioxidants.[103] After 8 months on the various dietary treatments, the activity of catecholamine uptake in brain synaptosomes was lower in groups I, II, and IV than in the control (Table 2). The data in Figure 5 further indicate that the level of norepinephrine and dopamine in the hypothalamus and caudate nucleus is higher in the antioxidant deficient group than in the control group. The level of dopamine in the caudate nucleus from the group fed a basal diet supplemented with BHT was also higher than the control. The decrease in norepinephrine uptake activity in the vitamin E and selenium deficient group suggests that some synaptosomal membrane

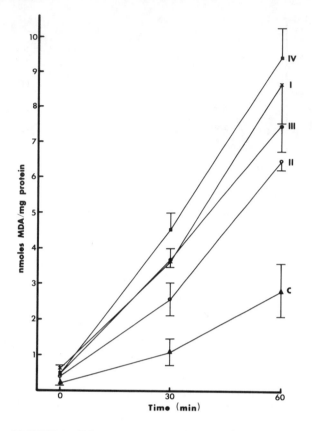

FIGURE 4.   Effect of dietary vitamin E, selenium, and BHT on lipid peroxidation of brain membranes. Lipid peroxidation was performed with brain homogenate in a medium containing 0.017 M FeSO$_4$, 0.3% KCl, and 0.1 M Tris-HCl buffered at pH 7.5. At the end of incubation at 37°C, triplicate aliquots of 3 ml were taken and malonyldialdehyde (MDA) formed was assayed by the thiobarbituric acid reaction. The dietary treatments for the various groups were same as described in Figure 3. Determinations were made at 8 months after initiation of the dietary treatments. Each point represents mean ± standard error of means.

functions may also be altered due to the dietary treatments. In fact, these changes are similar to those observed during aging.[99] The increase in norepinephrine level in hypothalamus and dopamine level in the caudate nucleus may be due to an activation of catecholamine biosynthesis through a feedback control mechanism. Catecholamines are known to play a very important role in the regulation of behavioral activities.[3] Therefore, a change in the biogenic amine metabolism may be related to a wide variety of neurological disorders. Although a dietary supplement of BHT has been shown to prolong the life span of some experimental animals,[16,39] and to retard the tissue damage due to the effects of X-ray and prooxidant compounds,[14,15] our results here indicate that the properties of brain membranes from rats given a BHT supplemented diet were not different from those which were deficient in dietary vitamin E and selenium. Possibly, BHT may act on body organs through a mechanism associated with the lipid solubility or the hydrophobic environment of the membranes.[65] Therefore, the prolonged life span observed by Harmon,[38] and Clapp and Satterfield,[16] and the decrease in fluorescent age pigment accumulation observed by Tappel et al.[129] after dietary BHT

Table 2
EFFECT OF DIETARY ANTIOXIDANT ON MEMBRANE-DEPENDENT PROCESSES

Group	Dietary treatment	No. of rats	NE-uptake (CPM/mg)	$(Na^+ + K^+)$-ATPase (μmole/mg)
C	Complete	(4)	3445 ± 326	3.78 ± 0.10
I	Basal	(4)	2982 ± 318	4.14 ± 0.17
II	Basal + Vit. E	(4)	2765 ± 194	3.86 ± 0.35
III	Basal + Se	(4)	3281 ± 420	3.91 ± 0.29
IV	Basal + BHT	(4)	2792 ± 343	4.23 ± 0.35

Note: Rats were on different dietary treatments for 8 months. NE-uptake activity was determined with synaptosomal particles isolated from the cerebral cortex of each rat. $(Na^+ + K^+)$-ATPase activity was assayed according to the method of Sun and Samorajski.[101] Data represents mean ± SEM.

From Sun, A. Y. and Sun, G. Y., *Adv. Exp. Med. Biol.,* 97, 285, 1978. With permission.

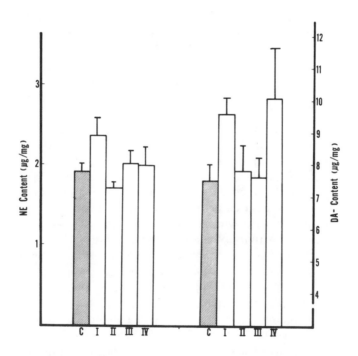

FIGURE 5.   Effect of dietary antioxidants on norepinephrine (NE) and dopamine (DA) content in hypothalamus and caudate nucleus of rat brain. Samples were taken from the hypothalamus and caudate nucleus of rats after 8 months of the dietary treatments (see Figure 3). NE and DA content was measured according to procedure described in Sun.[99] Data is expressed as μg NE or DA/mg protein in the sample.

treatment, may be due to a yet unknown type of antioxidant effect of this compound on body organs.

The $(Na^+ + K^+)$-ATPase in brain synaptic membranes is known to require a lipid environment for optimal functioning.[102] Previous studies in our laboratory have indicated that activity of this enzyme can be altered by chronic administration of

Table 3

ACYL GROUP COMPOSITION (%, WT) OF PHOSPHOLIPIDS FROM LIVER MITOCHONDRIA: A COMPARISON BETWEEN DIETARY VITAMIN E AND SELENIUM DEFICIENCY VERSUS CONTROLS

Fatty acids	PC[a]		PE		PI		CL	
	Con.	Def.	Con.	Def.	Con.	Def.	Con.	Def.
16:0	21.8	20.0	16.8	12.7	3.4	1.7	3.5	1.9
18:0	19.5	20.5	24.4	24.5	46.6	41.8	1.4	1.0
18:1	10.1	12.8	6.9	9.5	—	—	19.9	18.8
18:2	18.5	18.4	8.6	9.7	4.0	5.1	72.8	76.4
18:3	0.8	0.5	0.4	0.4	—	—	—	—
20:3	1.8	0.9	0.6	0.5	5.7	5.2	—	—
20:4	14.4	14.6	16.9	23.2	27.9	40.4	2.0	1.9
20:5	2.6	3.4	3.2	5.3	—	—	—	—
22:5	1.2	0.5	2.6	0.8	3.6	—	—	—
22:6	8.9	6.8	19.4	13.8	8.3	7.6	—	—

Note: Controls were given a basal diet supplemented with vitamin E and selenium. The mitochondrial lipids were separated by two-dimensional thin-layer chromatography as described in Table 1.

[a] Abbreviations: PC, diacyl-glycerophosphocholines; PE, diacyl-glycerophosphoethanolamines; PI, diacyl-glycerophosphoinositols; CL, cardiolipin.

alcohol,[106,107] and by feeding mice an essential fatty acid deficient diet.[122] When brain $(Na^+ + K^+)$-ATPase activity was compared among the various dietary groups, a higher activity was observed in the deficient group (I) and BHT-supplement group (IV) as compared to controls (Table 2). The change in ATPase activity is again regarded as an adaptive measure in order to compensate for the inhibitory effect due to the dietary insult. Sung et al.[123] also measured activity of enzymes involved in cholinergic transmission in brain using rats fed a vitamin E deficient diet for 7 to 8 weeks. They did not observe differences in activity of these enzymes in brain as compared to changes which occurred in muscle. Possibly, this is due to the fact that the brain is more resistant to dietary intervention than most other body organs, especially if the dietary treatment is only given over a relatively short period of time.

The cholesterol and cholesteryl ester content of rat adrenal gland was also affected by the various dietary treatments.[103] Rats reared on a vitamin E and selenium deficient diet indicated a higher level of cholesterol and cholesteryl ester in the adrenal as compared to controls. Also, rats which were reared on a basal diet supplemented with BHT were like the ones reared on a vitamin E and selenium deficient diet in indicating an elevated level of cholesterol in the adrenal.

We also determined the fatty acid composition of mitochondrial phospholipids from rat liver with respect to the various dietary treatments. When acyl group composition of mitochondria from the vitamin E and selenium deficient rats was compared to controls, results indicated a decrease in the (n-3) fatty acids, such as 22:6, and an increase in the (n-6) fatty acids, such as the 20:4, in the deficient animals as compared to controls (Table 3). On the other hand, the proportion of 18:2, which is a precursor for the (n-6) fatty acids, is not greatly altered. The decrease in (n-3) fatty acids in the group deficient in dietary antioxidants may reflect the result of peroxidative changes due to a lack of protection by the antioxidants. The increase in (n-6) fatty acids, however, is probably due to a compensative measure to maintain the polyunsaturated fatty

Table 4

ACYL GROUP COMPOSITION (%, WT) OF MAJOR
PHOSPHOLIPIDS FROM RAT LIVER
MITOCHONDRIA: A COMPARISON WITH RESPECT
TO DIETARY ANTIOXIDANT TREATMENTS[a]

Fatty acids	Control	Group I deficient	Group II + vit. E	Group III + selenium	Group IV + BHT
		Diacyl-glycerophosphocholines			
16:0	21.8	20.0	22.2	20.3	24.1
18:0	19.5	20.5	24.6	25.3	19.6
18:1	10.1	12.8	11.9	13.2	12.7
18:2	18.5	18.4	18.1	13.4	20.9
18:3	0.8	0.5	0.5	0.4	0.5
20:3	1.8	0.9	1.7	1.1	1.1
20:4	14.4	14.6	9.5	12.5	9.4
20:5	2.6	3.4	3.6	5.1	3.7
22:5	1.2	0.5	0.8	—	1.1
22:6	8.9	6.8	10.3	11.3	7.0
		Diacyl-glycerophosphoethanolamines			
16:0	16.8	12.7	17.8	18.9	20.3
18:0	24.4	24.5	25.2	23.5	26.0
18:1	6.9	9.5	7.8	8.5	8.8
18:2	8.6	9.7	8.2	6.0	10.3
18:3	0.4	0.4	—	0.4	—
20:3	0.6	0.5	0.7	0.5	0.5
20:4	16.9	23.2	12.6	14.6	14.3
20:5	3.2	5.3	3.7	5.7	3.7
22:5	2.6	0.8	1.4	1.4	1.9
22:6	19.4	13.8	21.7	20.4	15.4

Note: Rats in Control group were given a basal diet supplemented with vitamin E and selenium and those in the deficient group (I) were fed a basal diet deficient in both vitamin E and selenium. The rats in groups II, III, and IV were given a basal diet supplemented with either vitamin E, selenium or BHT. Fatty acid analysis was same as described in Table 1.

acid level in the membranes. This type of opposing response towards a single dietary treatment is not entirely surprising because several pathways are known to be responsible to their biosynthesis and metabolism.

We also made a comparison of the membrane acyl group composition from rats reared on diets which were supplemented with various types of antioxidants. As shown in Table 4, different types of dietary antioxidants seem to elicit a different response on the membrane fatty acids. For example, the group reared with a basal diet supplemented with vitamin E indicated a decrease in 20:4 and 22:5, whereas the group supplemented with selenium indicated a decrease in 18:2 and 22:5 instead. However, neither of these groups showed a decrease in 22:6, although such a change was observed in the group lacking both vitamin E and selenium in the diet. In fact, acyl group changes were most severe in the group fed a basal diet supplemented with BHT since the membrane phospholipids showed a decrease in almost all of the polyunsaturated fatty acids. Thus there is a difference in the tissue response towards the various types of dietary antioxidants. McCoy and Weswig[61] pointed out earlier that tissue responses towards selenium and vitamin E are different. Our results further show that BHT

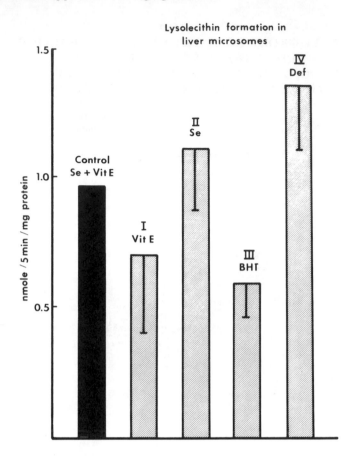

FIGURE 6.   Formation of endogenous lysolecithin in rat liver microsomes with respect to dietary antioxidant deficiencies. Dietary treatments were same as described in Figure 3. Lysolecithin level was determined by incubating liver microsomes with labeled oleoyl-CoA and
measuring the amount of radioactivity incorporated into phosphatidylcholines.

cannot be used as a biological antioxidant to replace vitamin E or selenium in protecting membrane fatty acids from oxidative changes.

Since the deacylation-reacylation process is important in regulating the membrane
fatty acid turnover,[54] an experiment was carried out to assess the endogenous lysolecithin content in rat liver microsomes with respect to the different dietary regimens.
Lysolecithin is the product of phospholipase A-mediated deacylation and the substrate
of the acyltransferase-mediated reacylation activity. As shown in Figure 6, endogenous
lysolecithin level of liver microsomes was highest in the vitamin E and selenium deficient group as compared to controls and other dietary groups. Surprisingly, the groups
given a vitamin E or BHT supplement to the deficient diet were both lower in the
endogenous lysolecithin content as compared to controls. One can conclude from these
results that the deacylation-reacylation activity in rat liver microsomes is also under
the influence of dietary antioxidants. However, the exact implication of this type of
response to the cellular lipid metabolism remains to be investigated.

Wilson et al.[141] have studied the effects of dietary supplement of a high level of
vitamin E and antioxidants such as butylated hydroxyanisole (BHA) and butylated
hydroxytoluene (BHT) to rabbits which were fed a low cholesterol atherogenic diet.
Their results indicated that aortic and coronary atherosclerosis were more frequent

and extensive in rabbits fed the basal atherogenic diet (containing butter) and the basal diet supplemented with BHA and BHT as compared to those fed the basal diet supplemented with 1% vitamin E. Furthermore, the level of serum cholesterol and phospholipids from the vitamin E supplemented group was low and actually resembled the group fed a corn-oil control diet, whereas serum lipids from the group reared on the basal atherogenic diet and the BHA and BHT supplemented diets were obviously higher than controls.

Little information is available regarding the effects of vitamin E and selenium deficiency on tissue lipid composition. Farnsworth et al.[28] reported that such dietary deficiencies may or may not produce a change in tissue lipid composition depending on the type of tissue analyzed. Thus even within the retinal tissues, a decrease in the (n-3) polyunsaturated fatty acid level due to dietary vitamin E and selenium deficiency was observed only in the retinal pigment epithelium but not in other types of retinal tissue. The small increase in the level of 20:4 in the susceptible retinal tissues is actually similar to what we have observed with liver mitochondria.

Several investigators have shown that liver microsomes[60,82] isolated from animals given a vitamin E deficient diet were more prone to peroxidation in vitro than those from controls. Other studies also indicate that this type of dietary deficiency can elicit changes in microsomal membrane phospholipids and fatty acids,[36] age pigment formation[135] as well as activity of some membrane enzymes.[30,36,140] Some of these changes are similar to those observed during aging. However, the results of an extensive study by Grinna[35] seem to indicate that the requirement of dietary tocopherol may decrease with age and that the age-related alterations in membrane compositional and functional parameters may not be correlated with dietary vitamin E. Indeed, the effects of dietary antioxidants on the cellular aging process are complex functions which cannot be evaluated by simple biochemical parameters alone.

VI. CONCLUDING REMARKS

Lipid peroxidation in body organs is an ongoing biological process involving the participation of a number of enzymic and nonenzymic systems.[31] Lipid peroxidation has also been implicated in various organ injuries due to ingestion of organic halides, ethanol, and other prooxidant compounds.[24] Condition such as overexposure to ultraviolet rays and air pollutants may also elicit an increase in the peroxidation reactions in body tissues.[13] Consequently, propagation of free radical reactions in the biological systems can be destructive if they are not properly controlled. Membrane polyunsaturated fatty acids are the primary target of free radical attack, and this process has been demonstrated in body organs through detection of various end-products such as formation of malonydialdehyde and hydrocarbon gases evolved from humans and animals. The appearance of fluorescent age-pigments is another positive evidence of the peroxidation process.

Superoxide dismutase and glutathione peroxidase are two known enzymic systems which can convert the superoxide anions and hydroperoxides to more stable and less destructive compounds. Selenium is an integral component of glutathione peroxidase and thus is required by the enzyme for activity. However, the exact mechanism underlying the role of glutathione peroxidase is not well understood and awaits further investigation.

Vitamin E is a naturally occurring antioxidant which can quench free radical reactions and reduce lipid peroxidation. This compound is probably the most important biological antioxidant with respect to membrane lipids due to its lipid solubility which can penetrate the hydrophobic region of membranes. From the results of our experiments as well as those from McCoy and Weswig,[61] it is obvious that the action of vitamin E is different from that exerted by selenium. Animals reared on a vitamin E-deficient diet were inhibited in body growth and exhibited a number of deficiency symptoms similar to those described in premature organ aging.

Some of the peroxidative processes in the biological systems may also be prevented by synthetic antioxidants such as BHT and BHA. Mice given a diet supplement of BHT seem to have a longer life span. However, our results indicate that these compounds do not exert a similar protective effect to the cell membranes as shown by the naturally occurring antioxidants. The exact mode of action of these synthetic antioxidants on cell membrane composition and metabolism is not well understood. From the results of our studies, we have concluded that BHT is not a suitable substitute for vitamin E.

Cellular membranes are important in the biological system because they not only serve as a permeability barrier but also regulate the active transport of substances across the cell boundary and respond to hormonal and immunological action. Alteration of the membrane structure due to premature aging or dietary insult can cause malfunctioning of the entire organ system and produce diseases affecting the well-being of the individual. Therefore, it is important to provide proper protection mechanism in order to maintain a healthy membrane system for proper functioning.

A number of the membrane changes due to dietary vitamin E deficiency are in fact similar to those in aging. Dietary antioxidants have been shown to protect the cellular membranes from peroxidative changes. However, whether a supplement of the dietary antioxidants may retard the complex process of aging remains to be demonstrated.[50] Normally, the human individual is rarely afflicted with vitamin E or selenium deficiency. It is doubtful that a dietary supplement of the antioxidants can elicit a beneficial effect in improving sexual potency and fertility of the individual. Nevertheless, vitamin E in therapeutic amounts may be useful in certain clinical situations such as encephalopathies, myopathies, erythrocyte abnormalities, certain hereditary deficiencies, and cardiovascular disease.[50] Wilson et al.[141] also showed that a high dietary level of vitamin E may help to reduce mortality and inhibit organ abnormalities in rabbits reared on an atherogenic diet. These results suggest that when individuals are exposed to agents which may cause excessive peroxidative damage, a short-term intake of vitamin E may be beneficial in preserving the integrity of cellular membranes and in preventing premature aging.

ACKNOWLEDGMENTS

The assistance of Dr. L. Foudin in various aspects of this research project is gratefully acknowledged. We also thank Mrs. D. Torres for her excellent secretarial assistance in the preparation of this manuscript. This work was supported in part from USPHS Research Grants NS12752 and NS 12960 from NIH.

REFERENCES

1. **Badger, C. R., Foudin, L. L., Sun, G. Y., and Sun, A. Y.**, Effect of antioxidants on acyl group composition of phosphoglyceride from rat liver mitochondria, *Fed. Proc.,* 37, 1707, 1978.
2. **Behnke, J. A., Finch, C. E., and Moment, G. B.**, *The Biology of Aging,* Plenum Press, N. Y., 1978, 1.
3. **Bender, A. D.**, The influence of age on the activity of catecholaminos and related therapeutic agents, *J. Am. Gerontol. Soc.,* 18, 220, 1970.
4. **Berlet, H. H. and Volk, B.**, Age-related microheterogeneity of myelin basic protein isolated from human brain, in *Aging of the Brain and Dementia,* Amaducci, L., Davison, A. N., and Antuono, P., Eds., Raven Press, N. Y., 1980.

5. Boag, J. W., Overlapping effects of ultraviolet and ionizing radiations, *Br. J. Radiol.,* 41, 879, 1968.
6. Bowen, D. M., Smith, C. B., and Davison, A. N., Molecular changes in senile dementia, *Brain,* 96, 849, 1973.
7. Bowen, D. M., Smith, C. B., White, P., Goodhart, M. J., Spillane, J. A., Flack, R. H. A., and Davison, A. N., Chemical pathology of the organic dementias, *Brain,* 100, 397, 1977.
8. Brody, H., The deposition of aging pigment in the human cerebral cortex, *J. Gerontol.,* 15, 258, 1960.
9. Budowski, P., Bartov, I., Dror, Y., and Frankel, E. N., Lipid oxidation products and chick nutritional encephalopathy, *Lipids,* 14, 768, 1979.
10. Casselman, W. G. B., The *in vitro* preparation and histochemical properties of substances resembling ceroid, *J. Exp. Med.,* 94, 549, 1951.
11. Chio, K. S. and Tappel, A. L., Synthesis and characterization of the fluorescent products derived from malonaldehyde and amino acid, *Biochemistry,* 8, 2821, 1969.
12. Chio, K. S., Reiss, U., Fletcher, B., and Tappel, A. L., Peroxidation of subcellular organelles, formation of lipofuscin like fluorescent pigments, *Science,* 166, 1535, 1969.
13. Chow, C. K. and Tappel, A., An enzymatic protection mechanism against lipid peroxidation damage to lungs of ozone-exposed rats, *Lipids,* 7, 518, 1972.
14. Clapp, N. K., Interaction of ionizing radiation, nitrosamines, sulfonoxyalkanes and antioxidants as they affect carcinogenesis and survival in mice, *Am. Ind. Hyg. Assoc. J.,* 39, 448, 1978.
15. Clapp, N. K. and Satterfield, L. C., Modification of radiation lethality by previous treatment with butylated hydroxytoluene, *Rad. Res.,* 64, 388, 1975.
16. Clapp, N. K., Satterfield, L. C., and Bowles, N. D., Effect of the antioxidant butylated hydroxytoluene (BHT) on mortality in BALB/c mice, *J. Gerontol.,* 34, 497, 1979.
17. Combs, G. F., Naguchi, T., and Scott, M. L., Mechanisms of selenium and vitamin E in protection of biological membranes, *Fed. Proc.,* 34, 2090, 1975.
18. Combs, G. F., Jr. and Scott M. L., Antioxidants effects on selenium and vitamin E function in the chick, *J. Nutr.,* 104, 1297, 1974.
19. Cornwell, D. G., Huttner, J. J., Milo, G. E., Panganamala, R. V., Sharma, H. M., and Geer, J. C., Polyunsaturated fatty acids, vitamin E, and the proliferation of aortic smooth muscle cells, *Lipids,* 14, 194, 1979.
20. Csallany, A. S., Ayaz, K. L., and Su, L. C., Effect of dietary vitamin E and aging on tissue lipofuscin pigment concentration in mice, *J. Nutr.,* 107, 1792, 1977.
21. Dillard, C. J., Dumelin, E. E., and Tappel, A. L., Effect of dietary vitamin E on expiration of pentane and ethane by the rat, *Lipids,* 12, 109, 1977.
22. Dillard, C. J., Litov, R. E., and Tappel, A. L., Effect of dietary vitamin E, selenium and polyunsaturated fats on *in vivo* lipid peroxidation in the rat as measured by pentane production, *Lipids,* 13, 396, 1978.
23. Di Luzio, N. R., The role of lipid peroxidation and antioxidants in ethanol-induced lipid peroxidation, *Exp. Mol. Pathol.,* 8, 394, 1968.
24. Di Luzio, N. R., Antioxidants, lipid peroxidation, and chemical-induced liver injury, *Fed. Proc.,* 32, 1875, 1973.
25. Di Luzio, N. R. and Hartman, A. D., Role of lipid peroxidation in the pathogenesis of the ethanol-induced fatty liver, *Fed. Proc.,* 26, 1436, 1967.
26. Downey, J. E., Irving, D. H., and Tappel A. L., Effects of dietary antioxidants on *in vivo* lipid peroxidation in the rat as measured by pentane production, *Lipids,* 13, 403, 1978.
27. Dumelin, E. E. and Tappel, A. L., Hydrocarbon gases produced during *in vivo* peroxidation of polyunsaturated fatty acids and decomposition of preformed hydroperoxides, *Lipids,* 12, 894, 1977.
28. Farnsworth, C. C., Stone, W. L., and Dratz, E. A., Effects of vitamin E and selenium deficiency on the fatty acid composition of rat retinal tissues, *Biochim. Biophys. Acta,* 552, 281, 1979.
29. Ferber, E. and Resch, K., Phospholipid metabolism of stimulated lymphocytes: activation of acyl-CoA: lysolecithin acyltransferases in microsomal membranes, *Biochim. Biophys. Acta,* 296, 335, 1976.
30. Finch, C. E., Enzyme activities, gene function, and aging in mammals, *Exp. Gerontol.,* 7, 53, 1972.
31. Fong, K. L., McCay, P. B., Poyer, J. L., Keele, B. B., and Misra, H., Evidence that peroxidation of lysosomal membranes is initiated by hydroxyl free radicals produced during flavin enzyme activity, *J. Biol. Chem.,* 248, 7792, 1973.
32. Foudin, L. L., Seaman, R. N., Sun, G. Y., and Sun, A. Y., Dietary antioxidants and mitochondria functions, *Fed. Proc.,* 37, 759, 1978.
33. Gabrielsen, B. O. and Opstvedt, J., A biological assay for determination of availability of selenium for restoring blood plasma glutathione peroxidase activity in selenium depleted chicks, *J. Nutr.,* 110, 1089, 1980.
34. Greenberg, J. H. and Mellors, A., Specific inhibition of an acyltransferase by Δ^9-tetrahydrocannabinol, *Biochem. Pharmacol.,* 27, 329, 1978.

35. Grinna, L. S., Effect of dietary α-tocopherol in liver microsomes and mitochondria of aging rats, *J. Nutr.*, 106, 918, 1976.

36. Grinna, L. S. and Barber, A. A., Age-related changes in membrane lipid content and enzyme activities, *Biochim. Biophys. Acta*, 288, 347, 1972.

37. Hafeman, D. G. and Hoekstra, W. G., Lipid peroxidation *in vivo* during vitamin E and selenium deficiency in the rat as monitored by ethane evolution, *J. Nutr.*, 107, 666, 1977.

38. Harmon, D., Free radical theory of aging: effect of free radical reaction inhibitors on the mortality rate of male LAF mice, *J. Gerontol.*, 23, 476, 1968.

39. Harmon, D., Prolongation of life: role of free radical reactions in aging, *J. Am. Geriatr. Soc.*, 17, 721, 1969.

40. Harmon, D., Free radical theory of aging, *Triangle*, 12, 153, 1973.

41. Harmon, D., Free radical theory of aging: nutritional implications, *Age*, 1, 145, 1978.

42. Hatman, L. J. and Kayden, H. J., A high-performance liquid chromatographic method for the determination of tocopherol in plasma and cellular elements of the blood, *J. Lipid Res.*, 20, 639, 1979.

43. Hennacy, D. M. and Horrocks, L. A., Recent developments in the turnover of proteins and lipids in myelin and other plasma membranes in the central nervous system, *Bull. Mol. Biol. Med.*, 3, 207, 1978.

44. Henriksen, T., Effect of oxygen on radiation-induced free radicals in protein, *Radiat. Res.*, 32, 892, 1967.

45. Hochstein, P. and Ernster, L., ADP-activated lipid peroxidation coupled to the TPNH oxidase system of microsomes, *Biochem. Biophys. Res. Commun.*, 12, 388, 1963.

46. Hoekstra, W. G., Biochemical role of selenium, in *Trace Element Metabolism in Animals*, Vol. 2, Hoekstra, W. G., Suthi, J. W., Ganther, H. E., and Mutz, W., Eds., University Press, Baltimore, Md., 1972, 61.

47. Horrocks, L. A., Composition and metabolism of myelin phosphoglycerides during maturation and aging, *Prog. Brain Res.*, 40, 383, 1973.

48. Horrocks, L. A. and Sun, G. Y., Ethanolamine plasmalogens, in *Research Methods in Neurochemistry*, Vol. 1, Marks, N. and Rodnight, R., Eds., Plenum Press, N.Y., 1972, 223.

49. Horrocks, L. A., Van Rollins, M., and Yates, A. J., Lipid changes in the ageing brain, in *The Molecular Basis of Neuropathology*, Thompson, R. H. S. and Davison, A. N., Eds., Edward Arnold, London, 1980, chap. 23.

50. Horwitt, M. K., Therapeutic uses of vitamin E in medicine, *Nutr. Rev.*, 38, 105, 1980.

51. Katz, M. L., Stone, W. L., and Dratz, E. A., Fluorescent pigment accumulation in retinal pigment epithelium of antioxidant-deficient rats, *Invest. Opthalmol. Visual Sci.*, 17, 1049, 1978.

52. King, M. M., Lai, E. K., and McCay, P. B., Singlet oxygen production associated with enzyme-catalyzed lipid peroxidation in liver microsomes, *J. Biol. Chem.*, 250, 6496, 1975.

53. Lands, W. E. M., The biosynthesis and metabolism of prostaglandins, *Ann. Rev. Physiol.*, 41, 633, 1979.

54. Lands, W. E. M. and Crawford, C. G., Enzymes of membrane phospholipid metabolism in animals, in *The Enzymes of Biological Membranes*, Vol. 2, Martonosi, A., Ed., Plenum Press, N.Y., 1976, 3.

55. Leibovitz, B. E. and Siegel, B. V., Aspects of free radical reactions in biological systems: aging, *J. Gerontol.*, 35, 45, 1980.

56. Litov, R. E., Irving, D. H., Downey, J. E., and Tappel, A. L., Lipid peroxidation: a mechanism involved in acute ethanol toxicity as demonstrated by *in vivo* pentane production in the rat, *Lipids*, 13, 305, 1978.

57. Logani, M. K. and Davies, R. E., Lipid oxidation: biologic effects and antioxidants — a review, *Lipids*, 15, 485, 1980.

58. Makinodan, T., Biology of aging: retrospect and prospect, in *Immunology and Aging*, Makinodan, T. and Yunis, E., Eds., Plenum Press, N.Y., 1977, 1.

59. McCay, P. B., Gibson, D. D., Fong, K. L., and Hornbrook, K. R., Effect of glutathione peroxidase activity on lipid peroxidation in biological membrane, *Biochim. Biophys. Acta*, 431, 459, 1976.

60. McCay, P. B., Poyer, J. L., Pfeifer, P. M., May, H. E., and Gilliam, J. M., A function for α-tocopherol: stabilization of the microsomal membrane from radical attack during TPNH-dependent oxidations, *Lipids*, 6, 297, 1971.

61. McCoy, K. E. M. and Weswig, P. H., Some selenium responses in the rat not related to vitamin E, *J. Nutr.*, 98, 383, 1969.

62. Mcknight, R. C., Hunter, F. E., Jr., and Oehlert, W. H., Mitochondrial membrane ghosts produced by lipid peroxidation by ferrous ion, *J. Biol. Chem.*, 240, 3439, 1965.

63. Mead, J. F., Free radical mechanisms of lipid damage and consequences for cellular membranes, in *Free Radicals in Biology*, Pryor, W. A., Ed., Academic Press, N.Y., 1976.

64. Menzel, D. B., The role of free radicals in the toxicity of oxidizing air pollutants (nitrogen oxides and ozone), in *Free Radicals in Biology*, Vol. 2, Pryor, W. A., Ed., Academic Press, New York, 1977, 181.

65. Metcalfe, S. M., Cell culture as a test system for toxicity, *J. Pharm. Pharmacol.*, 23, 817, 1971.

66. Murty, H. S., Caasi, P. I., Brooks, S. K., and Nair, P. P., Biosynthesis of heme in the vitamin E deficient rat, *J. Biol. Chem.*, 245, 5498, 1970.

67. Nielson, H., Reaction between peroxidized phospholipid and protein. II. Molecular weight and phosphorus content of albumin after reaction with peroxidized cardiolipin, *Lipids*, 14, 900, 1979.

68. Omaye, S. T. and Tappel, A. L., Effect of dietary selenium on glutathione peroxidase in the chick, *J. Nutr.*, 104, 747, 1974.

69. Packer, L., Dreamer, D. N., and Heath, R. L., Regulation and deterioration of structure in membranes, *Adv. Gerontol. Res.*, 2, 77, 1967.

70. Parce, J. W., Cunningham, C. C., and Waite, M., Mitochondrial phospholipase A_2 activity and mitochondrial aging, *Biochemistry*, 17, 1634, 1978.

71. Pfeifer, P. M. and McCay, P. B., Reduced triphosphopyridine nucleotides oxidase alteration of membrane phospholipids. VI. Structural changes in mitochondria associated in activation of election transport activity, *J. Biol. Chem.*, 247, 6763, 1972.

72. Porta, E. A. and Hartroft, W. S., in *Wolman, Pigment in Pathology*, Academic Press, New York, 1969, 191.

73. Pryor, W. A., The role of free radical reactions in biological systems, in *Free Radicals in Biology*, Vol. 1, Pryor, W. A., Ed., Academic Press, N.Y., 1976, 1.

74. Rechnagel, R. O., Glende, E. A., Jr., and Hruszkewyca, A. M., Free radicals in biology, in *Free Radicals in Biology*, Vol. 3, Pryor, W. A., Ed., Academic Press, N.Y., 1977, 97.

75. Reiss, U. and Gershon, D., Rat liver superoxide dismutase: purification and age-related modifications, *Eur. J. Biochem.*, 63, 617, 1976.

76. Reiss, U. and Tappel, A. L., Decreased activity in protein synthesis systems from liver of vitamin E deficient rats, *Biochim. Biophys. Acta*, 12, 608, 1973.

77. Rotruck, J. T., Hoekstra, W. G., and Pope, A. L., Glucose-dependent protection by dietary selenium against haemolysis of rat erythrocytes *in vitro*, *Nat. New Biol.*, 231, 223, 1971.

78. Rotruck, J. T., Pope, A. L., Ganther, H. E., and Hoekstra, W. G., Prevention of oxidative damage to rat erythrocytes by dietary selenium, *J. Nutr.*, 102, 689, 1972.

79. Rotruck, J. T., Pope, A. L., Ganther, H. E., Swanson, A. B., Hafeman, D. G., and Hoekstra, W. G., Selenium: biochemical role as a component of glutathione peroxidase, *Science*, 179, 588, 1973.

80. Rouser, G. and Yamamoto, A., Curvilinear regression course of human brain lipid composition changes with age, *Lipids*, 3, 284, 1968.

81. Rouser, G. and Yamamoto, A., Lipids, in *Handbook of Neurochemistry*, Vol. 1, Lajtha, A., Ed., Plenum Press, N.Y., 1969, 121.

82. Rowe, L. and Wills, E. D., Effects of dietary lipids and vitamin E on lipid peroxide formation; cytochrome P-450 and oxidative demethylation in the endoplasmic reticulum, *Biochem. Pharmacol.*, 25, 175, 1976.

83. Samorajski, T., Ordy, J. M., and Keefe, J. R., The fine structure of lipofuscin age pigment in the nervous system of aged mice, *J. Cell Biol.*, 26, 779, 1965.

84. Samorajski, T., Ordy, J. M., and Rady, P., Lipofuscin pigment accumulation in the nervous system of aging mice, *Anat. Rec.*, 160, 555, 1968.

85. Samuelsson, B., Goldyne, M., Granstrom, E., Hamberg, M., Hammarstrom, S., and Malmsten, C., Prostaglandins and thromboxanes, *Ann. Rev. Biochem.*, 47, 997, 1978.

86. Scott, M. L., *Handbook of Lipid Research*, Vol. 2, De Luca, H. F., Ed., Plenum Press, New York, 1978, 133.

87. Seregi, A., Schaefer, A., and Komlos, M., Protective role of brain ascorbic acid content against lipid peroxidation, *Experientia*, 34, 1056, 1978.

88. Sharma, O. P., Peroxidation of rat brain mitochondrial lipids, *J. Neurochem.*, 28, 1377, 1977.

89. Sharma, O. P. and Krishna-Murti, C. R., Ascorbic acid — a naturally occurring mediator of lipid peroxide formation in rat brain, *J. Neurochem.*, 27, 299, 1976.

90. Shier, W. T., Inhibition of acyl Coenzyme A: lysolecithin acyltransferases by local anesthetics, detergents and inhibitors of cyclic nucleotide phosphodiesterases, *Biochem. Biophys. Res. Commun.*, 75, 186, 1977.

91. Shimasaki, H., Ueta, N., and Puvett, O. S., Isolation and analysis of age-related fluorescent substances in rat testes, *Lipids*, 15, 236, 1980.

92. Silbert, D. F., Cronan, J. E., Jr., Beacham, I. R., and Harder, M. E., Genetic engineering of membrane lipid, *Fed. Proc.*, 33, 1725, 1974.

93. Sipes, I. G., Krishna, G., and Gillette, J. R., Bioactivation of carbon tetrachloride, chloroform and bromotrichloromethane: role of cytochrome P-450, *Life Sci.*, 20, 1541, 1977.

94. Strehler, B. L., On the histochemistry and ultrastructure of age pigment, *Adv. Gerontol. Res.*, 1, 343, 1964.

95. Strehler, B. L., Mark, D. D., Milovan, A. S., and Gee, M. V., Rate and magnitude of age pigment accumulation in the human myocardium, *J. Gerontol.*, 14, 430, 1959.

96. Sulkin, N. M., The occurrence and duration of 'senile' pigments experimentally induced in the nerve cells of the young rat, *Anat. Rec.*, 130, 377, 1958.

97. Sulkin, N. M. and Srivary, P., The experimental production of senile pigments in the nerve cells of young rats, *J. Gerontol.*, 15, 2, 1960.

98. Sun, A. Y., The effect of lipoxidation on synaptosomal $(Na^+ + K^+)$-ATPase isolated from the cerebral cortex of squirrel monkey, *Biochim. Biophys. Acta*, 266, 350, 1972.

99. Sun, A. Y., Aging and in vivo NE-uptake in mammalian brain, *Exp. Aging Res.*, 2, 207, 1976.

100. Sun, A. Y. and Samorajski, T., Effects of ethanol on the activity of adenosine triphosphatase and acetylcholinesterase in synaptosomes isolated from guinea pig brain, *J. Neurochem.*, 17, 1365, 1970.

101. Sun, A. Y. and Samorajski, T., The effects of age and alcohol on $(Na^+ + K^+)$-ATPase activity of whole homogenate and synaptosomes prepared from mouse and human brain, *J. Neurochem.*, 24, 161, 1975.

102. Sun, A. Y. and Sun, G. Y., Functional roles of phospholipids of synaptosomal membrane, in *Functions and Metabolism of Phospholipids in CNS and PNS*, Porcellati, G., Amaducci, L., and Galli, C., Eds.,Plenum Press, New York, 1976, 169.

103. Sun, A. Y. and Sun, G. Y., Effects of dietary vitamin E and other antioxidants on aging process in rat brain, *Adv. Exp. Med. Biol.*, 97, 285, 1978.

104. Sun, A. Y. and Sun, G. Y., Neurochemical aspects of the membrane hypothesis of aging, *Interdiscipl. Top. Gerontol.*, 15, 34, 1979.

105. Sun, A. Y., Badger, C. R., Jr., and Foudin, L. L., Vulnerability of brain membranes to lipid peroxidation, *Trans. Am. Soc. Neurochem.*, 9, 165, 1978.

106. Sun, A. Y., Ordy, J. M. and Samorajski, T., Effect of alcohol on aging in the nervous system, *Adv. Behav. Biol.*, 16, 505, 1975.

107. Sun, A. Y., Sun, G. Y., and Middleton, C. C., Alcohol-membrane interaction in the brain. Effect of chronic ethanol administration, *Curr. Alcoholism*, 1, 81, 1977.

108. Sun. G. Y., The metabolism of palmitic acid in mouse brain: an age study, *Neurobiology*, 1, 232, 1971.

109. Sun, G. Y., The turnover of phosphoglycerides in the subcellular fractions of mouse brain. A study using $[^{14}C]$-oleic acid as precursor, *J. Neurochem.*, 21, 1083, 1973.

110. Sun, G. Y., On the membrane phospholipids and their acyl group profiles of adrenal gland, *Lipids*, 14, 918, 1979.

111. Sun, G. Y. and Horrocks , L. A., The fatty acid and aldehyde composition of the major phospholipids of mouse brain, *Lipids*, 3, 91, 1968.

112. Sun, G. Y. and Horrocks, L. A., The acyl and alk-1-enyl groups of the major phosphoglycerides from ox brain myelin and mouse brain microsomal, mitochondrial and myelin fraction, *Lipids*, 5, 1006, 1970.

113. Sun, G. Y. and Horrocks, L. S., The metabolism of palmitic acid in the subcellular fractions of mouse brain, *J. Lipid Res.*, 14, 206, 1973.

114. Sun, G. Y. and Leung, B. S., Phospholipids and acyl groups of subcellular membrane fractions from human intracranial tumors, *J. Lipid Res.*, 15, 423, 1974.

115. Sun, G. Y. and Samorajski, T., Age change in the lipid composition of whole homogenates and isolated myelin fractions of mouse brain, *J. Neurochem.*, 12, 629, 1972.

116. Sun, G. Y. and Samorajski, T., Age differences in the acyl group composition of phosphoglycerides in myelin isolated from the brain of the rhesus monkey, *Biochim. Biophys. Acta*, 316, 19, 1973.

117. Sun, G. Y., Creech, D. M., Corbin, D. R., and Sun, A. Y., The effect of chronic ethanol administration on arachidonoyl transfer to 1-acyl-glycerophosphorylcholine in rat brain synaptosomal fraction, *Res. Comm. Chem. Path. Pharm.*, 16, 753, 1977.

118. Sun, G. Y., Hallett, D., and Ho, I. K., Effect of morphine on hepatic lipid metabolism, *Biochem. Pharmacol.*, 27, 1779, 1978.

119. Sun, G. Y. and Su, K. L., Metabolism of arachidonoyl phosphoglycerides in mouse brain subcellular fractions, *J. Neurochem.*, 32, 1053, 1979.

120. Sun, G. Y., Su, K. L., Der, O. M., and Tang, W., Enzymic regulation of arachidonate metabolism in brain membrane phosphoglycerides, *Lipids*, 14, 229, 1979.

121. Sun, G. Y. and Sun, A. Y., Phospholipids and acyl groups of synaptosomal and myelin membranes isolated from the cerebral cortex of squirrel monkey *(Saimiri sciureus)*, *Biochim. Biophys. Acta*, 280, 306, 1972.

122. Sun, G. Y. and Sun, A. Y., Synaptosomal plasma membranes: acyl group composition of phosphoglycerides and Na^+K^+-ATPase activity during fatty acid deficient, *J. Neurochem.*, 22, 15, 1974.

123. Sung, S. C., Sanberg, P. R., and McGeer, E. G., Cholinergic systems in muscle and brain in vitamin E-deficient rats, *Neurochem. Res.*, 3, 815, 1978.

124. Svingen, B. A., Buege, J. A., O'Neal, F. O., and Aust, S. D., The mechanism of NADPH-dependent lipid peroxidation, *J. Biol. Chem.*, 254, 5892, 1979.

125. Takeuchi, N., Matsumiya, K., Takahashi, Y., Higashino, K., Tanaka, F., and Katayama, Y., Thiobarbituric acid reactive substances and lipid metabolism in alpha-tocopherol deficient rats, *Exp. Gerontol.*, 12, 67, 1977.

126. Tappel, A. L., Lipid peroxidation damage to cell components, *Fed. Proc.*, 32, 1870, 1973.

127. Tappel, A. L., *Pathological Aspects of Cell Membranes*, Vol. 1, Trumps, B. F. and Artila, A., Eds., Academic Press, New York, 1975, 145.

128. Tappel, A. L., Protection against free radical lipid peroxidation reactions, *Adv. Exp. Med. Biol.*, 97, 111, 1978.

129. Tappel, A. L., Fletcher, B., and Deamer, D., Effect of antioxidants and nutrients on lipid peroxidation fluorescent products and aging parameters in the mouse, *J. Gerontol.*, 28, 415, 1973.

130. Taylor, S. L., Lamden, M. P., and Tappel, A. L., Sensitive fluorometric method for tissue tocopherol analysis, *Lipids*, 11, 530, 1976.

131. Thomson, C. D., Rea, H., Robinson, M. F., and Chapman, O. W., Low blood selenium concentrations and glutathione peroxidase activities in elderly people, *Proc. Univ. Otago Med. Sch.*, 35, 18, 1977.

132. Thompson, J. N. and Scott, M. L., Role of selenium in the nutritions of the chick, *J. Nutr.*, 97, 335, 1969.

133. Thompson, J. N., and Scott, M. L., Impaired lipid and vitamin E absorption related to atrophy of the pancreas in selenium deficient chick, *J. Nutr.*, 100, 797, 1970.

134. Toews, A. D., Horrocks, L. A., and King, J. S., Simultaneous isolation of purified microsomal and myelin fractions from rat spinal cord, *J. Neurochem.*, 27, 25, 1976.

135. Toth, S. E., The origin of lipofuscin age pigment, *Exp. Gerontol.*, 3, 19, 1968.

136. Triggle, D. J., Functional role for phospholipids, *J. Theor. Biol.*, 25, 499, 1970.

137. Vahouny, G. V., Hodges, V. A., and Treadwell, C. R., Essential fatty acid deficiency and adrenal cortical function in vitro, *J. Lipid Res.*, 20, 154, 1979.

138. Van Deenen, L. L. M. and de Gier, J., *The Red Blood Cell*, Bishop, Ch. and Surgenov, D. M., Eds., Academic Press, New York, 1964, chap. 7.

139. Weltzien, H. U., Cytolytic and membrane-perturbing properties of lysophosphatidylcholine, *Biochim. Biophys. Acta*, 559, 259, 1979.

140. Wilson, P. D., Enzyme changes in aging mammals, *Gerontology*, 19, 79, 1973.

141. Wilson, R. B., Middleton, C. C., and Sun, G. Y., Vitamin E, antioxidants, and lipid peroxidation in experimental atherosclerosis of rabbits, *J. Nutr.*, 108, 1858, 1978.

142. Wisniewski, H. M. and Terry R. D., Morphology of the aging brain, human and animal, *Prog. Brain Res.*, 40, 167, 1973.

143. Wolman, M. and Zaidel, L., Hyperoxia and formation of chromolipid pigments, *Experientia*, 18, 323, 1962.

144. Yeh, Y. Y. and Johnson, R. M., Vitamin E deficiency in the rats: alteration in mitochondrial membranes and its relation to respiratory decline, *Arch. Biochem. Biophys.*, 159, 821, 1973.

145. Young, V. R., Nutrition and aging, *Adv. Exp. Med. Biol.*, 97, 85, 1978.

Chapter 8

EFFECTS OF AGING UPON INTESTINAL ABSORPTION

Peter R. Holt

TABLE OF CONTENTS

I. INTRODUCTION

The gastrointestinal tract as an absorptive organ is known to have considerable functional reserve. Since the loss of baseline organ function is relatively modest with advancing age, one would anticipate that overall absorptive functions would generally be well maintained in the elderly. Furthermore, the clinical consequences of mild impairment of absorption are quite covert and, in addition, commonly used laboratory tests are not sensitive indicators of intestinal malabsorption. It is not surprising therefore that little attention has been given to intestinal disorders with advancing age. Two approaches that can be used to gain an initial appraisal of the magnitude of the problem of intestinal malabsorption in an aging population are (1) to perform a clinical evaluation of small intestinal function in an unselected group of well, elderly subjects and (2) to determine whether there is evidence of progressive nutritional impairment with advancing age.

A. Clinical Studies

Each of the last four decades has spawned a group of clinical studies on the aging human gut. All the authors of these studies have expected to detect clinical disorders in their older subjects and each has had difficulties in finding major problems. Meyer, Necheles, and co-workers first described impaired secretion of accessory gastrointestinal organs with advanced age[1,2] — they subsequently suggested that sugar (galactose) absorption might be reduced in their older subjects.[3] Kirsner's group was satisfied that advanced age did not create major clinical problems related to malabsorption.[4] On the other hand, Pelz and co-workers carefully studied 50 subjects, of which 9 had shown severe weight loss and a progressive wasting syndrome culminating in death and found increased stool fat (as a percent of stool dry weight), reduced urine xylose excretion after a standard oral load and hypoalbuminemia in their elderly subjects.[5] More recently, Montgomery, et al.[6] studied 50 elderly people consisting of 33 subjects with "anemia" and 17 "healthy controls". They found malabsorption in 13 of the 33 anemic subjects, of which two had a partial gastrectomy, one pancreatic calcification, and three jejunal diverticulosis. Two of their "healthy" controls showed malabsorption. Their conclusions were that covert malabsorption could occur in an apparently healthy older group. A review of the problem of malabsorption in older patients by a research group headed by Dawson suggested that subtle pancreatic insufficiency might occur more commonly than generally anticipated in the elderly.[7] In summary, these and other clinical studies have not provided satisfactory answers to the question of whether uniform deterioration of gastrointestinal function occurs or whether particular clinical disorders develop commonly with advancing age.

B. Is There Evidence of Progressive Caloric Malnutrition with Advancing Age?

In order to answer the question — is undernutrition common in the elderly? — one needs to have an estimate of the caloric intake and energy expenditure of older subjects. As man ages, a reduction in caloric intake of most nutrients occurs which some have calculated to be on the order of 35 to 40%.[8] This reduced intake appears to be due to a decrease in basal metabolic rate and the marked reduction in physical activity that occurs in later years. Food intake may be further reduced in the elderly by disinterest in cooking, impaired taste sensitivity, dental status, and the unavailability of reasonable foods. Recommended dietary allowances are usually met in high economic groups and rarely are any deficiencies manifested as chemical or physiologic changes. However, as income decreases to or below poverty level, nutritional deficiencies become more frequent and more severe, particularly in the free living elderly population and in single-person households.

Another approach to estimate the incidence of progressive malnutrition might be to determine changes in body weight. For example, does the frequency of obesity decrease with advancing age? Published studies suggest that obesity decreases after the age of 50.[9] Such changes in the incidence of obesity might occur because very obese subjects die earlier than age matched normal weight subjects or because the obese become progressively thinner with advancing age. Body composition studies have shown that the percent of total weight present as fat tissue even in normal weight subjects increases with advancing age, at least in the economically favored Westerners.[10] If obesity is defined as excessive fat, then although subjects might lose total body weight as they grow older, they may still be obese. An excellent summary of these data is available.[11] Although considerable attention has recently been given to defining nutritional disorders in the elderly, it is presently unclear whether there are slowly progressive changes in body tissues and body weight that might reflect subtly impaired digestive function. Such data from longitudinal studies are badly needed.

II. ABSORPTION OF MACRONUTRIENTS

A. Fat

Dietary fat comprises 45% of the caloric density of the American diet and the digestion and absorption of fat is complex. Therefore, one would anticipate that malabsorption of lipids might be relatively pronounced if gastrointestinal function fails with advancing age and also that the nutritional impact of fat malabsorption would be severe.

In early experimental work measuring blood chylomicron curves following a standard meal, higher and delayed chylomicron counts were demonstrated in aged subjects when compared to younger controls.[12] The changes were ameliorated by administration of pancreatic lipase or Tween® concomitant with the meal. These findings were confirmed in a subsequent study[13] but the indirect methods used were unsatisfactory to permit firm conclusions. The same objections apply to the study of Citi and Salvini[14] who found decreased absorption of ^{131}I triolein compared to ^{131}I oleic acid in older test subjects. Webster et al.[15] also used nephelometry to study postprandial plasma chylomicron appearance, but by better controlled methods, and again suggested that modest fat malabsorption might occur late in life. The methods used in all of these studies were indirect and were dependent in part upon the vagaries of gastric emptying,[16] but they all suggest the presence of digestive defects due to pancreatic disease.

Clinical observations of fat malabsorption emphasize that people develop the same diseases in old age as when younger,[17] though they indicate the frequency of multiple jejunal diverticulosis[6] and pancreatic insufficiency.[7,18] To summarize, direct testing methods have not been used to determine the frequency of fat malabsorption in aging. Such baseline studies are needed, as are carefully conducted investigations on the importance of altered pancreatic lipolysis and intraluminal bacterial overgrowth syndromes — both readily treatable conditions — in causing lipid malabsorption.

In general, the concentration of serum cholesterol is said to increase with advancing age[13] although most studies suggest that serum concentrations level off after age 60.[19] Hollander and Morgan have studied cholesterol absorption in old and young rats and suggested that cholesterol absorption increases with advancing age.[20] Their data were calculated on the basis of small intestinal length. As discussed below, the best method of comparing intestinal absorption rates in aged and younger animals is unclear. For this reason, the interesting observations of Hollander and Morgan must await further research.

B. Protein

The same problem that has beset other absorptive studies in elderly subjects — contradictory results for no obvious reason — is found when one reviews nitrogen balance data in the aged. Older subjects were found to be in positive nitrogen balance,[21] to require increased protein intake compared to young adults to maintain nitrogen balance,[22,23] or to be no different from a younger population.[24,25] Blood isotope determinations and urine collections following ingestion of ^{131}I labeled albumin solubilized in glucose water indicated no difference in digestion and absorption between older and younger subjects.[26] In old rats, enhanced methionine,[27] lysine, and cysteine[28] absorption has been described. Although the authors of these studies suggest that enhanced absorption must reflect tissue needs in the aged animals, the conclusions of these rat studies are uncertain since gut weight is so different in younger and older animals.

It is clear that research studies exploring the effect of the aging process upon human protein digestion and absorption have been negligible. An important reason is the absence of acceptable techniques that can be employed readily in older volunteer subjects. One approach to the study of intestinal protein digestion in the elderly is the utilization of newer synthetic peptides with prosthetic groups that are hydrolyzed by pancreatic proteolytic enzymes, are quantitatively excreted in urine and are readily measured.[29]

C. Carbohydrate

Approximately 65% of dietary carbohydrate consists of polysaccharides that require digestion to monosaccharides prior to intestinal absorption. Salivary and pancreatic amylase hydrolyze the endo-α-1,4 glucosyl units of polysaccharides so rapidly that digestive defects due to enzyme depletion rarely occur. On the other hand, the final hydrolysis of tri- and disaccharides depends upon enzymes present on the surface of the small intestinal mucosa, therefore the concentration of these enzymes reflects the integrity of the intestine. There is no evidence that intestinal lactase concentrations fall with advancing age,[30] but studies of carbohydrate digestive capacity in older subjects have not been performed.

Oral glucose tolerance tests are different in the elderly possibly due to altered intestinal glucose absorption. However, intravenous glucose tolerance tests also change with age,[31] so that defects in glucose metabolism and delayed gastric emptying might be responsible for altered oral tolerance tests. Human intestinal glucose absorption can only be measured directly by the use of complex intraduodenal perfusion techniques. Investigators have been reluctant to apply such techniques in older subjects. As a result, studies of the effect of age upon glucose absorption have been performed in experimental animals. The majority of this research in animals implies that glucose absorption falls with advancing age when calculated on the basis of total body surface area of the test animal.[32,33] Contradictory data were presented by Klimas,[34] who found no change in glucose absorption from rat intestinal loops after the age of 12 months. In another study, following incubation of aged male mouse intestinal slices with 6-deoxy-D-glucose, increased accumulation was found in older animals.[35] These data were interpreted as indicating greater carbohydrate absorption with age.

An alternative mechanism for altering normal intestinal absorption of monosaccharides might involve a change in enzymes concerned with intestinal mucosal sugar metabolism. One preliminary study described a fall in V_{max} and no change in K_m of 34-month-old mouse mucosal phosphomonoesterases compared to enzyme activities in 11-month-old animals.[36] Glycolytic enzyme activities in liver and gut need to adapt rapidly to changes in substrates.[37] One-year-old rats demonstrated a blunted adaptive response of hepatic glycolytic enzymes to feeding of test carbohydrates.[38] Parallel studies in the small bowel were inconclusive.[39] Since a loss of rapid adaptation is one of the characteristic defects of the aging process, further studies of intestinal adaptation to carbohydrates and other substrates are needed.

Because of the difficulty in the measurement of human glucose absorption, many investigators have substituted xylose, a pentose which is not metabolized significantly in the body and which is rapidly excreted in the urine. The consensus of extensive work indicates that xylose absorption decreases gradually with advancing age[40] when renal excretion of xylose is normalized by the use of both intravenous and oral xylose tolerance tests.[41,42]

In this laboratory, we have used a different approach to the measurement of intestinal absorption of carbohydrates. The excretion of excess hydrogen in expired air following a carbohydrate-containing meal reflects the passage of unabsorbed carbohydrate substrate into the colon.[43] Using this technique of breath hydrogen analysis, we have studied the capacity of aging subjects to absorb carbohydrates following standardized meals containing 25 to 200 g carbohydrate. The data indicate that one third of active, clinically well individuals over the age of 65 malabsorbed a portion of a 100-g carbohydrate meal.[44] Furthermore, mean carbohydrate absorptive capacity fell progressively from age 65 to 85 plus. In our preliminary study, such subtle absorptive defects were not associated with gastrointestinal symptoms or with anthropometric indices of malnutrition.

III. ABSORPTION OF MICRONUTRIENTS

Whether deficiencies or diseases occur in the elderly as a result of altered gastrointestinal handling of the micronutrients, the vitamins, or minerals is unclear. Such uncertainty exists despite extensive reviews concerned with the vitamin needs of the elderly.[45] Some of the reasons for the lack of clarity about this important topic are outlined below.

A. Problems with Measurement of Body Content of Micronutrients

The preclinical stage of vitamin depletion is marked by a progressive reduction in body vitamin stores.[46] Most investigators seeking evidence of vitamin depletion with age have measured the plasma or serum concentration of the vitamin under study. Blood concentrations usually reflect only the most recent dietary intake and may be maintained while organ stores are greatly diminished. The plasma concentrations of lipophilic vitamins or their active metabolites are controlled in some cases by the plasma content of specific binding proteins. In order to determine that age per se has a specific influence upon changes in blood concentration of vitamins, data from well individuals of each sex and at different ages should be calculated using statistical methods of linear regression. When this was done with serum carotene, alpha and beta carotene, vitamin A, thiamine, total blood ascorbic acid, and alpha tocopherol, only the results for blood ascorbic acid showed a statistically significant age-associated difference.[47-49]

The tissues most commonly used for an estimate of cellular vitamin concentration are red cells or white cells. In general, the use of blood cell components gives a better index of body micronutrient stores than measurement of plasma concentrations. However, an example of the problem of using red cells to measure body stores is seen with red cell folate concentrations which are determined at the reticulocyte stage and thus do not reflect current folacin stores. Hair and nails have been used extensively to determine the tissue concentration of several minerals. This is a very sensitive analytic technique if care is taken to exclude contamination with chemical applicants.

B. Accurate Measurement of Dietary Intake

Accurate measurement of the dietary intake for many vitamins is still not possible since methods for determining food vitamin content are very imperfect. In addition, foods may contain different chemical forms of a vitamin, e.g., folate polyglutamates, and furthermore, the destructive effects of cooking are poorly quantitated. On the other hand, an accurate index of intake is needed if the balance technique is to be used to evaluate the presence of intestinal malabsorption.

C. Urinary Excretion of Vitamins as Index of Absorption

The urinary excretion of vitamins can be used as an index of vitamin body stores if one assumes that fecal losses are constant. The sensitivity of the urinary excretion technique to quantitate body stores can be greatly enhanced if urinary excretion is measured during administration of gradually increasing doses of the vitamin. This technique uses the assumption that, as body stores are saturated, excess vitamins will be excreted and detectable in the urine. Such experimental approaches cannot be used to study lipophilic vitamins which are sequestered in fat stores when excess amounts are administered. These relatively simple techniques have not been widely used for the study of vitamin stores in the elderly.

D. Micronutrient Absorption

The most accurate measure of the rate of intestinal absorption is the balance technique. In general, this techinque has not been used for the study of changes in micronutrient absorption because analytic methods were cumbersome or unavailable. Furthermore, absorption rate is dependent upon the dose and upon the form in which the vitamin is administered, e.g., in a pure crystalline form or incorporated into food, and on whether the vitamin is administered fasting or together with a meal. In general, if the intestinal absorption of passively or actively transported substances is found to be depressed with advancing age, one expects that this holds also for the water-soluble vitamins. If dietary fat absorption is impaired in the elderly, then the absorption of fat-soluble vitamins also would be affected.

E. Methods of Measuring Human Micronutrient Status

Human micronutrient status can be determined also by measuring the consequences of physiologic depletion or the effects of dietary supplementation upon function. As an example of the former, serum transketolase activity has been used to assess thiamin stores and glutamic oxaloacetic acid transaminase for pyridoxal activity. Few other functional studies in the elderly have been published. Although pharmacological vitamin and mineral supplementation has been employed for many years in order to evaluate body vitamin needs with aging, most studies have not been double-blind and have used subjective and not objective criteria.

F. Specific Vitamin Problems in the Aged

1. Vitamin A

Some surveys of serum vitamin A concentration demonstrate a small number of elderly subjects with levels below the lower limit of normal.[50] Other surveys show no effect of age upon vitamin A levels.[51] No significant age trends were found for fasting serum vitamin A or carotene levels in the studies of Yiengst and Shock.[52] The response curve of serum vitamin A to an oral dose of 100,000 units of vitamin A demonstrated no significant difference in the peak concentrations attained but a definite delay in the timing of the peak and the decay. Since vitamin A concentration curves following a pharmacological dose probably reflect lipoprotein concentrations in addition to quantitating the mass absorbed, it is possible that the changes found by Yiengst and Shock may indicate a distinctly altered absorption pattern. In the rat, vitamin A absorption was stated to gradually increase with advancing age when determined on the basis of intestinal length.[53] Visual sensitivity, revealed by measuring light threshold, falls with advancing age, but improvement could not be detected in a group of elderly subjects treated with large doses of vitamin A for several months.[54]

2. Thiamin

Based upon determination of serum concentrations, the presence of thiamin depletion in older subjects has been reported.[55] Rafsky and Newman, measuring urinary thiamin excretion, found that a larger oral dose was needed in elderly subjects to produce a constant urinary output than in a younger control group.[56] Although this study suggested that thiamin malabsorption might occur in the aged, Thomson found no evidence of malabsorption after oral doses of ^{35}S labeled thiamin in studies in 24 elderly individuals.[57]

3. Riboflavin and Niacin

Riboflavin and niacin depletion appear to be uncommon with advancing age[58,59] and no age-dependent studies of their absorption were found. On the other hand, there is evidence for age-wise differences in tissue pyridoxine content as judged by determination of the activity of pyridoxal-dependent serum glutamic oxoloacetic acid transaminase.[60,61] It is possible that older people have a larger dietary requirement for pyridoxine than the young.[62]

The consensus from many clinical studies is that if malabsorption of vitamin B_{12} occurs during the process of aging, then it is of minor degree and importance. The evidence for this view is discussed below in Section IV, as are the data on folacin depletion and malabsorption.

4. Vitamin C

It has been suggested that ascorbic acid deficiency makes an important contribution to ill-health in elderly people.[63] A careful analysis of leukocyte vitamin C levels suggested that dietary fruit intake and smoking were of greater import than the age of the test subjects.[64] One recent study demonstrated that supplemental vitamin C (1 g/day) given to a group of hospitalized elderly with low plasma and leukocyte ascorbic acid concentrations resulted in a small but significant rise in weight and in some improvement in the sense of well being.[65] These and other data do not clarify whether intestinal vitamin C malabsorption may occur with advancing age.

5. Vitamin D

The evidence for altered intestinal calcium absorption as a mechanism for the osteopenia of advancing age is described below (Section V). Experimental studies of the results of vitamin D supplementation imply that increased oral doses of this vitamin may be needed in older well subjects to maintain homeostasis.[66] Plasma 25-hydroxy-cholecalciferol concentrations in geriatric patients were only marginally greater on 2000 IU of vitamin D daily than on 500 IU.[67] Our own intestinal perfusion studies in the rat demonstrated impaired intestinal absorption of vitamin D_3.[68] In an excellent study of ^{3}H cholecalciferol absorption administered with and without a high fat meal vehicle, Barragry, et al.[69] showed, in elderly well females, significantly lower plasma levels of unchanged ^{3}H cholecalciferol and its metabolites, indicating impaired absorption of this vitamin.

6. Other Micronutrients

Little data on vitamin E and vitamin K depletion were found in the literature. It is likely that the absorption of their lipophilic vitamins would parallel that of other lipids.

The human nutritional requirements of trace metals or microminerals has only recently been determined for adults and for young children.[70] Deficiencies usually occur only in patients being treated with total parenteral nutrition.[71] No special requirements have been reported for the elderly. One survey found a low percentage of subjects with reduced plasma concentrations of zinc, copper, and magnesium.[72] Special attention has been given to possible zinc depletion in the elderly because of the relationship between this trace metal and taste acuity. An extensive recent study found little evidence for tissue depletion of either zinc or copper.[73] In addition, in one double-blind study, dietary zinc supplementation did not result in a significant improvement in taste acuity in a group of elderly subjects in a nursing home setting.[74]

IV. ABSORPTION OF HEMATINICS

Anemia, defined as reduced hemoglobin or hematocrit compared to a younger population, occurs quite commonly in the elderly. The usual explanation for such anemia is a reduction of the intake or impaired absorption of hematinics.

A. Iron

A decrease in *iron* absorption has been reported in old age,[75,76] but the selection of control subjects was not adequate. On the other hand, an *increase* in bone marrow iron stores has been found with advancing age[77] and serum ferritin levels rise,[78] findings which do not correlate with potential iron malabsorption. Marx[79] conducted a comprehensive study of iron absorption in 40 active aged and 25 young healthy controls plus a group of iron deficient patients of all ages. This investigator used a double-isotope technique to separately measure mucosal uptake, mucosal transfer and long-term body retention of iron. Young male subjects in this study had 25% greater mucosal uptake of iron than males over age 60 but the difference was not statistically significant and there was no difference with age in females. Total iron transfer into the body was unimpaired, suggesting that overall iron absorption in the elderly was adequate. An important aspect of this study was the demonstration that iron absorption in six aged patients with iron deficiency was similar to that in younger iron-deficient subjects, suggesting that the absorptive response to iron depletion was not impaired in the older subjects. The amount of radiolabeled iron incorporated into red cells was also investigated in this excellent study and this was found to decrease with age. Thus the data of Marx's study imply that any defect in the handling of iron in the elderly was due to ineffective erythroporesis. Studies of human iron absorption are usually performed using labeled inorganic iron as the test substrate. Therefore, such experiments do not exclude the possibility that food iron malabsorption might occur but they make it most unlikely. The demonstration that many older subjects have increased total body iron stores[80] discounts iron malabsorption as a major cause of anemia in the elderly.

B. Serum Vitamin B_{12}

Serum vitamin B_{12} levels may decrease with advancing age.[81,82] Reduced serum vitamin B_{12} concentrations are usually ascribed to reduced dietary content or to vitamin B_{12} malabsorption. One mechanism for malabsorption of vitamin B_{12} would involve reduced secretion of intrinsic factor which would accompany the frequent findings of atrophic gastritis in the aged.[83] Alternatively, the active absorption of this vitamin, mediated by specific receptors in the distal small intestine, could be reduced. Although vitamin B_{12} malabsorption was suggested in early experimental studies[84,85] of older subjects, the data of Hyams,[86] indicate that the intestinal uptake of a test dose of ^{58}CO labeled vitamin was not different from that in young controls. The data in this excellent study were based upon the fecal excretion of vitamin B_{12} following an oral bolus of radiolabeled B_{12} and does not exclude subtly reduced absorption rate nor malabsorption of protein-bound vitamin B_{12}.[87] One experimental approach to the detection of milder degrees of vitamin B_{12} malabsorption would be to measure the decrease in total body B_{12} label after an initial ^{57}CO vitamin B_{12} dose.[88] Such a study has not been performed in the elderly.

C. Folacin

Folacin concentrations in the serum and red cells are low in elderly subjects as compared to younger controls[89] in some studies but not in others.[90] These changes have been invoked to imply that there is a significant total body depletion of folacin in the aged.[91] An alternative possibility — that one reason for reduced serum folacin levels might be a reduction in the number of serum or tissue folacin binding sites — is presently under study in this laboratory. Folate malabsorption could occur:

1. because gastric acid secretion falls with advancing age, causing a higher pH in upper intestinal contents in older than younger subjects and resulting in impairment of intestinal folate absorption;[92]
2. because of impaired secretion of intestinal folate conjugase — an enzyme necessary to hydrolyze food folate polyglutamates;[93] or
3. reduced active intestinal absorption of folic acid.[94]

One study suggested that conjugated folacin absorption was reduced in elderly subjects more than the absorption of folic acid[95] but the methods used in this interesting work were imperfect. Because the incidence of low serum folate levels is so common in elderly subjects and folacin has a crucial role in many metabolic processes in addition to its action as a hematinic, further studies appear to be mandatory.

V. ABSORPTION OF MACROMINERALS

A. Calcium

A well recognized and well described loss of body function with advancing age is the reduction of bone calcium. The histologic changes characteristic of both osteoporosis and of osteomalacia have been found in older subjects in the absence of overt diseases that disturb calcium homeostasis.[96] Other studies have suggested that the development of osteoporosis does not relate to a change in calcium intake with age. Therefore, changes in intestinal calcium absorption and in vitamin D metabolism have been the focus of attention.

Young growing animals absorb more calcium than mature rats[97,98] and intestinal calcium absorption is enhanced by a low calcium diet.[99] In humans, a bolus of isotopic calcium is absorbed less well in older than younger people[100,101] and balance techniques demonstrate calcium conservation following reduced calcium intake.[102] In a study of bidirectional calcium flux into an intestinal perfusate by Ireland and Fordtran[103] calcium absorption was found to be lower in subjects over age 60 compared to a young control group and, importantly, the calcium conservation response to a 4- to 8-week period on a low calcium diet was severely blunted. Such a poor response to dietary calcium has also been found in in vitro studies in the rat.[104] Intestinal malabsorption of vitamin D or cholecalciferol may be important.[69] Some investigators have suggested that renal 1,25 hydroxylase activity falls in older subjects.[105] However, overall recent studies do not suggest that 1,25-hydroxycholecalciferol or parathormone formation is significantly blunted in the elderly. Therefore, the present experimental data support the possibility of impaired intestinal responsiveness to either 1,25-hydroxycholecalciferol or to parathormone with advancing age. If this hypothesis is proven to be correct, and poor intestinal response to hormones is found to parallel bone calcium losses, then there will be a place for therapeutic supplementation with calciferol metabolites or hormone substitutes in the aged.

B. Phosphorus

There are no known effective physiologic mechanisms regulating human intestinal phosphate absorption. Control of body phosphate needs generally is achieved by changes in dietary intake and renal excretion.[106] Similar to calcium, there is probably a flux of phosphate secreted into the intestinal lumen as well as absorption by the mucosa from the lumen. No information on changes in phosphate metabolism with aging was found in a review of the literature.

C. Magnesium

There is little data on magnesium needs of the elderly. However, during experimental magnesium depletion, the exchangeable stores of magnesium available to older rats is very much smaller than to young rats.[107]

In a review of the literature, no satisfactory studies were found concerned with the importance of gastrointestinal function in the maintenance of magnesium stores in the elderly.

VI. ALTERED PHYSIOLOGIC PROCESSES THAT MAY UNDERLIE ABSORPTIVE DISORDERS IN THE ELDERLY

In order to clarify potentially important effects of advancing age upon the function of the gastrointestinal tract, it will be necessary to answer some basic questions related to normal gastrointestinal physiology.

A. Is There a Reduction in Intestinal Absorbing Surface with Advancing Age?

The rate of transfer of passively absorbed substrates is dependent upon the mucosal surface dimensions functionally exposed to luminal contents. This functional surface consists of the area of the microvillus membrane absorbing surface, the proportion of the length of the villus that is exposed to the substrate from bulk luminal contents, and the characteristics of the barrier to diffusion created by the unstirred water layer.

Several pieces of evidence suggest that the villus absorbing surface is reduced with advancing age. In the rat and the mouse, age-related changes in structure examined under the light microscope[108] and in ultrastructure[109] have been described. These observed changes would be expected to reduce the villus absorbing surface in older animals. Jejunal villus height was decreased but villus width and mucosal cell height were unchanged in a biopsy study of 16 aged subjects.[110] The nutritional status of the subjects of this study was undefined, casting doubt on the importance of the observations as age related. In another study, preliminary observations indicate a progressive reduction in mucosal surface area, as calculated by Chalkley's template method, in intestinal biopsies, between age 10 and 75.[111] No studies were found which attempted to quantitate the amount of the intestinal villus exposed to bulk luminal content in younger and older animals. One experimental study demonstrated a reduced barrier to diffusion of glucose in 12-month-old rabbits when compared to neonatal animals.[112]

If the transfer of any substrate from the bulk phase of intestinal contents to and through the intestinal mucosal membrane is reduced during the process of aging, then this would be a major cause for impaired intestinal substrate absorption. It is clear that critical studies that measure the diffusion kinetics and uptake rates of passively transported substrates are crucially needed.

Because of uncertainty about the best method of measuring the intestinal absorbing surface, it has been difficult to interpret many of the results of studies that attempt to compare intestinal absorption rates in younger and older animals. In contrast to man, the weight and protein content of the whole intestine and of the mucosa in experimental animals increases into old age. Intestinal absorption rates in animals generally have been related either to mucosal or intestinal wet weight or protein content or to total body weight or surface area. One recent study has related the absorption rate of cholesterol to gut length.[20] It is clear that the interpretation of rates of absorption is dependent upon the denominator used for the calculation. Our own unpublished studies in the Sprague-Dawley rat indicate that between 5 and 22 months, body weight increases by about 70%, intestinal length by 20%, and intestinal or mucosal weight by over 100%. If the total absorption rate of a substrate were found to be 20% higher in a 22-month- than a 5-month-old animal, such a transport rate would be relatively depressed in the older rat on the basis of intestinal or body growth rates. It is clear that research studies in experimental animals must consider these differences in depth before concluding that aging has an effect upon intestinal absorption rate.

B. Is There a Generalized Impairment of Responsiveness of End Organs to Hormonal Stimulation Related to the Gastrointestinal Tract?

Many of the functions of the gastrointestinal tract are mediated through the action of gastrointestinal hormones. The interaction between these hormones and the effect on end organs which results in a physiologic response involves a series of individual steps. Any of these steps may be altered with advancing age and thereby might result in an impaired response including

1. a reduction in the number of hormone synthesizing cells;
2. a reduction in the synthesis rate of the hormone;
3. a reduction in the release of the hormone from the synthesis site resulting in a suboptimal hormone response to a standard stimulus;
4. an inadequate end organ response to the hormone due to a reduction in the number of hormone-sensitive receptors;
5. impaired synthesis or release of the physiologic products of the hormone action in the end organ.

Surprisingly, essentially no data were found in the literature concerning hormonal stimuli in the aging gastrointestinal tract. There is accumulating general evidence of changes in tissue responsiveness to hormones with aging.[113] However, the results are not sufficiently consistent to permit a unifying hypothesis of changes with age. For example, an important human study of the secretion of corticotropin and somatotropin by the adenohypophysis in senescent man concludes that its functional status was not impaired in old age.[114]

Even the fall in the gastric acid secretion rate which occurs during aging has not been adequately studied. It certainly would be feasible to investigate whether gastric secretion in older individuals is reduced because of the destruction of parietal cells that occurs with atrophic gastritis, a common condition in the elderly, is due to a reduction in gastrin-producing cells in the antrum, or to impaired release of gastrin from these cells, or due to poor gastric parietal cell responsiveness to a gastrin stimulus. More directly related to the problem of intestinal absorption, the availability of newer radioimmunoassay procedures for the measurement of gastrointestinal hormones should permit evaluation of the responsiveness of hormone-secreting organs to physiologic stimuli. For example, data should be sought on the plasma response curve for cholecystokinin, to specific stimuli such as protein meals, or duodenal perfusion with amino acids.

C. Is There a Generalized Reduction in the Number of Mucosal Receptors for Active Absorption from Intestinal Lumen?

One of the manifestations of advancing age is a reduction in the basal number of protein receptors in several endocrine organs. In addition, the recruitment or synthesis of receptors in response to appropriate stimuli also may fall. During intestinal absorption, the active transport of many substrates occurs through the functioning of specific receptors. Research work in this area is in its infancy so that no information is available as to the effects of advancing age. However, now that mucosal receptor assays are being developed, e.g., the ileal vitamin B_{12} receptor, studies should be extended to normal aging humans.

D. Is Pancreatic Function Reduced Sufficiently During Aging to Impair Digestion?

The pancreas has a truly enormous reserve capacity for the secretion of pancreatic enzymes into the intestinal lumen for the digestion of lipids[115] and of carbohydrates.[116] It has been calculated that as little as 10% of the usual rate of pancreatic enzyme secretion after a meal is necessary to maintain normal absorption of these dietary substrates. For this reason, defects in pancreatic enzyme secretion would appear to be an unlikely cause for malabsorption in the elderly. However, little data on pancreatic function with advancing age are available. It has been reported that pancreatic weight decreases gradually with advancing age.[117,118] Furthermore, histologic studies suggest that parenchymal cell number per unit weight of the pancreas falls as one ages, to be replaced by fat and fibrous tissue. Pancreatic enzyme output was shown to decrease with age using older methods.[1] On the other hand, a retrospective review of the results of secretin stimulation tests by the Mount Sinai group[119] failed to show any consistent trend in their older subjects. One study has described a group of elderly patients with painless chronic idiopathic pancreatitis resulting in weight loss and steatorrhea thought to be due to vascular disease.[120] If the elderly have a generalized insensitivity to hormonal stimuli, then pancreatic enzyme secretion controlled by cholecystokinin would likely be affected. Quantitatively accurate pancreatic function tests require the passage of a triple lumen tube into the duodenum and the prolonged perfusion of a water soluble marker during the digestion of a meal.[121] These techniques are quite difficult for older subjects to endure and newer techniques evaluating pancreatic function are badly needed. Indirect methods, such as the measurement of trypsin by radioimmunoassay,[122] or the measurement of the capacity for protein digestion by the use of synthetic substrate, may be more acceptable measures. Furthermore, since cholecystokinin also stimulates gallbladder contraction, recently developed methods for the measurement of gallbladder emptying by ultrasound techniques[123] might be applied to detect hormone defects in the aged.

E. Is There Sufficient Reduction in Mucosal Blood Supply in the Elderly to Affect Mucosal Function?

Mucosal cell function critically depends upon a good splanchnic vascular supply. Approximately 30% of the cardiac output supplies the splanchnic bed in the resting state. Postprandially, there is believed to be up to a 25% increase in total mesenteric blood flow.[124] However, such changes in total blood flow probably are not the most important in the maintenance of intestinal mucosal cell oxygenation. More crucial is the redistribution of mesenteric blood flow from the submucosa to intestinal mucosal capillaries. In general, major clinical problems due to intestinal vascular insufficiency (intestinal angina) rarely occur in the elderly. However, this fact does not exclude the possibility that more subtle vascular changes are very important in altering absorptive function during aging.

The methods presently available for the study of functional mucosal blood supply in humans are too inadequate and cumbersome to be applied to the aging process. Therefore, critical research on the importance of changes in intestinal blood supply upon intestinal function awaits the development of simpler experimental techniques.

F. Are There Sufficient Changes in Intestinal Mucosal Defenses Against External Stimuli to Lead to Mucosal Cell Injury and Dysfunction?

Several mechanisms maintain the integrity of the intestinal cell. The mucosa minimizes the intestinal uptake of potentially injurious macromolecules by maintaining a relatively impenetrable barrier to particulate transport. Increased intestinal permeability to large molecules from dietary or microbial components may lead to local and distal dysfunction. Methods have recently been developed for the accurate study of the intestinal barrier and have demonstrated that chronic inflammatory disease allows the permeation of macromolecules.[125] Such methods can readily be applied to the study of the permeability of the aging gut since they do not involve complex invasive tests. The small intestinal mucosa also maintains its integrity by the production of a mucous glycocolyx barrier. There is evidence for biochemical changes in gastric mucus in old age and similar changes might occur in the small intestine. In addition, the small intestine has an effective local immunological response which impedes entry through the gut by foreign proteins.[126] In general, the aging process is felt to be accompanied by gradual impairment in immune functioning. Studies of the IgA-mediated immune system of the small intestine have not been performed in older subjects. Studies of the mucosal defenses to the entry of potentially pathogenic molecules are important not only for research on mechanisms causing impaired absorption but also on ways that oncogenic chemicals and organisms might gain entry to the body in the aged.

G. Is Altered Intestinal Proliferation Important in Absorptive Dysfunction in the Elderly?

The small intestinal mucosa is an organ that demonstrates very active cell proliferation. Rat mucosal renewal occurs every 36 hr and human small intestinal mucosa proliferates in less than 3 days.[127] Two factors suggest that an alteration of mucosal cell turnover might contribute to intestinal dysfunction in old age. When cell turnover is accelerated by intestinal resection[128] or is delayed by starvation,[129] mucosal cell metabolism and absorptive function are affected. Cell proliferation rates generally fall in aging animals.[130] The most detailed studies that investigated small intestinal turnover with aging were performed in the mouse[131,132] and the authors concluded that duodenal and jejunal epithelial transit time was increased in older animals due principally to a longer crypt stem cell generation time. In contrast, the ileum of aged mice did not show such changes.[133] Further studies of the relationship between altered mucosal cell turnover, structure, and function are needed to determine the importance of such changes in cell renewal rates in intestinal dysfunction in the elderly.

H. Do Changes in the Gastrointestinal Tract Combine to Create Conditions Permitting the Syndrome of Small Intestinal Bacterial Overgrowth?

Small intestinal bacterial overgrowth syndrome results in impaired digestion of fats, in bacterial utilization of carbohydrates, in interference with vitamin B_{12}-intrinsic factor association and perhaps in histologic damage to the small bowel. Factors that prevent bacterial proliferation in the small intestine include the gastric acid barrier,[134] normal gastrointestinal motility,[135] the absence of anatomic changes that create blind loops, and local mucosal immunologic factors. In the elderly, an increased incidence of multiple jejunal diverticulosis has been described which may be accompanied by overt malabsorption. In addition, preliminary evidence suggests that some older patients presenting with a syndrome of slow weight loss and debility had biochemical evidence for malabsorption, no radiologic evidence for any intestinal anatomic abnormality, but had abnormal ^{14}C glycocholate breath tests,[136] suggesting the presence of intestinal bacterial overgrowth. No other cause for malabsorption was found in these patients and they improved after the administration of broad spectrum antibiotics. In the elderly, there is a progressive increase in the incidence of hypochlorhydria and there is a tendency toward immunoincompetence, both of which might contribute to intestinal bacterial overgrowth. A change in the population of the intestinal microflora also occurs during aging.[137] However, the most important factor preventing bacterial proliferation in the small intestine is normal intestinal motility. A review of the literature failed to reveal any definitive intestinal motility studies in the elderly. Impaired bowel motility is susceptible to treatment, by metaclopramide, for example, so that such studies in older subjects are urgently needed.

VII. SUMMARY

In summary, this review has considered much of the pertinent data that relates to changes in normal intestinal absorption that may occur with advancing age. It must be very clear that the information base that is available does not permit scientifically solid conclusions about the effects of age per se upon the physiologic processes that lead to normal digestion and absorption. The National Institute of Aging has made as one of its important research goals improved information about the nutritional needs of the elderly. It will be difficult to set dietary goals without knowing whether the food components that are eaten are well digested and absorbed. Therefore, this review has also pointed out the research areas that should be the subject of investigation. One initial need is the development of simple and noninvasive test methods for measuring intestinal absorption and malabsorption of a variety of substances in elderly subjects. It is hoped that this review can be a stimulus toward new and incisive research into the subject of intestinal absorption during the process of aging.

REFERENCES

1. Meyer, J. and Necheles, H., IV. The clinical significance of salivary, gastric, and pancreatic secretion in the aged, *JAMA*, 115, 2050, 1940.
2. Necheles, H., Plotke, F., and Meyer, J., Studies in old age. V. Active pancreatic secretion in the aged, *Am. J. Dig. Dis.*, 9, 157, 1942.

3. Meyer, J., Sorter, H., Oliver, J., and Necheles, H., Studies in old age. VII. Intestinal absorption in old age, *Gastroenterology,* 1, 876, 1943.

4. Sklar, M., Kirsner, J. B., and Palmer, W. L., Gastrointestinal disease in the aged, *Med. Clin. North Am.,* 40, 223, 1956.

5. Pelz, K. S., Gottfried, S. P., and Soos, E., Intestinal absorption studies in the aged, *Geriatrics,* 23, 149, 1968.

6. Montgomery, R. D., Haeney, M. R., Ross, I. N., Sammons, H. G., Barford, A. V., Balakrishnan, S., Mayer, P. P., Culank, L. S., Field, J., and Gosling, P., The ageing gut: a study of intestinal absorption in relation to nutrition in the elderly, *Q. J. Med.,* 47, 197, 1978.

7. Price, H. L., Gazzard, B. G., and Dawson, A. M., Steatorrhoea in the elderly, *Br. Med. J.,* 1, 1582, 1977.

8. Abraham, S., Carroll, M. D., Dresser, C. M., and Johnson, C. L., Dietary intake source data, *Vital and Health Statistics,* National Center for Health Statistics, U.S. Department of Health, Education and Welfare, Hyattsville, Md., Publication No. (PHS) 79-1221, 1979.

9. Abraham, S. and Johnson, C. L., Overweight adults 20-74 years of age: United States, 1971-74, *Vital and Health Statistics,* Advance Data No. 51, Public Health Service, U.S. Department of Health, Education and Welfare, Hyattsville, Md., 1975.

10. Bourlière, F. and Parot, S., Le vieillissement de deux populations blanches vivant dans des conditions écologiques très différentes, étude comparative, *Rev. France Etud. Clin. Bio.,* 7, 629, 1962.

11. Rossman, I., Anatomic and body composition changes with aging, in *Handbook of the Biology of Aging,* Finch, C. E. and Hayflick, L., Eds., Van Nostrand Reinhold, New York, 1977, 189.

12. Becker, G. H., Meyer, J., and Necheles, H., Fat absorption in young and old age, *Gastroenterology,* 14, 80, 1950.

13. Garcia, P., Roderuck, C., and Swanson, P., The relation of age to fat absorption in adult women together with observations on concentration of serum cholesterol, Journal paper J-2578, Iowa Agricultural Experiment Station, Ames Iowa, Project 1028, 1954, 601.

14. Citi, S. and Salvini, L., The intestinal absorption of ^{131}I labeled olein and triolein, of ^{58}CO vit. B12 and ^{59}FE, in the aged subjects, *Giorn. Gerontol.,* 12, 123, 1964.

15. Webster, S. G. P., Wilkinson, E. M., and Gowland, E., A comparison of fat absorption in young and old subjects, *Age and Ageing,* 6, 113, 1977.

16. Van Liere, E. J. and Northup, D. W., The emptying time of the stomach of old people, *Am. J. Physiol.,* 134, 719, 1941.

17. Ryder, J. B., Steatorrhea in the elderly, *Gerontol. Clin.,* 5, 30, 1963.

18. Ammann, R. and Sulser, H., Die "senile" chronische Pankreatitis — eine neue nosologische Einheit? *Schweiz. Med. Wochenschr.,* 106, 429, 1976.

19. Justice, C. L., Howe, J. M., and Clarke, H. E., Dietary intakes and nutritional status of elderly patients, *J. Am. Diet. Assoc.,* 65, 639, 1974.

20. Hollander, D. and Morgan, D., Increase in cholesterol intestinal absorption with aging in the rat, *Exp. Gerontol.,* 14, 201, 1979.

21. Bogdonoff, M. D., Shock, N. W., and Nichols, M. P., Calcium, phosphorus, nitrogen and potassium balance studies in the aged male, *J. Gerontol.,* 8, 272, 1953.

22. Kountz, W. B., Hofstatter, L., and Ackermann, P. G., Nitrogen balance studies on elderly people, *Geriatrics,* 2, 173, 1947.

23. Kountz, W. B., Hofstatter, L., Ackermann, P. G., Nitrogen balance studies in four elderly men, *J. Gerontol.,* 6, 20, 1951.

24. Cheng, A. H. R., Gomez, A., Bergan, J. G., Lee, T. C., Monckeberg, F., and Chichester, C. O., Comparative nitrogen balance study between young and aged adults using three levels of protein intake from a combination wheat-soy-milk mixture, *Am. J. Clin. Nutr.,* 31, 12, 1978.

25. Zanni, E., Calloway, D. H., and Zezulka, A. Y., Protein requirements of elderly men, *J. Nutr.,* 109, 513, 1979.

26. Chinn, A. B., Lavik, P. S., and Cameron, D. B., Measurement of protein digestion and absorption in aged persons by a test meal of I^{131}-labeled protein, *J. Gerontol.,* 11, 151, 1956.

27. Penzes, L., Simon, G., and Winter, M., Effect of concentration on the intestinal absorption and utilization of radiomethionine in old age, *Exp. Gerontol.,* 3, 257, 1968.

28. Winter, D., Dobre, V., and Oeriu, S., Cystein-S^{35} absorption in old rats, *Exp. Gerontol.,* 6, 367, 1971.

29. Imondi, A. R. and Wolgemuth, R. L., Improved sensitivity of the BTPABA pancreatic function test in animals with meals of raw egg white, *Dig. Dis. Sci.,* 24, 214, 1979.

30. Welsh, J. D., Poley, J. R., Bhatia, M., and Stevenson, D. E., Intestinal disaccharidase activities in relation to age, race, and mucosal damage, *Gastroenterology,* 75, 847, 1978.

31. Hofstatter, L., Sonnenberg, A., and Kountz, W. B., The glucose tolerance in elderly patients, *Biol. Symp.,* 11, 87, 1945.

32. Phillips, R. A. and Gilder, H., Metabolism studies in the albino rat: the relation of age, nutrition and hypophysectomy on the absorption of dextrose from the gastrointestinal tract, *Endocrinology,* 27, 601, 1940.

33. Sapp, O. L., III, Sessions, J. T., Jr., and Rose, J. W., Jr., Effect of aging on intestinal absorption of sugars, *Clin. Res.,* 12, 31, 1964.

34. Klimas, J. E., Intestinal glucose absorption during the life-span of a colony of rats, *J. Gerontol.,* 23, 529, 1968.

35. Calingaert, A. and Zorzoli, A., The influence of age on 6-deoxy-D-glucose accumulation by mouse intestine, *J. Gerontol.,* 20, 211, 1965.

36. Sayeed, M., Age-related changes in intestinal phosphomonoesterases, *Fed. Proc.,* 26, 259, 1967.

37. Stifel, F. B., Herman, R. H., and Rosensweig, N. S., Dietary regulation of glycolytic enzymes. III. Adaptive changes in rat jejunal pyruvate kinase; phosphofructokinase; fructose diphosphatase and glycerol-3-phosphate dehydrogenase, *Biochim. Biophys. Acta,* 184, 29, 1969.

38. Espinoza, J. and Rosensweig, N., Effect of aging on the response of rat hepatic glycolytic enzyme activities to dietary sugars, *Am. J. Clin. Nutr.,* 26, 608, 1973.

39. Rosensweig, N. S., personal communication, 1980.

40. Guth, P. H., Physiologic alterations in small bowel function with age: the absorption of D-xylose, *Am. J. Dig. Dis.,* 13, 565, 1968.

41. Kendall, M. J., The influence of age on the xylose absorption test, *Gut,* 11, 498, 1970.

42. Webster, S. G. P. and Leeming, J. T., Assessment of small bowel function in the elderly using a modified xylose tolerance test, *Gut,* 16, 109, 1975.

43. Bond, J. H., Jr. and Levitt, M. D., Use of pulmonary hydrogen (H_2) measurements to quantitate carbohydrate absorption; study of partially gastrectomized patients, *J. Clin. Invest.,* 51, 1219, 1972.

44. Feibusch, J. and Holt, P. R., Impaired absorptive capacity for carbohydrates in the elderly, *Am. J. Clin. Nutr.,* 32, 942, 1979.

45. Brin, M. and Bauernfeind, J. C., Vitamin needs of the elderly, *Postgrad. Med.,* 63, 155, 1978.

46. Brin, M., Erythrocyte as a biopsy tissue for functional evaluation of thiamine adequacy, *JAMA,* 187, 762, 1964.

47. Kirk, J. E. and Chieffi, M., Vitamin studies in middle-aged and old individuals. I. The vitamin A, total carotene and $\alpha + \beta$ carotene concentrations in plasma, *J. Nutr.,* 36, 315, 1948.

48. Kirk, J. E. and Chieffi, M., Vitamin studies in middle-aged and old individuals. III. Thiamine and pyruvic acid blood concentrations, *J. Nutr.,* 38, 353, 1949.

49. Kirk, J. E. and Chieffi, M., Vitamin studies in middle-aged and old individuals. XI. The concentration of total ascorbic acid in whole blood, *J. Gerontol.,* 8, 301, 1953.

50. Harril, I. and Cervone, N., Vitamin status of older women, *Am. J. Clin. Nutr.,* 30, 431, 1977.

51. Gillum, H. L., Morgan, A. F., and Sailer, F., Nutritional status of the ageing. V. Vitamin A and carotene, *J. Nutr.,* 55, 655, 1955.

52. Yiengst, M. J. and Shock, N. W., Effect of oral administration of vitamin A on plasma levels of vitamin A and carotene in the aged males, *J. Gerontol.,* 4, 205, 1949.

53. Hollander, D. and Morgan, D., Aging: its influence on vitamin A intestinal absorption in vivo by the rat, *Exp. Gerontol.,* 14, 301, 1979.

54. Birrin, J. E., Bick, M. W., and Yiengst, M. J., Relation of structural changes of the eye and vitamin A to elevation of the light threshold on later life, *J. Exp. Psychol.,* 40, 260, 1950.

55. Brin, M., Dibble, M. V., Peel, A., McMullen, E., Bourquin, A., and Chen, N., Some preliminary findings on the nutritional status of the aged in Onondaga County, New York, *Am. J. Clin. Nutr.,* 17, 240, 1965.

56. Rafsky, H. A. and Newman, B., Vitamin B_1 excretion in the aged, *Gastroenterology,* 1, 737, 1943.

57. Thomson, A. D., Thiamine absorption in old age, *Gerontol. Clin.,* 8, 354, 1966.

58. Horwitt, M., Dietary requirements of the aged, *J. Am. Diet. Assoc.,* 29, 443, 1953.

59. Morgan, A. G., Kelleher, J., Walker, B. E., Losowsky, M. S., Droller, H., and Middleton, R. S. W., A nutritional survey in the elderly: blood and urine vitamin levels, *Int. J. Vitam. Nutr. Res.,* 45, 448, 1975.

60. Ranke, E., Tauber, S. A., Horonick, A., Ranke, B., Goodhart, R. S., and Chow, B. F., Vitamin B_6 deficiency in the aged, *J. Gerontol.,* 15, 41, 1960.

61. Rose, C. S., Gyorgy, P., Spiegel, H., Brin, M., Butler, M., and Shock, N. W., Vitamin B_6 status of American adult males, *Fed. Proc.,* 33, 697, 1974.

62. Vir, S. C. and Love, A. H. G., Vitamin B_6 status of the hospitalized aged, *Am. J. Clin. Nutr.,* 31, 1383, 1978.

63. Kataria, M. S., Rao, D. B., and Curtis, R. C., Vitamin C levels in the elderly, *Gerontol. Clin.,* 7, 189, 1965.

64. Burr, M. L., Elwood, P. C., Hole, D. J., Hurley, R. J., and Hughes, R. E., Plasma and leukocyte ascorbic acid levels in the elderly , *Am. J. Clin. Nutr.,* 27, 144, 1974.

65. Schorah, C. J., Newill, A., Scott, D. L., and Morgan, D. B., Clinical effects of vitamin C in elderly inpatients with low blood-vitamin-C levels, *Lancet*, 1, 403, 1979.

66. Lester, E., Skinner, R. K., and Wills, M. R., Seasonal variation in serum 25-hydroxyvitamin D concentrations in the elderly in Britain, *Lancet*, 1, 979, 1977.

67. MacLennan, W. J. and Hamilton, J. C., Vitamin D supplements and 25-hydroxyvitamin D concentrations in the elderly, *Br. Med. J.*, 2, 859, 1977.

68. Holt, P. R. and Dominguez, A. A., Intestinal absorption of triglyceride and vitamin D_3 in aged and young rats, *Dis. Dis. Sci.*, in press.

69. Barragary, J. M., France, M. W., Corless, D., Gupta, S. P., Switala, S., Boucher, B. J., and Cohen, R. D., Intestinal cholecalciferol absorption in the elderly and in younger adults, *Clin. Sci. Mol. Med.*, 55, 213, 1978.

70. U.S recommended daily allowances (U.S. RDA) and permissible compositional ranges for dietary supplements of vitamins and minerals, *Federal Register*, 41, 46172, October 19, 1976, Washington, D.C.

71. Burch, R. E. and Hahn, H. K. J., Trace elements in human nutrition, *Med. Clin. North Am.*, 63, 1057, 1979.

72. Fisher, S., Hendricks, D. G., and Mahoney, A. W., Nutritional assessment of senior rural Utahns by biochemical and physical measurements, *Am. J. Clin. Nutr.*, 31, 667, 1978.

73. Vir, S. C. and Love, A. H. G., Zinc and copper status of the elderly, *Am. J. Clin. Nutr.*, 32, 1472, 1979.

74. Greger, J. L. and Geissler, A. H., Effect of zinc supplementation on taste acuity of the aged, *Am. J. Clin. Nutr.*, 31, 633, 1978.

75. Freiman, H. D., Tauber, S. A., and Tulsky, E. G., Iron absorption in the healthy aged, *Geriatrics*, 18, 716, 1963.

76. Jacobs, A. and Owen, G. M., The effect of age on iron absorption, *J. Gerontol.*, 24, 95, 1969.

77. Benzie, R. M., The influence of age upon the iron content of bone marrow, *Lancet*, 1, 1074, 1963.

78. Loria, A., Hershko, C., and Konijn, A. M., Serum ferritin in an elderly population, *J. Gerontol.*, 34, 521, 1979.

79. Marx, J. J. M., Normal iron absorption and decreased red cell iron uptake in the aged, *Blood*, 53, 204, 1979.

80. Burkhardt, R., Iron overload of bone marrow and bone, in *Iron Metabolism and its Disorders*, ICS 366, Kief, H., Ed., Excerpta Medica, Amsterdam, 1975, 264.

81. Elsborg, L., Lund, V., and Bastrup-Madsen, P., Serum vitamin B_{12} levels in the aged, *Acta Med. Scand.*, 200, 309, 1976.

82. Bailey, L. B., Wagner, P. A., Christakis, G. J., Araujo, P. E., Appledorf, H., Davis, C. G., Dorsey, E., and Dinning, J. S., Vitamin B_{12} status of elderly persons from urban low-income households, *J. Am. Geriatr. Soc.*, 28, 276, 1980.

83. Joske, R. A., Finckh, E. S., and Wood, I. J., Gastric biopsy: a study of 1,000 consecutive successful gastric biopsies, *Q. J. Med.*, 24, 269, 1955.

84. Glass, G. B. J., Goldbloom, A. A., Boyd, L. J., Laughton, R., Rosen, S., and Rich, M., Intestinal absorption and hepatic uptake of radioactive vitamin B_{12} in various age groups and the effect of intrinsic factor preparations, *Am. J. Clin. Nutr.*, 4, 124, 1956.

85. Chow, B. F., Gilbert, J. P., Okuda, K., and Rosenblum, C., The urinary excretion test for absorption of vitamin B_{12}. I. Reproducibility of results and agewise variation, *Am. J. Clin. Nutr.*, 4, 142, 1956.

86. Hyams, D. E., The absorption of vitamin B_{12} in the elderly, *Gerontol. Clin.*, 6, 193, 1964.

87. Streeter, A. M., Balasubramanian, D., Boyle, R., O'Neill, B. J., and Pheills, M. T., Malabsorption of vitamin B_{12} after vagotomy, *Am. J. Surg.*, 128, 340, 1974.

88. Amin, S., Spinks, T., Ranicar, A., Short, M. D., and Hoffbrand, A. V., Long-term clearance of (^{57}Co)cyanocobalamin in vegans and pernicious anaemia, *Clin. Sci.*, 58, 101, 1980.

89. Hurdle, A. D. F. and Picton Williams, T. C., Folic-acid deficiency in elderly patients admitted to hospital, *Br. Med. J.*, 2, 202, 1966.

90. Girdwood, R. H., Thomson, A. D., and Williamson, J., Folate status in the elderly, *Br. Med. J.*, 2, 670, 1967.

91. Baker, H., Frank, O., Thind, I. S., Jaslow, S. P., and Louria, D. B., Vitamin profile in elderly persons living at home or in nursing homes versus profile in healthy young subjects, *J. Am. Geriatr. Soc.*, 27, 444, 1979.

92. MacKenzie, J. F. and Russell, R. I., The effect of pH on folic acid absorption in man, *Clin. Sci. Mol. Med.*, 51, 363, 1976.

93. Rosenberg, I. H. and Neumann, H., Multistep mechanism in the hydrolysis of pteroylpolyglutamate by chicken intestine, *J. Biol. Chem.*, 249, 5126, 1974.

94. Bhanthumnavin, K., Wright, J. R., and Halsted, C. H., Intestinal transport of tritiated folic acid (^{3}H-PGA) in the everted gut sac of different aged rats, *Johns Hopkins Med. J.*, 135, 152, 1974.

95. Baker, H., Jaslow, S. P., and Frank, O., Severe impairment of dietary folate utilization in the elderly, *J. Am. Geriatr. Soc.*, 26, 218, 1978.

96. Nordin, B. E. C., Osteoporosis, osteomalacia and calcium deficiency, *Clin. Orthop.*, 17, 235, 1960.

97. Schachter, D., Dowdle, E. B., and Schenker, H., Active transport of calcium by the small intestine of the rat, *Am. J. Physiol.*, 198, 263, 1960.

98. Walling, M. W. and Rothman, S. S., Phosphate-independent, carrier-mediated active transport of calcium by rat intestine, *Am. J. Physiol.*, 217, 1144, 1969.

99. Walling, M. W. and Rothman, S. S., Apparent increase in carrier affinity for intestinal calcium transport following dietary calcium restriction, *J. Biol. Chem.*, 245, 5007, 1970.

100. Avioli, L. V., McDonald, J. E., and Lee, S. W., The influence of age on the intestinal absorption of ^{47}Ca in women and its relation to ^{47}Ca absorption in postmenopausal osteoporosis, *J. Clin. Invest.*, 44, 1960, 1965.

101. Bullamore, J. R., Wilkinson, R., Gallagher, B. E., Nordin, C., and Marshall, D. H., Effect of age on calcium absorption, *Lancet*, 2, 535, 1970.

102. Nordin, B. E. C., Wilkinson, R., Marshall, D. H., Gallagher, J. C., Williams, A., and Peacock, M., Calcium absorption in the elderly, *Calc. Tis. Res.*, 21, 442, 1976.

103. Ireland, P. and Fordtran, J. S., Effect of dietary calcium and age on jejunal calcium absorption in humans studied by intestinal perfusion, *J. Clin. Invest.*, 52, 2672, 1973.

104. Armbrecht, H. J., Zenser, T. V., Bruns, M. E. H., and Davis, B. B., Effect of age on intestinal calcium absorption and adaptation to dietary calcium, *Am. J. Physiol.*, 236, E769, 1979.

105. Gallagher, J. C., Riggs, B. L., and DeLuca, H. F., Effect of age on calcium absorption and serum 1,25(OH)$_2$D, *Clin. Res.*, 26, 680A, 1978.

106. Massry, S. G., Friedler, R. M., and Coburn, J. W., Excretion of phosphate and calcium. Physiology of their renal handling and relationship to clinical medicine, *Arch. Int. Med.*, 131, 828, 1973.

107. Breibart, S., Lee, J. S., McCoord, A., and Forbes, G. B., Relation of age to radiomagnesium exchange in bone, *Proc. Soc. Exp. Biol. Med.*, 105, 361, 1960.

108. Moog, F., The small intestine in old mice: growth, alkaline phosphatase and disaccharidase activities, and deposition of amyloid, *Exp. Gerontol.*, 12, 223, 1977.

109. Hohn, P., Gabbert, H., and Wagner, R., Differentiation and aging of the rat intestinal mucosa, *Mech. Ageing Dev.*, 7, 217, 1978.

110. Webster, S. G. P. and Leeming, J. T., The appearance of the small bowel mucosa in old age, *Age Ageing*, 4, 168, 1975.

111. Warren, P. M., Pepperman, M. A., and Montgomery, R. D., Age changes in small-intestinal mucosa, *Lancet*, 2, 849, 1978.

112. Thomson, A. B. R., Unstirred water layer and age-dependent changes in rabbit jejunal D-glucose transport, *Am. J. Physiol.*, 236, E685, 1979.

113. Roth, G. S. and Adelman, R. C., Age-related changes in hormone binding by target cells and tissues. Possible role in altered adaptive responsiveness, *Exp. Gerontol.*, 10, 1, 1975.

114. Blichert-Toft, M., Secretion of corticotrophin and somatotrophin by the senescent adenohypophysis in man, *Acta Endocrinol.*, (Suppl.), 78, 15, 1975.

115. DiMagno, E. P., Go, V. L. W., and Summerskill, W. H. J., Relations between pancreatic enzyme outputs and malabsorption in severe pancreatic insufficiency, *N. Engl. J. Med.*, 288, 813, 1973.

116. Gray, G. M., Carbohydrate digestion and absorption, *N. Engl. J. Med.*, 292, 1225, 1975.

117. Kurtz, S. M., *Structural Aspects of Ageing*, Bourne, G. F., Ed., Pitman, London, 1961, 79.

118. McKeown, F., *Pathology of the Aged*, Butterworth's, London, 1965, 219.

119. Rosenberg, I. R., Friedland, N., Janowitz, H. D., and Dreiling, D. A., The effect of age and sex upon human pancreatic secretion of fluid and bicarbonate, *Gastroenterology*, 50, 191, 1966.

120. Ammann, R., Zur vaskularen Genese der chronischen Pankreatitis, *Dtsch. Med. Wochenschr.*, 101, 867, 1976.

121. Go, V. L., Hofmann, W. A. F., and Summerskill, W. H. J., Simultaneous measurements of total pancreatic, biliary and gastric outputs in man using a perfusion technique, *Gastroenterology*, 58, 321, 1970.

122. Adrian, T. E., Besterman, H. S., Mallinson, C. N., Galarotis, C., and Bloom, S. R., Plasma trypsin in patients with steatorrhoea due to chronic pancreatitis, *Clin. Sci. Mol. Med.*, 54, 13P, 1978.

123. Everson, G. T., Braverman, D. Z., Johnson, M. L., and Kern, F., A critical evaluation of real-time ultrasonography for the study of gallbladder volume and contraction, *Gastroenterology*, 79, 40, 1980.

124. Brandt, J. L., Castleman, L., Ruskin, H. D., Greenwald, J., and Kelly, J. J., Jr., The effect of oral protein and glucose feeding on splanchnic blood flow and oxygen utilization in normal and cirrhotic subjects, *J. Clin. Invest.*, 34, 1017, 1955.

125. Sundqvist, T., Magnusson, K. E., Sjodahl, R., Stjernstrom, I., and Tagesson, C., Passage of molecules through the wall of the gastrointestinal tract. II. Application of low-molecular weight polyethyleneglycol and a deterministic mathematical model for determining intestinal permeability in man, *Gut*, 21, 208, 1980.

126. **Walker, W. A., Wu, M., Isselbacher, K. J., and Block, K. J.,** Intestinal uptake of macromolecules. III. Studies on the mechanism by which immunization interferes with antigen uptake, *J. Immunol.,* 115, 854, 1975.

127. **Eastwood, G. L.,** Gastrointestinal epithelial renewal, *Gastroenterology,* 72, 962, 1977.

128. **Hanson, W. R., Osborne, J. W., and Sharp, J. G.,** Compensation by the residual intestine after intestinal resection in the rat. I. Influence of amount of tissue removed, *Gastroenterology,* 72, 692, 1977.

129. **Lohrs, U., Wiebecke, B., Heybowitz, R., and Eder, M.,** Cell turnover in intestinal epithelium during experimental starvation, in *Intestinal Adaptation — Proceedings of an International Conference on the Anatomy, Physiology and Biochemistry of Intestinal Adaptation,* Dowling, R. H. and Riecken, E. O., Eds., F. K. Schattauer Verlag, Stuttgart, Germany, 1974, 115.

130. **Cameron, I. L.,** Cell proliferation and renewal in aging mice, *J. Gerontol.,* 27, 162, 1972.

131. **Lesher, S., Fry, R. J. M., and Kohn, H. I.,** Influence of age on transit time of cells of mouse intestinal epithelium. I. Duodenum, *Lab. Invest.,* 10, 291, 1961.

132. **Fry, R. J. M., Lesher, S., and Kohn, H. I.,** Age effect on cell-transit time in mouse jejunal epithelium, *Am. J. Physiol.,* 201, 213, 1961.

133. **Fry, R. J. M., Lesher, S., and Kohn, H. I.,** Influence of age on the transit time of cells of the mouse intestinal epithelium. III. Ileum, *Lab. Invest.,* 11, 289, 1962.

134. **Frederiksen, W., Bruusgaard, A., and Thayser, E. H.,** Assessment of the relationship between gastric secretory capacity and jejunal bacteriology, *Scand. J. Gastroenterol.,* 8, 353, 1973.

135. **Vantrappen, G., Janssens, J., Hellemans, J., and Ghoos, Y.,** The interdigestive motor complex of normal subjects and patients with bacterial overgrowth of the small intestine, *J. Clin. Invest.,* 59, 1158, 1977.

136. **Roberts, S. H., Jarvis, E. H., and James, O.,** Bacterial overgrowth syndrome without 'blind loop': a cause for malnutrition in the elderly, *Gut,* 18, A969, 1977.

137. **Gorbach, S. L., Nahas, L., Lerner, P. I., and Weinstein, L.,** Studies of intestinal microflora. I. Effects of diet, age, and periodic sampling on numbers of fecal microorganisms in man, *Gastroenterology,* 53, 845, 1967.

Chapter 9

NUTRITION IN THE DEVELOPMENT AND AGING OF THE SKELETON

Agatha A. Rider

TABLE OF CONTENTS

I. ROLE OF SPECIFIC NUTRIENTS IN BONE FORMATION

Before the discovery of vitamins as essential nutrients it was evident that the ingestion of certain inorganic elements was essential for the formation of bone. In 1748 J. G. Gahn of Sweden determined that bones are composed largely of calcium and phosphorus, and thus these two elements were identified as dietary essentials.[1] It was also observed that bone contained an organic component which is protein in nature and so the necessity to provide protein precursors was realized.

A. Vitamin C

It had been observed for many years that certain disorders led to bone abnormalities and some of these disorders were later found to be attributable to dietary deficiencies. Among these is scurvy. Bone is formed and fractures are healed through the calcification of a collagen matrix. Any disorder in collagen formation or calcification, therefore, leads to faults in bone growth or fracture repair.

In 1748 Richard Walter, who was chaplain to Lord Anson's around-the-world expedition, reported that during attacks of scurvy old wounds broke open, thus observing (although he did not know it) the relationship between vitamin C and collagen.[2] Lind in 1753 recounted Ives' observation of delayed healing in a scorbutic seaman on HMS *Dragon* who had a "shattering of the humerus from a Spanish musket ball".[3] There are also accounts in the older literature of the reappearance of healed fractures during bouts with scurvy during the American Revolution.[3] During the 1914 to 1918 war the poor healing of wounds and fractures occurring in Turkish soldiers with scurvy was reported.[3]

Vitamin C is believed to exert its influence on the formation of collagen at the point of hydroxylation of the proline moiety of the molecule.[4] In the infant, interference with this process results in faulty endochondral bone growth with subperiosteal hemorrhages widely distributed throughout the skeleton and most marked in the areas of rapid growth such as the sternal end of the middle ribs, the lower end of the femur, the upper end of the humerus, both ends of the tibia and fibula, and the lower end of the radius and ulna.[5] Scurvy also retards the removal of the matrix of calcified cartilage, slows down new trabecular formation, and encourages the resorption of previously formed bone. Thus the ability of the bone to withstand mechanical stress is severely compromised.[6] Osteoporosis which is sometimes seen accompanying chronic vitamin C deficiency may be due in part to involuntary immobilization due to pain in the joints.[7]

B. Vitamin A

In 1921 Hess et al.[8] confirmed the 1913 observation of McCollum and Davis[9] that vitamin A was necessary for growth in the rat. Wolbach and Howe,[10] observing nervous lesions in rats on a vitamin A deficient diet, believed that the skeleton was normal and that the nervous lesions were due to a disproportionate growth of the central nervous system with a resultant crowding of that tissue. Mellanby in the 1940s[11] observed extensive nerve lesions in vitamin A deficient puppies. He noted that the skull cavity was greatly reduced in size due to a thickening of the skull itself. The spinal canal was narrowed due to thickening of the vertebrae and the marrow cavity in the femur was reduced because of a thickened shaft wall. These bony changes resulted in pressure on the cranial and spinal nerves as well as an overcrowding of the central nervous system tissue. Histological studies by Mellanby demonstrated that the bone defect in vitamin A deficiency is not so much a failure of bone growth as it is a breakdown in the resorption of previously formed bone as new bone is produced. This conclusion is supported by the observation that vitamin A deficiency leads to a deficit in the number and activity of osteoclasts which are responsible for bone resorption, especially marked on the inner surface of the skull adjacent to the central nervous system. In this case canals, such as the auditory meatus and the spinal canal, are narrowed and the skull cavity is shrunk although the outside dimensions of the skull are normal.[11]

In vitamin A deficiency there is also increased osteoblastic activity leading to increase in bone formation in certain sites such as the internal auditory meatus and the petrous bone.

The dog has been studied most thoroughly. Nervous lesions have also been observed in vitamin A deficient rats,[10] chicks,[12] ducks,[13] and rabbits.[14,15] There is very little information on skeletal changes in vitamin A deficiency in man.[16]

As might be expected, excessive doses of vitamin A also affect skeletal changes. Collazo and Sanchez-Rodriguez[17] observed fractures of distal limb bones in rats on diets containing a large excess of vitamin A. In hypervitaminosis A the activity of the osteoclasts is enhanced especially in sites of bone remodeling and osteoblastic activity is reduced. This results in bone fragility which is especially marked in the tibia and forearm.[16]

In chronic vitamin A poisoning in man, Caffey[18] has observed a tender swelling over the limbs with some impediment in movement. X-rays revealed smooth hyperostes in the central portion of long bones such as the ulnae and metatarsals. Similar changes were also seen by Bair in the skull.[19]

C. Vitamin D

It had been observed for many decades that the fault in the crippling disease of rickets lay in the failure of calcification of the cartilage at the growing end of the long bones. In 1919 Mellanby in England[20] reported the experimental production of rickets in dogs maintained on an oatmeal diet. In 1824, Scheutte[21] had used cod liver oil for the treatment of rickets and its use had continued. In 1913 McCollum had identified a substance in cod liver oil (vitamin A) which would promote growth and prevent xerophthalmia in rats.[9] Mellanby, therefore, dosed the oatmeal-consuming dogs with cod liver oil and in so doing prevented the symptoms of rickets. He thereby speculated that vitamin A possessed antirachitic properties. Concurrently McCollum and co-workers were producing rickets in rats by manipulating the calcium to phosphorus ratio in the diet. They discovered that cod liver oil would prevent rickets in rats on a dietary regimen which contained an imbalance of calcium to phosphorus, e.g., 4:1, 1:3, etc. They further showed that when the vitamin A in the cod liver oil was oxidized, the oil still possessed antirachitic properties. They thus established the existence of a second fat soluble micronutrient which they labeled vitamin D.[22]

The peculiar geographic distribution of rickets, however, still posed unsolved questions. Its wide prevalence in temperate regions as compared to tropical regions seemed to argue against a dietary deficiency as a causative factor. In addition, Kassowitz in 1906 had noted a progressive rise in rickets in the winter months and Hansemann had observed that the bones of infants born in the spring and dying in the fall showed no evidence of rickets, whereas the bones of those born in the fall and dying in the spring were rachitic.[23] Palm in 1890 believed that light was a therapeutic agent for rickets[22] and certain European physicians used sunlight as a curative agent. The demonstration by Goldblatt and Soames[24] of the presence of an antirachitic factor in the livers of rats which had been irradiated with ultraviolet light and its absence in nonirradiated rats led Steenbock and Black to speculate that ultraviolet irradiation changed a precursor of vitamin D into its active form.[25] Furthermore, this irradiation was effective not only when applied to animals but also when applied to their food.

In 1931 Askew et al.[26] elucidated the structure of vitamin D_2, which is formed by ultraviolet irradiation of the plant sterol, ergosterol. Windaus and colleagues[27] pre-

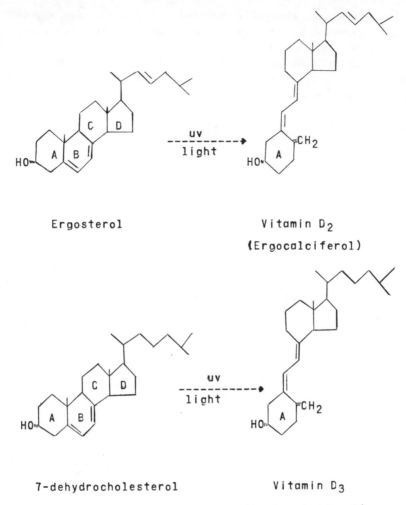

FIGURE 1.   Products of UV irradiation of ergosterol and of 7-dehydrocholecalciferol.

pared an analogue of ergosterol, 7-dehydrocholesterol, which on ultraviolet irradiation is transformed into vitamin D_3. It is this form of the vitamin which was later found to occur naturally upon irradiation of the skin.[28,29] Figure 1 shows the relationships of these compounds.

The fault in rickets lies in the failure in calcification of the collagen at the growing ends of the long bones and rib cage. As a result the bones are unable to support the weight of the body and bowed legs or knock knees result. A lack of dietary calcium or a faulty absorption of calcium from the intestine can, therefore, lead to rickets. This malabsorption may be caused by an unphysiological calcium to phosphorus ratio,[30] or the presence of oxalates or phytates which form insoluble calcium salts in the diet, or by a deficiency of vitamin D. The question of how vitamin D functions to prevent rickets was answered partially when Shipley, Kramer, and Howland[31] demonstrated that rachitic bone or cartilage slices would calcify normally when incubated in normal blood containing adequate amounts of calcium and phosphorus but not in blood from rachitic rats, which is low in these two elements. This led them to the conclusion that the defect in rickets lay in the blood, not in the bone. They further showed that the administration of vitamin D to rachitic rats led to an increase in the blood levels of calcium and phosphorus to a level adequate to support calcification of the cartilage. As DeLuca has pointed out[32] these findings pointed to a role of vitamin D in calcium and phosphorus absorption but did not rule out the possibility of an additional action of vitamin D on the bone itself.

The importance of the role of vitamin D in the absorption of calcium and phosphorus differs in different species. In their early work, McCollum et al. had noted that in rats a diet containing adequate amounts of calcium and phosphorus in a ratio of close to 1:1 did not produce rickets even in the absence of vitamin D, but that vitamin D was required for proper bone formation in the presence of unphysiological ratios of these two elements.[33-36] Recently Howard and Baylink[37] have confirmed these earlier observations in rats.

In other species studied (including man) vitamin D is required for the active transport of calcium across the intestinal mucosa.[38] An exception to this is in the absorption of calcium by the suckling infant.[39]

Nicolaysen in 1937 proved that vitamin D directly aids in the absorption of calcium[40] and that it is required when the needs for increased calcium absorption are high.[41] He put forth the idea that an endogenous factor produced by the bone is responsible for informing the intestinal mucosa of the need of the skeletal tissue for calcium. He speculated that this endogenous factor required vitamin D for its expression. Furthermore, the Harrisons[42] in the 1960s demonstrated that vitamin D also plays a key role in the absorption of phosphorus.

Vitamin D acts not only to aid in the absorption of calcium but also facilitates removal of calcium and phosphorus from bone when the serum calcium level falls sufficiently to pose a danger of tetany. This was first shown by Carlsson in 1952.[43] Rasmussen et al.[44] in 1963 showed that this action is mediated through the parathyroid hormone.

Within the last decade our understanding of the mode of action of vitamin D has been greatly enlarged by the brilliant work of H. F. DeLuca and associates of the University of Wisconsin, and of other workers in the U.S. and England. Intrigued by the observation that in the rat there is a time lag of about 12 hr between the administration of vitamin D and a rise in serum calcium levels, they sought active metabolites of the vitamin.[32] Through a series of fractionations of lipid components of serum, liver, kidney, and intestine, they followed the fate of radioactively labeled vitamin D. They have conclusively shown that vitamin D is carried by means of a vitamin D binding protein to the liver where it undergoes a hydroxylation in the 25 position.[45-47] Experiments of groups led by DeLuca,[48] Fraser and Kodicek,[49] and Norman[50] established that this metabolite is then carried to the kidney where it undergoes another hydroxylation to form the 1α-25-dihydroxyvitamin D as shown in Figure 2. This dihydroxy derivative then initiates in the intestinal mucosa the formation of a calcium binding protein which is responsible for the active transport of calcium across the intestinal wall. A phosphate binding protein is similarly produced to facilitate the absorption of phosphate. The dihydroxy metabolite is also the form of the vitamin which is active in bone mobilization when the occasion demands it.

DeLuca[32] considers the active metabolite of vitamin D_3 a hormone since it is manufactured in one organ (the kidney) and functions in another (intestine and bone). As a hormone its production must be regulated in some way by the levels of calcium and phosphorus in the serum. Boyle,[51] Omdahl,[52] and Henry,[53] have shown that the production of the dihydroxy form of the vitamin is enhanced when hypocalcemia occurs and diminished when the serum calcium is elevated. The picture was further clarified by Garabedian,[54] who showed that thyroparathyroidectomized rats no longer produced 1,25-dihydroxyvitamin D_3 when serum calcium fell, but that injection of parathyroid

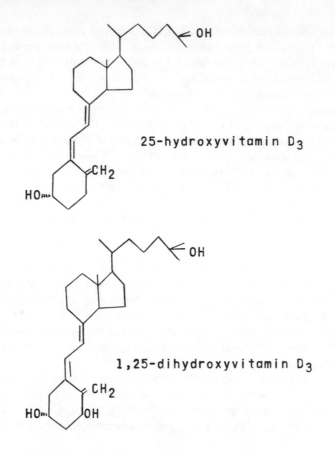

FIGURE 2.   Metabolites of vitamin D₃ formed from vitamin
D₃ in liver (upper) and from 25-hydroxyvitamin D₃ in kidney
(lower).

hormone restored this ability. We can therefore conclude that a fall in serum calcium
stimulates the secretion of parathyroid hormone which in turn stimulates the biosynthesis of 1,25-dihydroxyvitamin D₃. These two hormones then act in concert to stimulate renal reabsorption of calcium and mobilization of calcium from bone.[32]

D. Inorganic Elements

The mineral of bone resembles that of hydroxyapatite ($Ca_{10} [PO_4]_6[OH]_2$). Calcium
and phosphate, however, may form amorphous salts on the way to becoming crystalline and many other ions such as carbonate, sodium, potassium, and magnesium may
become a part of the hydration shell.[55] Fluoride also may become part of the structure,
replacing the hydroxyl group in the hydroxyapatite crystal. In areas with extremely
high levels of fluoride in the drinking water and where fluorosis occurs, osteosclerosis
is also endemic. The incorporation of fluoride into tooth enamel produces a tooth
which, because of the decreased solubility of the mineral structure, is more resistant
to dental caries. The bones are also more dense and studies have shown a lower incidence of vertebral fractures in women 55 years of age or older in areas with high as
compared to those with low fluoride content in the water. A denser bone is not necessarily stronger than one less dense and rats dosed with excessive amounts of fluoride
have shown abnormal bone structures.[56]

Zinc deficiency leads to impairment in collagen synthesis and crosslinking and in
the incorporation of methionine into protein.[57] Thus it could exert an effect on bone
formation and healing.

In 1972 two papers appeared which reported the essentiality of silicon for the chick[58] and for the rat.[59] Later it was shown that silicon plays a role in cartilage formation,[60] and most recently a very careful study by Carlisle indicates a requirement of silicon for normal skull and long bone formation in the chick.[61,62] Whether silicon is essential for man is not proven and its ubiquity makes studies on silicon deficiency extremely difficult.

E. Protein

Severe protein deficiency such as occurs with kwashiorkor can lead to retardation of bone development. In a study using monkeys, protein deficiency led to a lack of matrix deposition and a decrease in endochondral bone formation as well as a decreased cortical thickness.[63] Such a bone, then, would be less dense at maturity and so, perhaps, be more susceptible to osteoporosis.

Many nutrients which are essential for proper bone formation, such as vitamin A, vitamin D, calcium, zinc, etc. rely on binding proteins in the serum for their transport. A deficiency of protein may therefore decrease the utilization of these substances.

II. CHANGES IN THE SKELETON WITH AGE

In a recent paper Vogel[64] recounts some of the history of studies on the changes which occur in aging bones. In 1876 Rauber demonstrated a decrease in bone strength with increasing age and others since then have corroborated and extended these observations. Lindahl and Lindgren[65] studied the tensile strength of bones from humans ages 20 to 80 years and found a decrease with age. In his recent work, Vogel has demonstrated that the changes which occur in rat bone with maturation and with aging are distinct from each other. The content of insoluble collagen increases with maturation and then decreases with aging concurrently with the changes in tensile strength, thus emphasizing the importance of the organic as well as the inorganic constituents of bone.

Bone is a constantly renewing tissue and it has been estimated that normally 400 to 600 mg of calcium per day are turned over in bone resorption and remodeling. The turnover occurs most rapidly in the ribs, vertebrae, and long bones, and at a somewhat slower rate in the mandible and skull.[66] As long as bone formation equals bone resorption, the skeleton retains its mass. If, however, bone resorption is greater than bone formation, the condition known as osteoporosis results. Avioli has defined this as ''a reduction in bone mass below that which normally characterizes the skeleton for the age, sex, and race of an individual.''[66] Beginning with the fourth decade of life, bone density begins to decrease so that bone density at age 80 may be only one half that at age 40. This occurs somewhat earlier and proceeds more rapidly in the female than in the male.[54] The estimated rates of bone loss are 4% per decade for males and 8% for females.[66] In addition, in early adulthood the female skeleton is lighter than that of the male, the ratio of cortical area to body weight being 20% lower in females as compared to males.[66] As bone mass diminishes, fractures of the vertebrae, femur, and wrist occur. It is estimated that the incidence of vertebral fractures is about four times more frequent in women than in men and that femoral neck fractures occur 2.4 times more often in women.[63]

Changes in mandibular bone also occur with age, leading to a lessening of tooth support, a fenestration of roots, and eventual loss of teeth as is seen in periodontal disease.[66]

Skillman[67] speculates that clinical osteoporosis occurs most frequently in small-statured persons who therefore approach later years with a smaller bone mass than do their larger boned peers. Even though they may not be losing bone at a more rapid pace, more fragile bones will result at a younger age.

It is evident that postmenopausal women are at the highest risk for osteoporosis. In 1940 Albright et al.[68] speculated that estrogen decline led to a decline in osteoblastic function. While this has not been proven, it has been shown that estrogen secretion and bone mass decline concurrently. Bone remodeling has been found to increase somewhat after menopause but bone resorption also increases and at a greater rate, thus leading to a decrease in the skeletal mass.[69,70] Since an increase in bone resorption occurs with age, it is expected that levels of parathyroid hormone might also be found to increase and this has indeed been shown.[71] This increase is associated with a significantly lower serum ionized calcium and inorganic phosphate. Older women, in whom the rate of occurrence of osteoporosis is higher than that occurring in men, also show a higher level of serum parathyroid hormone.

It has been demonstrated that the efficiency of calcium absorption declines with age.[72] This is accompanied by lower levels of serum 1,25-dihydroxyvitamin D,[73] the efficiency of calcium absorption having been shown to be positively correlated ($r = 0.50$) with serum levels of the dihydroxyvitamin D metabolite.[74] Osteoporotic women show a greatly decreased absorption of calcium when compared with nonosteoporotic subjects matched for years since the menopause.[73] These differences occur in the presence of normal serum levels of 25-hydroxyvitamin D, suggesting a defect in the production of the dihydroxy metabolite. DeLuca speculates that since in his studies the serum level of parathyroid hormone in osteoporotic subjects was either normal or low, even with low levels of serum calcium, the defect could be due to the failure of the parathyroid to produce the hormone, although an actual defect in the metabolism of 25-hydroxyvitamin D to the 1,25-dihydroxy form (such as occurs in old rats) is also a possibility.[74]

It has been seen that parathyroid hormone stimulates the production of 1,25-dihydroxyvitamin D by the kidney. Recently the treatment of thyroparathyroidectomized rats with parathyroid extract resulted in a fourfold increase in the conversion of ^{3}H-25-hydroxyvitamin D to 1,25-dihydroxyvitamin D over that occurring in similar rats which did not receive the injection.[75] Aarskog and Aksnes[76] infused parathyroid hormone extract in three children presenting with different disorders of calcium metabolism and observed a 32 to 64% rise in serum levels of 1,25-dihydroxyvitamin D. Such a rise as a result of parathyroid hormone treatment has also been seen in adults.[77]

In a study using Japanese quail, Castillo and associates[78] found that the administration of estradiol stimulated the formation of 1,25-dihydroxyvitamin D from its monohydroxy precursor to a greater extent than did the injection of parathyroid hormone and that the effect of the administration of both hormones was additive. Thus a mechanism for a postmenopausal decrease in calcium absorption becomes evident.

In the face of the evidence, then, it would seem that osteoporosis could result either from increased levels of parathyroid hormone which could lead to increased mobilization of calcium from bone or to decreased levels of parathyroid hormone which would lead to decreased circulating levels of 1,25-dihydroxyvitamin D and a resulting faulty absorption of dietary calcium. Either condition could be accompanied by a low estrogen level.

As with many of the diseases which are more common in the older population, osteoporosis is likely to be multicausal. Observations on the occurrence of osteoporosis have shown differences between various population groups. For example, in a study of hospital admissions of patients 75 years of age and older, the incidence of hip fractures in white women exceeded that in black women by a ratio of about 3:1.[79] This difference was not attributable to socioeconomic status or to age. Jowsey[63] states that blacks have a larger skeletal mass at maturity and that, as was pointed out earlier, males possess a heavier skeleton than females. In addition, blacks lose bone less rapidly than do whites.[80] Jowsey[63] speculates that this is due to a slower rate of bone resorption.

It has been shown that just as stress will result in a larger muscle mass, so stress on the skeleton results in heavier bones. Saville in comparing individuals with and without osteoporosis found that a greater proportion of osteoporotic subjects than nonosteoporotics weighed less than 140 lbs.[81] Jowsey[63] points out that this protective effect of heavier body weight could occur because of the increased stress on the bone as well as due to an increased store of estrogens in the larger amount of fatty tissue which one would expect to find in heavier persons. Long distance runners (average age 55) have been shown to have a greater bone density than normal volunteers (average age 53).[82] Weight-bearing activities, such as walking, but not horizontal exercises, reversed the well-documented bone loss which occurs with immobilization.[63]

Increased loss of bone occurs with immobilization[63] and an immobilized limb will show a decrease in bone mass while the whole skeleton will retain its original amount of bone. Bone loss as reflected in a rise in serum ionized calcium levels and in hypercalciuria as well as in quantitative roentgenography is also seen in astronauts and other subjects who are maintained in a condition of zero gravity. Measurements of serum levels of parathyroid hormone show an increase which could be responsible for the increased bone resorption.[63]

III. ROLE OF NUTRITION IN THE ETIOLOGY OF OSTEOPOROSIS

We have discussed the importance of dietary sources of protein, of vitamins A, C, and D, and of the various mineral elements in the proper formation of bone. We have also considered the differences between the sexes and between various population groups in the skeletal mass at maturity and in the incidence of osteoporosis.

On the surface, it would seem reasonable to indict a low intake of calcium or a faulty calcium to phosphorus ratio or an inadequate supply of vitamin D as major factors in the etiology of osteoporosis. The picture is, however, more complicated. For example, black women show far less osteoporosis than do white women,[63] and yet data from HANES[83] show their intake of calcium to be lower than that of whites. The mean daily intake of calcium at age 1 to age 11 for white females increases from 956 to 1145 mg and for black females it goes from 689 to 775 mg. If we look at calcium intake during the postmenopausal years of 55 to 64, we see a consumption of 591 mg for white and 434 for black. Clearly calcium intake is not the whole story.

The HANES summary[83] does not indicate phosphorus or vitamin D intake, but if we take the prevalence of bowed legs and of knock-knees as an indicator of vitamin D nutriture, we find an increase in these two conditions in the blacks. For example, at age 45 to 49 the prevalence of bowed legs is 4.3% for whites of both sexes compared to 7.3% for blacks and of knock-knees it is 1.0% and 3.5% for whites and blacks, respectively. These parameters, of course, reflect nutrient intake in early life and tell us nothing about what happens in the later years.

A recent study in Yugoslavia[84] shows a difference in bone density and occurrence of wrist and femoral fractures between the populations of two areas of Yugoslavia which differ mainly in their calcium intake. In the high-calcium district the mean daily intake of calcium for males and females age 40 to 42 was 1087 and 940 mg, respectively, compared with 517 and 445 mg in the low-calcium area. Older residents of these areas (70 to 72 years) consumed 75 to 88% of the amount of calcium consumed by the younger group. The calcium:phosphorus ratio ranged from 0.45 to 0.68. In both sexes, bone density as measured by metacarpal cortical width was lower in the inhabitants of the low-calcium district and in both areas it was lower in older residents than in the younger ones, and lower in females than in males. An investigation of femoral fractures for the years 1968 to 73 showed an annual rate for women in the high-calcium district which ranged from 0.545/10,000 at ages 35 to 39 to 14.922 for those 75 and over. In the low-calcium area the values were 0.497 to 53.638, respectively. For males, the rates at ages 35 to 39 and at age 75 and over were 0.264 and 10.913, respectively, in the high-calcium area compared to 1.861 and 30.531 at those same ages in the low-calcium district. Thus age, sex, and calcium intake combined to determine the rate of femoral fractures. No significant difference in the occurrence of wrist fractures was found with differing calcium intake but women showed an incidence about twice that of the men. These data indicate a determining role for calcium in osteoporesis.

The inverse relationship seen in this study between the occurrence of bone fractures and the density of the bone when measured as early in life as at age 30, bolsters the contention of these workers and of others[85,86] that a larger bone mass at maturity exerts a protective effect against severe osteoporosis at a later age. In a further investigation of this, Mickelsen and co-workers[87] found no significant differences in cortical bone density of 200 lacto-ovo-vegetarian women in their third, fourth, and fifth decades of life and that of 71 Michigan omnivorous women of the same age. This finding is interesting in the light of their earlier finding that in similar groups of women in the same area who were 60 to 89 years of age, the bone density of the lacto-ovo-vegetarian women was significantly greater than that of the omnivores.[88] Since milk intake of the groups did not differ, the authors assume comparable calcium intake in the two groups of women and speculate, therefore, that the meat intake of the omnivorous women may play a role in increased bone loss seen after the menopause.

As long ago as 1920 Sherman[89] showed an increase in calcium excretion in the urine in human subjects as their meat intake increased. In 1931[90] it was suggested that increasing the acid ash producing substances in the diet would increase the urinary excretion of calcium, bone resorption acting as a buffering agent to maintain the proper pH of the blood. This finding has been verified by others.[91-93] Several workers[93-101] have also observed increased calcium excretion with increased protein intake in both rats and in man.

Recently Schuette, Zemel, and Linkswiler[102] studied the effect of high (110 to 113 g/day) and low (43 to 50 g/day) protein diets on renal function, calcium excretion, and the levels of circulating parathyroid hormone and of plasma 1,25-dihydroxyvitamin D in five men (ages 44 to 86) and six women (ages 65 to 79). There was no significant difference between the sexes in any of the parameters measured and so the data were pooled. An increase in protein intake resulted in a significant mean rise in urinary calcium (from 102 to 188 mg), all subjects responding to the dietary change with increased excretion. The mean value for calcium absorption did not change although five of the eleven subjects showed increased absorption. The mean calcium balance decreased significantly from 8 to −62 mg/day as protein intake increased. No effect of the level of protein in the diet on magnesium or phosphorus balance was observed. Urinary sulfate also increased with increased protein intake and correlated (r = 0.760) with urinary calcium. Serum parathyroid hormone was not modified by change in protein intake nor was the level of 1,25-dihydroxyvitamin D. The authors also found a mean decrease in the fractional renal tubular resorption of calcium with increased protein intake. They conclude that the level of protein intake influences the renal handling of calcium and that is what is responsible for the calciuria observed. This conclusion is in harmony with that of other studies showing an increase in glomerular filtration rate with a rise in protein intake.[103,104]

Since urinary sulfate and urinary calcium are positively correlated, it is of interest to compare the effects of proteins which differ in their content of sulfur-containing amino acids. Whiting and Draper[105] have studied urinary calcium in adult rats consuming diets high in lactalbumin, egg white, casein, or gelatin. These proteins contain 367, 395, 218, and 56 mg of sulfur amino acids per gram of total nitrogen, respectively.[106] The high protein diets were prepared by adding 24 g of nitrogen per kilogram of diet

Table 1

SULFUR-CONTAINING AMINO ACID CONTENT OF SELECTED PROTEINS

Protein	Sulfur-containing amino acids (mg/g of total nitrogen)[106]
Egg white	395
Egg yolk	265
Lactalbumin	367
Casein	218
Beef	234
Pork	229
Chicken	247
Lamb	232
Fish	266
Lima beans	136
Peas	118
Soy	195
Corn	226
Wheat	217

Data from Orr, M. L. and Watt, B. K., Amino Acid Content of Foods, Home Econ. Res. Rep. No. 4, U.S. Department of Agriculture, Washington, D.C., 1968.

in the form of the protein studied to a basal diet containing 24 g nitrogen per kilogram of diet as casein. If the amount of urinary calcium of rats on the basal diet was equated to 100, then the calcium excretion of rats on the high lactalbumin diet was 489; for high egg white, 429; for high casein, 340; and for high gelatin, 263. These were the peak values occurring at day 2. That adaptation to these high protein diets occurs is seen in the finding of relative urinary calcium values of 200, 183, 160, and 136, respectively, at the end of the 8-week experimental period. If the basal diet was supplemented with sulfur-containing amino acids in such a way as to make it equivalent to the high lactalbumin diet, a comparable level of calcium excretion occurred. Throughout these experiments, sulfate excretion paralleled that of calcium. From this series of experiments the authors conclude that the intake of sulfur-containing amino acids is the determining factor regulating the increased calcium excretion seen with high protein diets.

In the work cited above, the evidence is strong for a determining role of sulfur amino acids in the regulation of calcium excretion. Table 1 shows the content of these amino acids in some proteins commonly consumed by man. The vegetable proteins in general contain lesser amounts of the sulfur amino acids, legumes ranking among the lowest. It is the low level of these amino acids which is responsible for the poor quality of proteins derived from legumes, methionine being an essential ingredient of the human diet. Most animal proteins such as beef, pork, chicken, lamb, and fish fall in the same category as the cereal grains such as corn and wheat with a protein of milk (lactalbumin) and egg (white) containing the highest amounts of these substances. It is probable, therefore, that very high protein diets as are usually consumed will contain sulfur-containing amino acids at a level which could lead to an increased acid load and consequently to a heightened rate of bone resorption. It is likely that the level of protein intake at which this will occur varies with the individual as well as with the level of ingestion of other components of the diet. It must be recognized that conditions which lead to ketosis such as diabetes, fasting, and ketogenic reducing diets also call forth a buffering response and may, therefore, contribute to bone resorption.

IV. THERAPY OF OSTEOPOROSIS

It is beyond the scope of this chapter to evaluate in depth the various forms of therapy for osteoporosis. It should be noted, however, that most treatments are based on the findings reported above. Among the medications in use are estrogens, calcium, strontium, fluoride, phosphate, diphosphonates, calcitonin, growth hormone, vitamin D, vitamin C, and vitamin A, used singly or in combination.[63,107]

Among the forms of therapy currently under test is that which stems from the pioneering studies of Jowsey and co-workers at the Mayo Clinic, utilizing fluoride, calcium, and vitamin D[108] and based on the facts that fluoride will stimulate osteoblastic functions and calcium and vitamin D will aid in mineralization of the newly formed bone tissue. Results of this treatment indicate bone resorption is unchanged or slightly decreased accompanied by an increase in bone formation, resulting in an increase in bone mass. Riggs et al.[109] have recently reported a lower incidence of vertebral fractures in patients on this combination therapy.

Clinical trials are now underway utilizing 1,25-dihydroxyvitamin D or 1α-hydroxyvitamin D either with or without calcium supplementation to aid in the absorption of calcium.[73,74] If the ability to absorb calcium decreases with age and if it can be shown that the osteoporotic patient has a decreased circulating level of the dihydroxy metabolite of vitamin D, this approach should prove beneficial.

Recently Haas and co-workers[110] administered 1,25-dihydroxyvitamin D_3 for 6 months to 4 osteoporotic patients. In three of them they observed a change from a negative to a positive calcium balance and a rise in serum ionized calcium, accompanied by slight changes in bone resorption and formation.

Crilly and associates[73] compared six treatments for osteoporosis by measuring their effects on calcium balance, on total daily urinary hydroxyproline (a measure of collagen turnover and hence of bone turnover), and on the mean rates of metacarpal cortical bone loss in postmenopausal osteoporotic and nonosteoporotic women. All three measurements gave comparable results. The most successful treatments were estrogens, especially when combined with vitamin D metabolites, and calcium supplements. High doses of vitamin D combined with calcium were intermediate in effectiveness, and the least successful of the treatments studied were vitamin D and 1-α hydroxyvitamin D when given alone.

The well-known toxic effects of overdoses of fluoride, vitamin D, and of calcium[56] are factors which mandate caution in the use of these new therapies or indeed of any therapies designed to reverse the course of osteoporosis. Clearly this is not a field for "do-it-yourself" medicine and the public must be warned repeatedly about the dangers inherent in the overdosages of these substances.

V. PERSPECTIVE

Dr. R. N. Butler, Director of the National Institute of Aging, has pinpointed osteoporosis as one of the major problems of old age.[111] The resulting fractures cause at least temporary incapacitation. Vertebral fractures, in particular, immobilize many of the aged each year and the accompanying pain and restriction of physical activities contribute greatly to the frustrations of old age.

Methods for preventing osteoporosis must be found and followed. This however may not be easy to do. Certain conditions which frequently accompany old age have been shown to predispose to osteoporosis. Diabetics are reported to show a decrease in calcium absorption and increased loss when compared to nondiabetic controls and to suffer from vertebral and femoral fractures.[111-114] Schneider et al. have determined that the circulating level of 1,25-dihydroxyvitamin D but not of 25-hydroxyvitamin D is reduced by 65% in the experimentally diabetic rat.[115] Spencer and associates have shown this to be due to a defect in the synthesis of the hormone rather than its increased catabolism. The hormone level is restored upon administration of insulin.[116] As was noted previously, the ketosis which frequently accompanies diabetes may also lead to an increase in bone resorption, a condition which also is alleviated by insulin.

Although anticonvulsive drugs have been implicated as agents predisposing to bone loss due to their stimulatory effect on vitamin D metabolism by the hepatic microsomal enzyme systems, a recent study by Barden et al.[117] has shown no such effect. In 53 residents of a facility for the mentally disturbed, osteopenia was present equally in residents receiving anticonvulsant therapy and those who did not. This was corrected in both groups by multivitamin therapy. The hypocalcemia seen in anticonvulsive therapy, however, was not corrected by this supplementation.

If methods could be found for the early identification of those who are at high risk for osteoporosis, perhaps measures could be taken to slow the rate of bone loss. It has been suggested that since the loss of alveolar bone precedes by about one decade the reported occurrence of skeletal bone loss, that radiographic density of alveolar bone be measured by means of a microphotodensitometer to identify those who are at risk for serious osteoporosis in later life. A method for this has been developed by Albanese[118] who has applied it to 221 normal healthy females (15 to 75 years) and 105 males (15 to 78 years). He found an age-related correlation between the density of the alveolar bone and that of the phalanx measured at the same time. If such measurements were done along with periodic dental examinations, it might be possible to pick up early bone loss and then to institute preventive measures before severe osteoporosis occurs.

Since it is increasingly clear that prevention of osteoporosis is a matter of high priority, studies which more clearly delineate differences between those who show severe symptoms of the disease and those who don't must be undertaken. It is reasonable to assume that a bone which is thicker at maturity will be more resistant to fractures in later life as bone resorption sets in. Observations[87,88] on vegetarian and nonvegetarian women, however, have shown that thick bone may not be a necessary condition for relative resistance to osteoporosis. More attention should perhaps be paid to the calcium:phosphorus ratio in the diet.

During the course of an investigation for another study, we found in the female population an average dietary calcium to phosphorus ratio of 0.82 for Seventh-Day Adventist lacto-ovo-vegetarians, 0.96 for Seventh Day Adventist nonvegetarians, and 0.61 in a matched set from the general population. The mean daily calcium intake for these same groups was 833, 1151, and 659 mg, respectively, while the protein intake was 51, 71, and 66 g per day.[119] These values reflect different dietary patterns. If women such as these can be followed in a prospective study with concurrent assessment of nutrient intakes and of bone status, more clues regarding protective or predisposing factors for osteoporosis may be gathered.

Studies on the mechanisms underlying bone resorption are also needed. In recent times the observations that members of space crews have shown calciuria, rarefaction of trabecular bone, and increased risk of kidney stone formation have enlarged our understanding. That these changes were unaccompanied by changes in any of the hormones involved in osteoclastic or osteoblastic activity and were unaffected by diet, further emphasizes the complexity of the matter.[120] Animal studies may furnish some information on the effect of immobilization.

The supplementation of hypokinetic rats with physiological doses of 1-α-hydroxyvitamin D prevented hypocalcemia and bone demineralization but led to aortal calcination when the diet contained a calcium:phosphorus ratio of 1:3. Little effect was seen, however, with an optimal calcium:phosphorus ratio.[121]

If the trend to encourage the ingestion of high fiber diets which are high in phytates and oxalates continues, we must be aware of the hazard of decreased mineral absorption which may accompany this[122] and compensate for it by recommending higher intakes of calcium and other minerals. Some[123] advocate, in fact, discouraging the ingestion of substances such as these while encouraging the ingestion of calcium, phosphorus, vitamin D, vitamin C, and protein. They further suggest that the intake of calcium be spread out throughout the day since small amounts of calcium are absorbed more efficiently than are larger amounts.

HANES[80] and other studies both in Sweden[124] and the United States[125,126] have shown daily intakes of calcium by elderly women considerably lower than the 800-mg recommendation by the United States Food and Nutrition Board.[127] While no clear-cut evidence exists that this fact accounts for the incidence of osteoporosis, an attempt to correct this deficiency would seem to be in order.

In view of the findings discussed above that the ingestion of diets containing high levels of proteins composed of relatively large amounts of the sulfur-containing amino acids leads to increased urinary excretion of calcium, one is tempted to recommend diets low in such proteins. The proteins which are low in sulfur amino acids, however, are of poor quality since they are low in the essential amino acid, methionine. The diets of vegetarians, on the other hand, are frequently high in dairy products whose proteins are a rich source of the sulfur amino acids. They do, however, possess a favorable calcium to phosphorous ratio and there is evidence that the consumption of these diets may, in fact, protect against osteoporosis.[88]

It would seem wise, therefore, to consume a diet containing a mixture of proteins at a moderate level, an adequate but not excessive amount of fiber, and a reasonable quantity of dairy products while avoiding large intakes of those dietary ingredients, such as carbonated beverages, which are high in phosphorus.

VI. SUMMARY

The role of nutrition in skeletal development has been recognized for many years and the function of vitamins A, C, and D, certain inorganic elements, and protein have been thoroughly described. Severe deficiencies of these nutrients lead to well-recognized clinical symptoms while less severe deficiencies may result in bone which is less dense at maturity.

As the organism ages, bone resorption proceeds at a faster rate than bone formation resulting in a loss of bone tissue. The female skeleton is less dense at maturity than is the male skeleton and bone loss occurs at a more rapid rate. Thus osteoporosis occurs more frequently in females than in males. It is also more common in whites than in blacks.

The role played by nutrition in this process is not clearly defined. Dietary deficiencies of calcium, fluoride, and vitamin D, protein excess, and ketogenic diets have all been implicated. Osteoporosis is probably multicausal and so other conditions which commonly accompany aging such as low serum estrogen levels, decreased levels of circulating 1,25-dihydroxyvitamin D, reduced physical activity, and impairment of calcium absorption contribute to the syndrome.

Therapies for osteoporosis utilizing some or all of the above factors are being actively pursued in many centers. At the same time the search for methods to prevent the disease is continuing. Early identification of potential osteoporotics by routine X-ray of alveolar bone at the time of dental check-ups is being evaluated. Links between osteoporosis and other disorders of calcium metabolism such as kidney stones and bursitis are being sought. Basic studies on the mechanisms underlying bone resorption are being pursued.

The widespread occurrence of osteoporosis and the severity of the handicaps it imposes on the older members of our society give impetus to further research into its causes, cure, and, ultimately, its prevention.

REFERENCES

1. McCollum, E. V., *A History of Nutrition,* Houghton Mifflin, Boston, 1957, 323.
2. Bourne, G. H., Vitamin C and bone, in *The Biochemistry and Physiology of Bone,* Vol. 2, 2nd ed., Bourne, G. H., Ed., Academic Press, New York, 1972, 231.
3. Bourne, G. H., Vitamin C and bone, in *The Biochemistry and Physiology of Bone,* Vol. 2, 2nd ed., Bourne, G. H., Ed., Academic Press, New York, 1972, 232.
4. Hodges, R. E., Ascorbic acid, in *Present Knowledge of Nutrition,* 4th ed., Nutrition Foundation, New York, 1976, chap. 13.
5. Park, E. A., Guild, H. G., Jackson, D., and Bond, M., Recognition of scurvy with special reference to early X-ray changes, *Arch. Dis. Child,* 10, 263, 1935.
6. Watson, R. C., Grossman, H., and Meyers, M. A., Radiological findings in nutritional disturbances, in *Modern Nutrition in Health and Disease,* 6th ed., Goodhart, R. S. and Shils, M. E., Eds., Lea and Febiger, Philadelphia, 1980, 642.
7. Gordon, G. S. and Vaughan, C., *Clinical Management of the Osteoporoses,* Publishing Sciences Group, Acton, Massachusetts, 1976, 103.
8. Hess, A. F., McCann, G. F., and Pappenheimer, A. M., Experimental rickets in rats. II. The failure of rats to develop rickets on a diet deficient in vitamin A, *J. Biol. Chem.,* 47, 395, 1921.
9. McCollum, E. V. and Davis, M., The necessity of certain lipins during growth, *J. Biol. Chem.,* 151, 167, 1913.
10. Wolbach, S. B. and Howe, P. R., The epithelial tissues on experimental xerophthalmia, *Proc. Soc. Exp. Biol. Med.,* 22, 402, 1925.
11. Mellanby, E., *A Story of Nutritional Research,* Williams & Wilkins, Baltimore, 1950.
12. Wolbach, S. B. and Hegsted, D. M., Vitamin deficiency in chick: skeletal growth and central nervous system, *A.M.A. Arch. Pathol.,* 54, 13, 1952.
13. Wolbach, S. B. and Hegsted, D. M., Vitamin A deficiency in duck: skeletal growth and central nervous system, *A.M.A. Arch. Pathol.,* 54, 548, 1952.
14. Perlman, H. B. and Willard, J., Ear in experimental vitamin A deficiency, *J. Am. Otolaryngol. Rhinol. Laryngol.,* 50, 349, 1941.
15. Perlman, H. B., Effect on ear of vitamin A feeding after severe depletion, *Arch. Otolaryngol.,* 50, 20, 1949.
16. Barnicot, N. A. and Datta, S. P., Vitamin A and bone, in *The Biochemistry and Physiology of Bone,* Vol. 2, 2nd ed., Bourne, G. H., Ed., Academic Press, New York, 1972, 204.
17. Collazo, J. A. and Sanchez-Rodriguez, J., Die Symptomatologie der durch Fütterung von reinem A-Vitamin an jungen Ratten hervorgerufenen Hypervitaminose A, und Hypervitaminose A: exophthalmus und Spontanfrakturen, *Klin. Wochenschr.,* 12, 1732 und 1768, 1933.
18. Caffey, J., Chronic poisoning due to excess vitamin A, *J. Roentgenol. Radium Ther.,* 65, 12, 1951.
19. Bair, G., Chronic vitamin A poisoning; report of a case, *JAMA,* 146, 1573, 1951.
20. Mellanby, E., An experimental investigation on rickets, *Lancet,* 1, 407, 1919.
21. McCollum, E. V., The history of nutrition, *World Rev. Nutr. Diet.,* 1, 3, 1959.
22. McCollum, E. V., Simmonds, N., Becker, J. E., and Shipley, P. G., Studies on experimental rickets. XXI. An experimental demonstration of the existence of a vitamin which promotes calcium deposition, *J. Biol. Chem.,* 53, 293, 1922.
23. McCollum, E. V., *A History of Nutrition,* Houghton Mifflin, Boston, 1957, 277.
24. Goldblatt, H. and Soames, K. M., LIV. Studies on the fat-soluble growth promoting factor, *Biochem. J.,* 17, 446, 1923.
25. Steenbock, H. and Black, A., Fat soluble vitamin. XVII. The induction of growth-promoting and calcifying properties in a ration by exposure to ultraviolet ray, *J. Biol. Chem.,* 61, 405, 1924.
26. Askew, F. A., Bourdillon, R. B., Bruce, H. M., Jenkins, R. C. G., and Webster, T. A., The distillation of vitamin D, *Proc. R. Soc. B.,* 107, 76, 1931.
27. Windaus, A., Schenck, F., and von Werder, F., Über das antirachitisch wirksame Bestrahlungsprodukt aus 7-dehydrocholesterin, *Hoppe-Seyler's Z. Physiol. Chem.,* 241, 100, 1936.
28. Esvelt, R. P., Schnoes, H. K., and DeLuca, H. F., Vitamin D_3 from rat skins irradiated in vitro with ultraviolet light, *Arch. Biochem. Biophys.,* 188, 282, 1978.

29. Holick, M. F., Frommer, J. E., McNeill, S. C., Richland, N. M., Henley, J. W., and Potts, J. T., Jr., Photometabolism of 7-dehydrocholesterol to previtamin D_3 in skin, *Biochem. Biophys. Res. Comm.*, 76, 107, 1977.

30. McCollum, E. V., Orent-Keiles, E., and Day, H., *The Newer Knowledge of Nutrition*, 5th ed., MacMillan, New York, 1939, chap. 15.

31. Shipley, P. G., Kramer, B., and Howland, J., Calcification in vitro, *Biochem. J.*, 20, 379, 1926.

32. DeLuca, H. F., The vitamin D system in the regulation of calcium and phosphorus metabolism, Eleventh W. O. Atwater Memorial Lecture, *Nutr. Rev.*, 37, 161, 1979.

33. McCollum, E. V., Simmonds, N., Parsons, H. T., Shipley, P. G., and Park, E. A., Studies on experimental rickets. I. The production of rachitis and similar diseases in the rat by deficient diets, *J. Biol. Chem.*, 45, 333, 1921.

34. Shipley, P. G., Park, E. A., McCollum, E. V., Simmonds, N., and Parsons, H. T., II. The effect of cod liver oil administered to rats with experimental rickets, *J. Biol. Chem.*, 45, 343, 1921.

35. McCollum, E. V., Simmonds, N., Shipley, P. G., and Park, E. A., Studies on experimental rickets. IV. Cod liver oil as contrasted with butter fat in the protection against the effects of insufficient calcium in the diet, *Proc. Soc. Exp. Biol. Med.*, 18, 275, 1921.

36. McCollum, E. V., Simmonds, N., Shipley, P. G., and Park, E. A., Studies on experimental rickets. VIII. The production of rickets by diets low in phosphorus and fat-soluble A, *J. Biol. Chem.*, 47, 507, 1921.

37. Howard, G. A. and Baylink, D. J., Matrix formation and osteoid maturation in vitamin D-deficient rats made normocalcemic by dietary means, *Miner. Electrolyte Metab.*, 3, 44, 1980.

38. Linkswiler, H., Calcium, in *Present Knowledge in Nutrition*, 4th ed., Nutrition Foundation, New York, 1976, 233.

39. DeLuca, H. F., Some new studies emanating from a study of the metabolism and function of vitamin D (William C. Rose Lecture), *Nutr. Rev.*, 38, 169, 1980.

40. Nicolaysen, R., Studies upon mode of action of vitamin D: absorption of phosphates from isolated loops of small intestine in rat, *Biochem. J.*, 31, 122, 1937.

41. Nicolayson, R., Eeg-Larsen, N., and Malm, O. J., Physiology of calcium metabolism, *Physiol. Rev.*, 33, 424, 1953.

42. Harrison, H. E. and Harrison, H. C., Intestinal transport of phosphate, *Am. J. Physiol.*, 201, 1007, 1961.

43. Carlsson, A., On mechanism of skeletal turnover of lime salts, *Acta Physiol. Scand.*, 26, 212, 1952.

44. Rasmussen, H., DeLuca, H. F., Arnaud, C., Hawker, C., and von Stedingk, M., The relationship between vitamin D and parathyroid hormone, *J. Clin. Invest.*, 42, 1940, 1963.

45. Lund, J. and DeLuca, H. F., Biologically active metabolite of vitamin D_3 from bone, liver, and blood serum, *J. Lipid Res.*, 7, 739, 1966.

46. Morii, H., Lund, J., Neville, P. F., and DeLuca, H. F., Biological activity of a vitamin D metabolite, *Arch. Biochem. Biophys.*, 120, 508, 1967.

47. Blunt, J. W., DeLuca, H. F., Schnoes, H. K., 25-hydroxycholecalciferol, a biologically active metabolite of vitamin D, *Biochemistry*, 7, 3317, 1968.

48. Holick, M. F., Schnoes, H. K., and DeLuca, H. F., Identification of 1,25-dihydroxycholecalciferol, a form of vitamin D_3 metabolically active in the intestine, *Proc. Nat. Acad. Sci.*, 68, 803, 1971.

49. Lawson, D. E. M., Fraser, D. R., Kodicek, E., Morris, H. R., and Williams, D. H., Identification of 1,25-dihydroxycholecalciferol, a new kidney hormone controlling calcium metabolism, *Nature*, 230, 228, 1971.

50. Norman, A. W., Myrtle, J. F., Midgett, R. J., Nowicki, H. G., Williams, V., and Popjack, G., 1,25-dihydrocholecalciferol: identification of the proposed active form of vitamin D_3 in the intestine, *Science*, 173, 51, 1971.

51. Boyle, I. T., Gray, R. W., Omdahl, J. L., and DeLuca, H. F., *Endocrinology 1971* Proc. 3rd Int. Symp., Taylor, S., Ed., Wm. Heinemann Medical Books, London, 1972, 468.

52. Omdahl, J. L., Gray, R. W., Boyle, I. T., Knutson, J., and DeLuca, H. F., Regulation of metabolism of 25-hydroxycholecalciferol by kidney tissue in vitro by dietary calcium, *Nat. New Biol.*, 237, 63, 1972.

53. Henry, H. L., Midgett, R. J., and Norman, A. W., Regulation of 25-hydroxyvitamin D_3-1-hydroxylase in vivo, *J. Biol. Chem.*, 249, 7584, 1974.

54. Avioli, L. V., What to do with "Postmenopausal osteoporosis", *Am. J. Med.*, 65, 881, 1978.

55. Raisz, L. G., Bone metabolism and calcium regulation, in *Metabolic Bone Disease*, Avioli, L. and Krane, S. M., Eds., Academic Press, New York, 1977, chap. 1.

56. Gordan, G. S. and Vaughan, C., *Clinical Management of the Osteoporoses*, Publishing Sciences Group, Acton, Massachusetts, 1976, chap. 8.

57. Sandstead, H. H., Zinc, in *Present Knowledge in Nutrition*, 4th ed., Nutrition Foundation, New York, 1976, 292.

58. Carlisle, E. M., Silicon, an essential element for the chick, *Science*, 178, 619, 1972.

59. Schwarz, K. and Milne, D. B., Growth-promoting effect of silicon in rats, *Nature,* 239, 333, 1972.
60. Carlisle, E. M., In vivo requirements for silicon in articular cartilage and connective tissue formation in the chick, *J. Nutr.,* 106, 478, 1976.
61. Carlisle, E. M., A silicon requirement for normal skull formation in chicks, *J. Nutr.,* 110, 352, 1980.
62. Carlisle, E. M., Biochemical and morphological changes associated with long bone abnormalities in silicon deficiency, *J. Nutr.,* 110, 1046, 1980.
63. Jowsey, J., *Metabolic Diseases of Bone: Saunders Monograph in Clinical Orthopedics,* Vol. 1, W. B. Saunders, Philadelphia, 1977, 256.
64. Vogel, H. G., Influence of maturation and aging in mechanical and biochemical parameters of rat bone, *Gerontology,* 25, 16, 1979.
65. Lindahl, O. and Lindgren, G. H., Cortical bone mass, *Acta Orthop. Scand.,* 38, 133, 1967.
66. Avioli, L. V., Osteoporosis: pathogenesis and therapy, in *Metabolic Bone Disease,* Vol. 1, Avioli, L. V. and Krane, S. M., Eds., Academic Press, New York, 1977, 311ff.
67. Skillman, T. G., Can osteoporosis be prevented?, *Geriatrics,* 35, 95, 1980.
68. Albright, F., Bloomberg, E., and Smith, P. H., Postmenopausal osteoporosis, *Trans. Assoc. Am. Physicians,* 55, 298, 1940.
69. Heaney, R. P., Recker, R. R., and Saville, P. D., Menopausal changes in calcium balance performance, *J. Lab. Clin. Med.,* 92, 953, 1978.
70. Heaney, R. P., Recker, R. R., and Saville, P. D., Menopausal changes in bone remodeling, *J. Lab. Clin. Med.,* 92, 964, 1978.
71. Wiske, P. S., Epstein, S. I., and Bell, N. H., Increases in immunoreactive parathyroid hormone with age, *N. Engl. J. Med.,* 300, 1419, 1979.
72. Bullamore, J. R., Gallagher, J. C., Wilkinson, R., Nordin, B. E. C., and Marshall, T. H., Effect of age on calcium absorption, *Lancet,* 2, 252, 1970.
73. Crilly, R., Horsman, A., Marshall, D. H., and Nordin, B. E. C., Prevalence, pathogenesis, and treatment of postmenopausal osteoporosis, *Aust. N. Z. J. Med.,* 9, 24, 1979.
74. Gallagher, J. C., Riggs, B. L., Eisman, J., Hamstra, A., Arnaud, S. B., and DeLuca, H. F., Intestinal calcium absorption and serum vitamin D metabolites in normal subjects and osteoporotic patients, *J. Clin. Invest.,* 64, 729, 1979.
75. Rader, J. I., Howard, G. A., Feist, E., Turner, R. T., and Baylink, D. J., Bone mineralization and metabolism of ^{3}H-25-hydroxyvitamin D_3 in thyroparathyroidectomized rats treated with parathyroid extract, *Calcium Tissue Int.,* 29, 21, 1979.
76. Aarskog, D. and Aksnes, L., Acute response of plasma 1,25-dihydroxyvitamin D to parathyroid hormone, *Lancet,* 1, 362, 1980.
77. Eisman, J. A., Wark, J. D., Prince, R. L., and Moseley, J. M., Modulation of plasma 1,25-dihydroxyvitamin D in man by stimulation and suppression tests, *Lancet,* 2, 931, 1979.
78. Castillo, L., Tanaka, Y., DeLuca, H. F., and Sunde, M. L., The stimulation of 25-hydroxyvitamin D_3-1α-hydroxylase by estrogen, *Arch. Biochem. Biophys.,* 179, 211, 1977.
79. Moldawer, M., Zimmerman, S. J., and Collins, L. C., Incidence of osteoporosis in elderly whites and elderly negroes, *JAMA,* 194, 111, 1965.
80. Trotter, M., Broman, G. E., and Peterson, R. R., Densities of bone of white and negro skeletons, *J. Bone Jt. Surg.,* 42A, 50, 1960.
81. Saville, P. D., Observations on 80 women with osteoporotic spine fractures, in *Osteoporosis,* Marzel, U. S., Ed., Grune and Stratton, New York, 1970, 38.
82. Dalen, N. and Olsson, K. E., Bone mineral content and physical activity, *Acta Orthop. Scand.,* 45, 170, 1974.
83. Dietary Intake Source Data United States 1971-74, DHEW Publ. No. (PHS) 79-1221, U.S. Department of Health, Education, and Welfare, Hyattsville, Md., 1979.
84. Matković, V., Kostial, D., Simonović, I., Buzino, R. L., Brodarec, A., and Nordin, B. E. C., Bone status and fracture rates in two regions of Yugoslavia, *Am. J. Clin. Nutr.,* 32, 540, 1979.
85. Garn, S. M., Rohman, C. G., and Wagner, B., Bone loss as a general phenomenon in man, *Fed. Proc.,* 26, 1729, 1967.
86. Newton-John, H. F. and Morgan, D. B., The loss of bone with age, osteoporosis, and fractures, *Clin. Orthop.,* 71, 229, 1970.
87. Marsh, A. G., Sanchez, T. V., Mickelsen, O., Keiser, K., and Mayor, G., Cortical bone density of adult lacto-ovo-vegetarian and omnivorous women, *J. Am. Diet. Assoc.,* 76, 149, 1980.
88. Mickelsen, O., Personal communication, 1980.
89. Sherman, H. C., Calcium requirements for maintenance in man, *J. Biol. Chem.,* 44, 21, 1920.
90. Farquharson, R. F., Salter, W. T., and Aub, J. C., Studies of calcium and phosphorus metabolism. XIII. The effect of the ingestion of phosphates on the excretion of calcium, *J. Clin. Invest.,* 10, 251, 1931.
91. Lemann, J., Jr., Litzow, J. R., and Lennon, E. J., Studies of the mechanism by which chronic metabolic acidosis augments urinary calcium excretion in man, *J. Clin. Invest.,* 46, 1318, 1967.

92. Lennon, E. J. and Lemann, J., Jr., Decreased tubular calcium reabsorption during chronic metabolic acidosis in man, *J. Clin. Invest.,* 46, 1083, 1967.

93. Martin, H. E. and Jones, R., The effect of ammonium chloride and sodium bicarbonate on the urinary excretion of magnesium, calcium, and phosphate, *Am. Heart J.,* 62, 208, 1931.

94. Engstrom, G. W. and DeLuca, H. F., Effect of egg white diets on calcium metabolism in the rat, *J. Nutr.,* 81, 218, 1963.

95. Bell, R. R., Englemann, D. T., Sie, T. L., and Draper, H. H., Effect of a high protein intake on calcium metabolism in the rat, *J. Nutr.,* 105, 475, 1975.

96. Allen, L. H. and Hall, T. E., Calcium metabolism, intestinal calcium binding protein, and bone growth of rats fed high protein diets, *J. Nutr.,* 108, 967, 1978.

97. Lemann, J., Relman, A. S., and Conners, H. P., The relation of sulfur metabolism to acid base balance and electrolyte excretion: the effects of DL-methionine in normal man, *J. Clin. Invest.,* 38, 2215, 1959.

98. Johnson, N. E., Alcantara, E. N., and Linkswiler, H., Effect of level of protein intake on urinary and fecal calcium and calcium retention of young adult males, *J. Nutr.,* 100, 1423, 1970.

99. Walker, R. M. and Linkswiler, H. M., Calcium retention in the adult human male as affected by protein intake, *J. Nutr.,* 102, 1297, 1972.

100. Linkswiler, H. M., Joyce, C. L., and Anand, C. R., Calcium retention of young adult males as affected by level of protein and of calcium intake, *Trans. N.Y. Acad. Sci.,* Series II, 36, 333, 1974.

101. Kim, Y. and Linkswiler, H. M., Effect of level of protein intake on calcium metabolism and on parathyroid and renal function in the adult male, *J. Nutr.,* 109, 1399, 1979.

102. Schuette, S. A., Zemel, M. B., and Linkswiler, H. M., Studies on the mechanism of protein induced hypercalciuria in older men and women, *J. Nutr.,* 110, 305, 1980.

103. Pullman, T. N., Alving, A. S., Dern, R. J., and Landowne, M., The influence of dietary protein intake on specific renal function in normal man, *J. Lab. Clin. Med.,* 44, 320, 1954.

104. White, H. L. and Rolf, D., Effects of exercise and of some other influences on renal circulation in man, *Am. J. Physiol.,* 152, 505, 1948.

105. Whiting, S. J. and Draper, H. H., The role of sulfate in the calciuria of high protein diets in adult rats, *J. Nutr.,* 110, 212, 1980.

106. Orr, M. L. and Watt, B. K., Amino Acid Content of Foods, Home Econ. Res. Rep. No. 4, U.S. Department of Agriculture, Washington, D.C., 1968.

107. Gordan, G. S. and Vaughan, C., *Clinical Management of the Osteoporoses,* Publishing Sciences Group, Acton, Massachusetts, 1976, 101.

108. Jowsey, J., Riggs, B. L., Kelly, P. J., and Hoffman, D. L., Effect of combined therapy with sodium fluoride, vitamin D, and calcium in osteoporosis, *Am. J. Med.,* 53, 43, 1972.

109. Riggs, B. L., Hodgson, S. F., Hoffman, D. L., Kelly, P. J., Johnson, K. A., and Taves, D., Treatment of primary osteoporosis with fluoride and calcium, *JAMA,* 243, 446, 1980.

110. Haas, H. G., Dambacher, M. A., Guncaga, J., Lauffenberger, T., Lämmle, B., and Olah, J., 1,25-(OH)$_2$ vitamin D$_3$ in osteoporosis — a pilot study, *Horm. Metab. Res.,* 11, 168, 1979.

111. Butler, R. N., Research: the ultimate service, *Aging,* 303—304, 4, 1980.

112. Levin, M. E., Boisseau, V. C., and Avioli, L. V., Effects of diabetes mellitus on bone mass in juvenile and adult onset diabetes, *N. Engl. J. Med.,* 294, 241, 1976.

113. Jurist, J. M., In vivo determination of the elastic response of bone. II. Ulnar resonant frequency in osteoporotic, diabetic, and normal subjects, *Phys. Med. Biol.,* 15, 427, 1970.

114. Neuman, H. W., Arnold, W. D., and Hein, W., Das Vorkommen eines Diabetes mellitus bei 201 Patienten mit Schenkelhalsfrakturen und Wirbelkörperkompressionfrakturen, *Zentrabl. Chirurgie,* 97, 831, 1972.

115. Schneider, L. E., Schedl, H. P., McCain, T., and Haussler, M. R., Experimental diabetes reduces circulating 1,25-dihydroxy-vitamin D in the rat, *Science,* 196, 1452, 1977.

116. Spencer, E. M., Khalil, M., and Tobiassen, O., Experimental diabetes in the rat causes an insulin-reversible decrease in renal 25-hydroxyvitamin D$_3$-1α-hydroxylase activity, *Endocrinology,* 107, 300, 1980.

117. Barden, H. S., Mazess, R. B., Rose, P. G., and McArveeney, W., Bone mineral status as measured by direct photon absorptiometry in institutionalized adults receiving long-term anticonvulsant therapy and multivitamin supplementation, *Calcif. Tissue Int.,* 31, 117, 1980.

118. Albanese, A. A., Bone loss: causes, detection, and therapy, in *Current Topics in Nutrition and Disease,* Vol. 1, A. R. Liss, New York, 1977.

119. Rider, A. A., unpublished observations, 1980.

120. Editorial, Bones in space, *Br. Med. J.,* 280, 1288, 1980.

121. Ushakov, A. S., Spirichev, V. B., Balakovsky, M. S., Blazhejevich, N. V., and Posdnyakov, A. L., Effect of 1-alpha-hydroxy-cholecalciferol and varying phosphorus content in the diet on calcium phosphorus metabolism in hypokinetic rats, *Aviation Space, Environ. Med.,* 51, 24, 1980.

122. Kelsay, J. L., Behall, K. M., and Prather, E. S., Effect of fiber from fruits and vegetables on metabolic responses of human subjects. II. Calcium, magnesium, iron, and silicon balances, *Am. J. Clin. Nutr.*, 32, 1876, 1979.

123. Anon., Calcium in bone health, *Dairy Counc. Dig.*, 47, 31, 1976.

124. Abdulla, M., Jägerstad, M., Nordin, O., Qvist, I., and Svensson, S., Dietary intake of electrolytes and trace elements in the elderly, *Nutr. Metab.*, 21 (Suppl. 1), 41, 1977.

125. Grotkowski, M. L. and Sims, L., Nutritional knowledge, attitudes, and dietary practices of the elderly, *J. Am. Diet. Assoc.*, 72, 499, 1978.

126. Stiedemann, M., Jansen, C., and Harrill, I., Nutritional status of elderly men and women, *J. Am. Diet. Assoc.*, 73, 132, 1978.

127. Recommended Dietary Allowances, 9th ed., Food and Nutrition Board, National Academy of Sciences, Washington, D.C., 1980.

Chapter 10

AGING, ARTHRITIS, FOOD HYPERSENSITIVITIES, AND ALLERGIES: A RESEARCH OPPORTUNITY REVISITED

Gairdner B. Moment

TABLE OF CONTENTS

I. INTRODUCTION

In the course of organizing the present volume on nutritional approaches to aging research, it became apparent that almost no data were available on a possible relationship between nutrition and arthritis or any rheumatoid condition. Computer scans of several data banks including *Medline, Biosis, Excerpta Medica* and the U.S. Department of Agriculture's *Agricola* yield only one truly relevant title. An old-fashioned hand and eye search of the *Index Medicus* and several journals devoted to arthritis and related diseases was only slightly more successful.

This dearth of information seemed somewhat strange because the arthritis group of diseases is fully as much a characteristic of the second half of the human lifespan as are diabetes, cardiovascular ailments and other infirmities of aging about which there is an abundance of material relating to nutrition.

The reason for this lack of published information presumably lies in the failures of past efforts to uncover any link between diet and arthritis. The result has been a hardening of the dogma well expressed in the pronouncements of the Arthritis Foundation. "There is NO (their emphasis) special diet for arthritis. No specific food has anything to do with causing it." This statement appears in the Foundation's leaflet *Diet and Arthritis,* published in 1970 and still being distributed in July 1980. The Foundation goes even further in *Arthritis: The Basic Facts,* published in 1978 and currently being distributed. On page 22, in what must be some kind of a record for scientific naivete, is the claim that "If there was a relationship between diet and arthritis, it would have been discovered long ago." One does not have to be an historian of science to know that the history of science has been full of shattering surprises as the confident physicists of the late 19th century learned with the totally unexpected discovery of X-rays and then of atomic radiation.

II. STANDARD VIEW OF NUTRITIONISTS

Examination of recent editions of several standard textbooks of nutrition, both American and British, published during the last 3 years revealed a close agreement about diet and arthritis.[1-4] Many diets for treating arthritis, they point out, have been devised over the years, some have been high protein diets, others high in carbohydrates or have emphasized one or more vitamins. Others have been based on foods rich in potassium, sulfur, or some other component but none has been effective.

Most of the standard texts discuss food allergy, though not in relation to arthritis, and provide lists of foods most often involved. Wheat or milk usually head the lists followed by a wide variety of foods in apparently more or less random order, tomatoes, fish, eggs, beef, grapefruit, white potatoes, chocolate, oranges, strawberries, soybeans, celery, nuts, and the list continues.

However, it must be said at this point, that if food allergies of some sort should be causally related to arthritis in any way, the kind of studies undertaken by nutritionists of past decades could never detect it regardless of how well designed the experiments or how skillfully carried out. In the light of the tremendous advances in knowledge both of immunology and of the genes involved in immunological phenomena, it would seem worthwhile to reinvestigate this old problem.

III. POTATO FAMILY OF PLANTS: TOXINS OR ALLOGENS?

Recent studies on a possible relationship of food to arthritis take two different directions. Norman Childers[5] and associates believe that most arthritis is due to eating members of the nightshade family, the Solanaceae, because of a more or less toxic substance, solanine, these plants contain. A no-nightshade diet is a difficult one to follow because the Solanaceae include ubiquitous and staple foods such as the white potato, tomato, egg plant, tobacco and all peppers except the black which belongs to a very different group of plants.

Nevertheless, Childers and associates[5] have achieved a substantial though incomplete measure of success, ranging from complete remission of symptoms, to some amelioration to no positive results. As of September 6, 1979 they report, based on 763 replies, 28% marked improvement, 44% some improvement, and the remaining 27% no effect or a negative one. If those reporting some are added to those reporting marked improvement, the result is benefit in about 72% of the cases.

According to Healey, Wilske and Hansen,[21] the gold treatment for arthritis has been "effective" in about 50% of cases, takes about 2 or 3 months to be effective and, as is well known, is sometimes accompanied by deleterious side effects.

How the degree of success of the "no-nightshade" treatment compares with the gold chloride or any of the other standard treatments when studied in double blind tests with rigorous statistical analysis seems entirely unknown. To an objective observer they have to look equally effective until such a study is made. Such a program should have a high priority in any rational approach to the problem of this multibillion dollar disease.

It should be noted that a number of people on the no-nightshade diet reported that in addition to nightshades they had found it necessary to exclude several nonnightshade foods to be free of symptoms, chocolate, oranges, or coconut. Moreover, Childers and Russo place great emphasis on the importance of excluding even very small traces of tomatoes and peppers which are apt to be in such items as sauces and chowders. Both of these facts suggest an allergic reaction rather than a toxin. Moreover, Marshall Mandell[6,22] and associates, who are active in this area, found that of 15 people allergic to white potato only 9 were also allergic to tomatoes. Solanine, a glucoalkaloid, is a potent anticholinesterase and has other pharmacological effects. There is a widespread wasting and arthritis-like disease, discussed by Childers, of the bones, ligaments, and joints called enteque seco in cattle in South America which is brought on by eating a bush-like nightshade and which can be induced by placing some of this plant in the rumen of a cow. To a skeptical biologist who has been around for a long time, it appears that all these facts are consistent with a simple explanation. The exclusion of all the nightshades from the diet would benefit those who were allergic to one or more of the members of that group of plants or who were especially sensitive to solanine.

It is well known that many foods can cause, by whatever means, adverse reactions in some people. May and Bock[23] list a number of possible mechanisms which have nothing to do with allergies, e.g., a deficiency of disaccharidase in the intestine, noxious natural components of certain foods and psychological factors. Strong[25] has described a large number of "toxicants naturally occurring" in food plants.

Arthritis is such a diverse and large family of diseases that there is no necessity to postulate a single cause. It may be only the final, more or less common, pathway that is similar.

IV. FOOD ALLERGIES AS INCITANTS

The second direction taken in the search for a possible food-arthritis link is based on allergies. One of the older extant programs so based is the Albert Rowe[7] cereal-free and cereal and fruit-free dietary regimens. These diets have been published in great detail and some success has been reported. As in the Childers' program, "provocation" tests with suspected foods are used after remission of symptoms to determine if such foods would result in a return of symptoms. While such tests can tell much, they could not distinguish between a toxic effect and an allergy. Unhappily both of the Rowe diets include and exclude such a very wide variety of items that they have to be regarded as shotgun approaches.

More recently Lars Sköldstam[8] and associates in Sweden have used the shotgun more skilfully but it is still a shotgun. After a 7- to 10-day fast, which they report generally alleviates the symptoms of arthritis, they placed their patients on a "lactovegeterian" diet for 9 weeks with negative results. Since milk and many fruits and vegetables are high on the allergy lists, this can hardly be regarded as a completely surprising result to obtain from 16 patients.

In the U.S. there are presently a number of relatively new programs, it is difficult to determine how many, based on the food allergy hypothesis. At least some of them attempt to identify the foods suspected of being at fault by skin and other tests or by first excluding all foods and then feeding them back one at a time. The Mandell[6] and the associated Conte and Girsh group and the Theron Randolph[9] group have reported very encouraging results.

On reading Mandell[6] and Randolph[9] and their associates (though not Childers) it is easy to be reminded of the old "snake oil" and other panaceas, so many are the forms of arthritis and various other diseases that are blamed on food hypersensitivities, especially allergies. A more appropriate situation to recall is the very early days when the germ theory of contagious and infectious diseases was being established. It appeared incredible that such a vast array of diseases could all be due to essentially the same cause, bacteria. The number of forms of arthritis are not as numerous but still very diverse (see Christian and Paget[26]) and even the distinction between rheumatoid and osteoarthritis can be blurred.

V. GENETIC AND IMMUNOLOGICAL BASIS

A. Histocompatibility Gene Complex

The nonclinical side of the picture unequivocally points to an allergic base for arthritis and releated diseases. There is no longer any question that arthritis is closely linked to the immunological system through the histocompatibility gene complex, i.e., the HLA (human leukocyte antigen) system and the "rheumatoid factor", one of the IgM antibodies. McDevitt[10] gives an extensive and up-to-date presentation of this situation complete with gene maps. Of special interest is the circumstance that the B27 locus, which apparently confers susceptibility to arthritis, is a member of the histocompatibility group. The frequency of the B27 gene varies from one group of people to another but is found widely distributed (See Table 1). In the Haida Indians of the Pacific Northwest, they of the totem poles and big sea-going war canoes, it is rare in the general population. However, about 20% of the older men have ankylosing spondylitis and in them it is always present. Old men with that gene, but symptom free, can be found but are very few. Christiansen[11] and others have found that "B27 is almost an essential prerequisite for the development of classical ankylosing arthritis in Caucasoids." In addition, as Bodmer has shown,[24] rheumatoid arthritis is closely associated with the DR4 histocompatibility gene.

B. Immunological Dimensions of Standard Treatments

Significant also is the more or less recently demonstrated fact that some, and perhaps all, of the most widely used, and therefore presumably most effective, anti-arthritis compounds are highly active immunologically. Knowledge of this has recently been confirmed and extended by Rosenberg[12] in the case of the classic gold compound treatment. Miller[13] and associates and Goldstein[14] have demonstrated that levamisole acts like thymo-poietin, affecting many components of the immune system, and alters re-

Table 1
DISEASES ASSOCIATED WITH HLA
GENES

Disease	Racial group	HLA type
Ankylosing	Caucasian	B27
spondylitis	Japanese	B27
	Haida Indians	B27
	Bella Coola Indians	B27
	Pima Indians	B27
Reiters	Caucasian	B27
Yersinia-arthritis	Caucasian	B27
Salmonella-arthritis	Caucasian	B27
Psoriatic-arthritis	Caucasian	B13
Rheumatoid-arthritis	Caucasian	DR4

From McDevitt, H. O., *Arthritis and Allied Conditions,* 9th ed., McCarty, D. J., Jr., Ed., Lea & Febiger, Philadelphia, 1979. With permission.

sponses to tetanus and typhoid antigens as well as to the mitogenic lectins. Munthe[15] and associates have found the same kind of thing with penicillamine, a dimethyl cysteine, and remark how amazing, "so simple yet effective on such a complex disease".

Two additional relevant facts deserve some emphasis. One is the well-known production of arthritis in rats and other rodents by injection of Freund's complete adjuvant, a phenomenon recently reinvestigated by Chang[16] and others. The second is the deterioration with age in proper homeostatic abilities of the immune system so extensively investigated by Weindruch et al.,[17] Makinodan,[18] and by Vaughan[19] among others.

VI. CONCLUSIONS

In view of all these facts from so many different areas it would be surprising indeed if food allergies were not involved in one or more of the forms of arthritis from gout and lupus on down the line. It should be remembered, however, that science has been full of surprises in the past and there is no reason to imagine that the supply of surprises has been exhausted.

We are left with two certainties. There is a lot of smoke arising from the food allergy hypothesis, and there is an overwhelming need for relief from the burden of this family of diseases. The Arthritis Foundation estimates the *annual* cost in dollars at an all but incredible 13.4 billion! There is no way to quantify the human misery from which the road to escape is so baffling. There are at present a number of promising research programs on arthritis such as the Newcombe et al.[20] project on an analysis of the inflammatory process. Such programs warrant strong support. But in a billion dollar disease, no promising hypothesis should be overlooked. With the new knowledge of immunology and genetics, we are presented with an important opportunity for one or more teams of investigators to design and carry out experiments with adequate controls and statistical evaluations, which will dissect the essential elements of the problem, free from the great mass of irrelevant facts, the semantic noise of which now obscures the answers.

ACKNOWLEDGMENTS

It is a pleasure to acknowledge the help, the encouragement, and the criticisms of colleagues at Goucher College and in the Gerontology Research Center of the National Institute on Aging where I am privileged to be a Guest Scientist. I am also indebted to numerous knowledgeable and widely scattered individuals who, while not always agreeing with the point of view expressed, were yet very helpful.

REFERENCES

1. Davidson, S., Passmore, R., Brock, J. F., and Truswell, A. S., *Human Nutrition and Dietetics,* 7th ed., Churchill Livingstone, Edinburgh and London, 1979.
2. Krause, M. E. and Mahan, L. K., *Food, Nutrition and Diet Therapy,* 6th ed., W. B. Saunders, Philadelphia, 1979.
3. Robinson, C. H. and Lawler, M. R., *Normal and Therapeutic Nutrition,* 15th ed., Macmillan, New York, 1977.
4. Williams, S. R., *Nutrition and Diet Therapy,* 3rd ed., C. V., Mosby, St. Louis, 1977.
5. Childers, N. F. and Russo, G. M., *The Nightshades and Health,* Horticultural Publications, Somerset Press, Somerville, N.J., 1977.
6. Mandell, M., Study links rheumatic aches to food allergy, *Med. World News,* March 31, 1980.
7. Rowe, A. H. and Rowe, A., Jr., *Food Allergy,* Charles C Thomas, Springfield, Ill., 1972.
8. Sköldstam, L., Larsson, L., and Lindstrom, F. D., Effects of fasting and a lactovegetarian diet on rheumatoid arthritis, *Scand. J. Rheum.,* 8, 249, 1979.
9. Randolph, T. G., *Human Ecology and Susceptibility to the Chemical Environment,* Charles C Thomas, Springfield, Ill., 1978.
10. McDevitt, H. O., Genetic structure and functions of the major histocompatibility complex, in *Arthritis and Allied Conditions,* 9th ed., McCarty, D. J., Ed., Lea & Febiger, Philadelphia, 1979.
11. Christiansen, F. T., Hawkins, B. R., Dawkins, R. L., Owen, E. T., and Potter, R. M., The prevalence of ankylosing spondylitis among B27 positive normal individuals — a reassessment, *J. Rheum.,* 6, 713, 1979.
12. Rosenberg, S. A., Inhibition of pokeweed mitogen-induced immunoglobulin production in humans by gold compounds, *J. Rheum. Suppl.,* 5, 107, 1979.
13. Miller, B., DeMerieux, P., Srinivasan, R., Clements, P., Fan, P., Levy, J., and Paulus, H. E., Double-blind placebo controlled crossover evaluation of levamisole in rheumatoid arthritis, *Arth. Rheum.,* 23, 172, 1980.
14. Goldstein, G., Mode of action of levamisole, *J. Rheum. Suppl.,* 4, 143, 1978.
15. Munthe, E., Jellum, E., and Aaseth, J., Some aspects of the mechanism of penicillamine in rheumatoid arthritis, *Scand. J. Rheum. Suppl.,* 28, 6, 1979.
16. Chang, Y. H., Pearson, C. M., and Abe, C., Adjuvant polyarthritis. IV. Induction by a synthetic adjuvant, *Arth. Rheum.,* 23, 62, 1980.
17. Weindruch, R. H., Kristie, J. A., Cheney, K. E., and Walford, R. L., Influence of controlled dietary restriction on immunologic function and aging, *Fed. Proc.,* 38, 2007, 1979.
18. Makinodan, T., Good, R. A., and Kay, M. M. B., Cellular Basis of Immunosenescence, in *Immunology and Aging,* Makinodan, T. and Yunis, E., Eds., Plenum Press, New York, 1977.
19. Vaughan, J. H., Aging, Immunity, and Rheumatoid Arthritis, in *Aging, Immunity and Arthritic Disease,* Kay, M. M. B., Galpin, J., and Makinodan, T., Eds., Raven Press, New York, 1980.
20. Chang, J., Wigley, F., and Newcombe, D., Neural protease activation of peritoneal macrophage prostaglandin synthesis, *Proc. Natl. Acad. Sci. U.S.A.,* 77, 4736, 1980.
21. Healey, L. A., Wilske, K. R., and Hansen, B. H., *Beyond the Copper Bracelet: What You Should Know About Arthritis,* Charles C Thomas, Springfield, Ill., 1972.
22. Mandell, M. and Scanlon, L. W., *Five-Day Allergy Relief System,* Pocket Books-Nutri Books, New York, 1979.
23. May, C. D. and Bock, S. A., Adverse Reactions to Food Due to Hypersensitivity, in *Allergy: Principles and Practice,* Vol. 2, Middleton, E., Jr., Reed, C. E., and Ellis, E. F., Eds., C. V. Mosby, St. Louis, 1978, 1159.
24. Bodmer, W. F., A Super Supergene, in *The Harvey Lectures,* (72nd series), N.Y. Academy of Science, N.Y., 1976.
25. Strong, F., *Toxicants Occurring Naturally in Foods,* 2nd ed., National Academy of Sciences, Washington, D.C., 1973.
26. Christian, C. L. and Paget, S. A., Rheumatoid Arthritis, in *Immunological Diseases,* 3rd ed., Samter, M., Ed., Little, Brown, Boston, 1978.

Chapter 11

THE IMPORTANT INTERACTION OF ALCOHOLISM WITH NUTRITION IN THE ELDERLY

Frank L. Iber

TABLE OF CONTENTS

I. INTRODUCTION: DEFINITIONS AND INTERRELATIONS

The intake of alcohol in dependent persons rises as metabolic and neurological tolerance develop so that in alcoholics a substantial portion of the required calorie intake (rarely less than 600, usually about 1200 cal/day) is in the form of ethanol.[1] Alcoholic beverages rarely contain other nutrients in quantity so that the food that is replaced by the intake of alcoholic beverages frequently results in deficient intake of protein, trace minerals, water, and fat-soluble vitamins.[2]

Alcoholism* is usually associated with mild protein deficiency and frequent deficiencies of B vitamins, folate, zinc, and magnesium; and nearly always produces mild impairment of the efficiency of absorption by the small intestine and in intermediate metabolism by the liver.

Aging,** uncomplicated by specific disease or social problems affecting food availability, has few nutritional problems; arteriosclerosis, diabetes, and thin bones increase with age. Aging associated with severe disease of almost any sort, however, results in increasing malnutrition and the most severe problems in the elderly occur with combinations of poor intake and disease. In the elderly there are limited data and much is by deduction.

Figure 1 emphasizes that alcoholism, nutrition, and disease have important interactions with aging. Although these phenomena may be additive, most malnutrition occurs in areas of overlap with the other three in the Venn diagram.

II. ALCOHOL*** — ITS EFFECTS AT MODERATE DOSES AND AT HIGH DOSES

Ethanol is totally absorbed slowly from the stomach and more rapidly from the small intestine, passing in high concentration to the liver where it is eventually metabolized to acetate and then exported to other tissues for further oxidation. The hepatic oxidation of ethanol seems obligate and diminishes the intracellular NAD content which is replaced by NADH. There are many metabolic consequences of lowering the NAD/NADH ratio in the liver cells which appear in all drinking persons. Some of these are (A) increased production of lactic acid rather than pyruvate, (B) a mild acidosis and resultant retention by the kidney tubule of urate, i.e., the uric acid in the serum is higher in chronically drinking persons, (C) the metabolism of drugs or materials that require NAD almost ceases (conversion of galactose to glucose stops), and (D) the mobilization of stored folate from liver cells is slowed.[3,4]

Ethanol has enjoyed its great popularity as a beverage from its behavioral effects producing enhanced socialization, relaxation, and a perception of eloquence. Its use throughout the world has increased at least as fast as the population growth, and industrialization of a nation is almost invariably associated with an increased consumption of alcohol.[5]

A. Social Use of Alcohol

The social use of alcohol (i.e., regular or irregular use of ethanol below the level of five drinks daily to facilitate social communication and used only in the presence of

---

*   Alcoholism — will be used to indicate the usually poorly defined chronic use of ethanol to interfere with health, family, job or social relations or the quantitation of daily intake to exceed 50 g intake daily. Very high levels of intake when defined will be included in the description.

** Aging — aged or elderly indicate progressive ages beyond 60. Rarely are data available specifically looking at these subjects. Clear age trends even when extrapolated from lower level will be indicated as extrapolations.

***Alcohol — will be used in this paper interchangeably with ethanol; both will refer to ethyl alcohol.

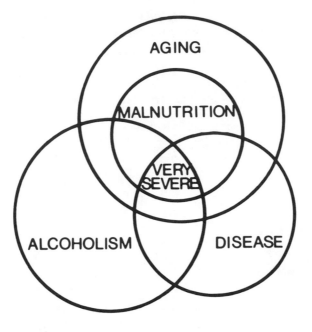

FIGURE 1.   Important interaction of alcoholism and nutrition in the elderly.

people), has many beneficial effects and a few harmful ones.[6-8] Reaction time and sequential decisions are slowed in the total time that it requires to make them in the drinking person. This is perceptible in a 70 kg person receiving at one time 30 g (two or three drinks) of pure ethanol and increases linearly with quantity of drinking thereafter. It is believed that this is the major factor, (delayed reaction time), that accounts for both increased industrial and increased automobile accidents.[9,10] Alcohol is an excellent soporific, but fires resulting from smoking in bed are not a feature of social drinking but alcoholic drinking.[11]

B. Alcoholism

Alcoholism and its habituation usually results in the frequent ingestion of an alcoholic beverage from the time of awakening until retirement and usually a portion is ingested each 2 to 3 hr, because it disappears so rapidly. Persons who drink very heavily, (10 to 15 portions, 150 g daily up), get major organ disease or die traumatic deaths and *do not reach older ages*.[12,13] Thus cirrhosis kills frequently in the 5th decade, pancreatitis has a similar age distribution, and the many severe neurological damages occur most often before 60. People drink heavily all of their lives (five to seven drinks daily) and have no substantive health problems even though they continue this problem into their older years. Some aspects of the elderly promote alcohol use. Among these are more free time, boredom, depression, bereavement, and occasionally the lack of dentition. Hearings before the U.S. Senate in 1976 estimated that there was a substantive alcohol problem in about 1 million persons over 65 or approximately the same 7 to 9% of adults at other ages.[14] Alcoholism is responsive to treatment. After a medically supervised 5 days of recovery from drinking (called detoxification), education in groups and behavior modification with Alcoholics Anonymous is highly effective and must continue for several years.[15,16]

C. Common Changes from Alcoholism

The vast majority of alcoholics show the common abnormalities indicated in Table 1. Although the gastritis contributes to poor intake of food, and the mild mental and

Table 1

ABNORMALITIES PRESENT IN MORE THAN 20% OF
ALCOHOLICS

Problem	Prevalence	Consequence
Small intestine malfunction	60—80%	Exaggerates trace nutrient deficiency
Memory and cogitative mental function	40%	
Gastritis	25%	Anorexia, may bleed
Increased lactate, urate liver NADH levels	50%	Acidosis Poor folate mobility
Increased drug metabolizing enzymes	60%	Altered drug sensitivity
Peripheral nerve damage	20%	Impaired sensation
Macronutrient deficiency		
Protein	20%	Impaired reserve
Calorie	50%	10-lb wt. loss
Micronutrient deficiency		
K$^+$	40%	May promote cardiac
Mg$^+$	20%	instability
Zn$^+$	20%	
Thiamine	40%	Peripheral and central
Riboflavin	40%	nervous damage
Pyridoxine	40%	
Folate	40%	Blood cells
Vitamin A	20%	Night blindness
Vitamin D	20%	

Table 2

SERIOUS DISEASES OF ALCOHOLICS

Disease	% of Alcoholics	Peak age of death
Accidents	1/year	20—40
Suicide	0.01/year	30
Homicide victim	0.01/year	30—50
Cirrhosis of liver	16	50
Alcoholic brain damage Wernicke-Korsakoff	6	40—60
Pancreatitis	1	40
Cardiomyopathy	0.2	45
Cancer (alcohol- or smoking-related)	4	50

peripheral nerve damage interferes with making a living, both are relatively unimportant to future health. The small intestine in alcoholism is damaged,[17] and many of the active transport enzymes for absorbing trace nutrients are impaired.

D. Major Organ Disease with Alcoholism

Table 2 indicates serious conditions that alcoholics develop, but it should be emphasized that only a minority of alcoholics ever develop these.[18] Most of these conditions shorten life and occur before age 60 or 65. However, elderly persons are seen with each of these conditions resulting from alcoholism. It is pertinent to inquire if these conditions are more prevalent in the elderly than in younger persons as a percentage of drinking persons. Data are well developed for cirrhosis of the liver. From the studies of Lelbach, it is clear that it requires less drinking over age 60 to produce cirrhosis than at age 40.[19] The common loss of memory found in alcoholism is quite similar to the loss of memory found in senility and therefore, it would be appropriate to suggest that these losses would be clinically more apparent from this additive effect.

Pancreatic function and heart function diminish with aging. Alcohol damage has few features that are unique, so there is little to support the view that the elderly are more susceptible — only that they have less reserve capacity in each of the organs that alcohol commonly attacks, therefore it is easier to become manifest.[20,21]

1. The Elderly

About 5% of the population over 65 (estimated 12 million in 1980), require institutionalization in hospitals and nursing homes and only this ill and disabled population show substandard dietary intake and frequent malnutrition. The calorie intake and needs progressively diminish by about 10% for each decade after age 60. For nutrients whose requirement is related to calorie intake (thiamin, niacin), this is less serious than for folate, vitamin A, and vitamin D where there seems an absolute requirement. There are no hard data to develop requirements in older persons. Although about 20% of elderly Americans in the Hanes survey[22] had diminished intakes of iron, vitamin A, ascorbic acid and protein, deficiencies approaching these frequencies were not observed suggesting that there is a reduction in some requirements. Nutritionists generally recommend that RDA levels be maintained even though there is a diminished total calorie intake. This means, in fact, that a careful choice of nutrients is required to get the RDA levels of the major nutrients while overall intake is diminished.[23] Needless to say, this is even more of a marked problem in the alcoholic.

III. ALCOHOL EFFECT IN ELDERLY

A. Behavior

Alcohol is a widely available nonprescription drug of great value and possesses great symbolism in most western societies. The drug gives pleasure, relieves stress, reduces pain, eliminates fears, raises self esteem, and induces sleep. Its symbolic use at nearly all family, religious, and most public celebration ceremonies enhances its image of importance and contributes to some placebo effect. The best descriptions of behavior effects comes from classical literature, but many aspects are now under study by newer psychological and statistical methods.

The behavioral effects of ethanol are quite similar to those of benzodiazepines, such as diazepam (Valium®) and chlordiazepoxide (Librium®), thus 20 g (two drinks) seem equivalent to 5 mg diazepam or 50 mg of chlordiazepoxide. It is, in fact, quite clear that the benzodiazepams substitute quite adequately for treating alcoholism withdrawal,[24] and the two alter one another's metabolism — an illustrative study by Ascione[25] indicates that diazepam levels rise twice as high and remain higher for 6 extra hours when given with ethanol instead of with water. Curiously, both diazepam and chlordiazepoxide decrease their metabolic clearance rate with ageing — this is not adequately studied for alcohol.[26,27] All measurements of behavioral effects are importantly modified by the subjects *expectation* regarding alcohol and sophisticated design to fully take this into account is not widespread, Lang and co-workers[28] administered tonic water with and without alcohol in a complex design which often provided alcohol with no expectation of its presence, and provided tonic water with assurances that alcohol was present. They showed clearly the relief of tension was more often based on *expectation* of relief rather than alcohol effect.

B. Anxiety

Wolff and co-workers[29] progressively increased heat applied to the forehead in a model that regularly produces anxiety and alarm, before it produces a severely painful sensation. The anxiety level was measured by skin resistance and was found regularly to be abnormal at a lower level of temperature elevation than the pain sensation. Alcohol in the amount of 0.4 g/kg (28 g or three drinks in a 70-kg person) significantly delayed the alarm sensation to a level above that of the pain sensation in the three subjects studied repetitively. Carpenter[30] used the skin resistance response to measure the "anxiety" of an unexpected loud and irritating noise superimposed on a basic task of concentration for card sorting, for which the study seemed primarily designed. Alcohol in a dose of 0.5 g/kg clearly lessened the skin response, lower doses had a partial effect.

C. Sleep Promoting

Alcohol has been known to have sleep producing effects as noted in the Bible.[31] A more modern scholar, Damrau[32] and associates, studied insomniacs in an open design using ethanol as a bottle of stout (18.6 g ethanol) compared to other treatments and no treatment. Improvement in sleep was almost uniform with alcohol, only 6 of 50 failed to have some improvement and persistence with repetitive study.

D. Sexual Function

Modern design methods have indicated in both men and women that the anticipated effect of alcohol is usually found; however when the anticipated effect is fully controlled it becomes clear that alcohol in men and women diminishes sexual arousal from identical stimuli.[33-35] Thus the admonition of the porter in *Macbeth* that (drink) provokes the desire but takes away the performance, is more than ever appropriate. Impotence in male alcoholics of all ages is a substantial problem.

IV. ALCOHOL BRAIN INJURY AND COMPARISON WITH CHANGES OF SENILITY

All subjects drinking more than five drinks daily for many months develop reversible changes in mentation that are widespread in the functions that are diminished, but conceptualization and abstract function are most impaired. As the alcohol injury becomes more prolonged and more severe, it reaches permanence.[36] When it is sufficiently marked as to interfere with behavior or function in society, it is often called the Korsakoff Syndrome. Chronic and irreversible brain impairment due to alcoholism occurs in about 6% of all alcoholics.[36]

Serial psychological tests have been widely applied to alcoholics.[37,38] Ryan and Butters[40] and Freund[39] have emphasized that there is only a limited recovery after the first 14 days, and that superficially there are many features in these persons in common with senile dementia. Both impair abstract function and conceptualization, but alcoholism leaves vocabulary functions much less impaired than ageing. With the passage of time (up to 5 years) alcoholic dementia remains stable if the person abstains, whereas senile dementia is measurably more advanced in each year of observation.

Although studies were not located, it seems safe to predict that the impairment to function promoted by the mental stages of either condition is additive, and that drinking in an alcoholic fashion in the older years will result in a higher incidence of mental impairment.

V. BENEFICIAL BEHAVIOR EFFECTS

Institutionalized elderly have been studied with and without alcohol. It must be fully understood that institutionalized elderly are often deprived of many aspects of power over their lives and the investigation nearly always adds new things besides alcohol. Similar data are not available on free living elderly. In an early study, Kastenbaum and Slater[41] studied two groups of 20 elderly institutionalized patients for 1 month giving one group one or two glasses of wine daily, and the other similar amounts of grape juice. The groups were then crossed over so that each group received the second beverage. Blinded-interview and psychological testing was performed at appropriate times before and during each treatment period. In both groups there was a *marked increase* in *social interaction* with a trend (not significant) to superior effect in the wine group. A much better study designed by Black[42] divided 34 senile hospitalized patients into two comparable groups based on pretesting for 75 behavioral characteristics. The groups were given either beer or fruit juice for 4 weeks and then crossed over to the other beverage. The beer groups were statistically more alert, friendly, and communicative; this improvement deteriorated when studied on fruit juice and the advantage of beer was statistically significant. This study and design seems excellent.

Mishara et al.[43,44] conducted two trials. In the first, 80 elderly patients were given wine in reward for good behavior or given wine regardless of behavior for a 10-week study period and a 6-month followup. Both groups showed immediate improvement in sleep patterns and reduction in the amounts of sleeping medication and an improvement in interpersonal communication over the control period. Neither pattern of offering wine showed a clear advantage. In the second study, nicely controlled in either nursing homes or in residence homes, 2 oz. of 80 proof beverage alcohol was given 5 days a week for 18 weeks in the alcohol groups and nonalcoholic beverages in the control group. No adverse effects of alcohol were observed and positive effects included improved cognitive performance, increased morale, less worrying and less difficulty in falling asleep. All in all, these studies show support of a beneficial effect of moderate intake on behavior in the elderly in the quality of life, the enhancement of social interactions with no adverse effects in these amounts (maximum of two portions of alcohol daily).

VI. METABOLIC CHANGES OF ALCOHOL IN ELDERLY

A. Absorption

Table 3 illustrates the major metabolic interferences from alcoholism that will be discussed in this section. Nearly every known substance that is transported from low to high concentration in the intestines is impaired in its absorption by chronic alcoholism.[17] Thus transport of water soluble vitamins, amino acids, sugars, and some drugs are impaired. The absorption of thiamine utilizes a membrane bound Na, K activated ATPase, which is specifically inhibited and the absorption for thiamine is interfered with by the concommitant administration of ethanol.[17] A similar inhibition occurs with ascorbic acid.

The diminished food intake of the alcoholic amplifies this impaired absorption. No specific studies on the elderly have been found to suggest the impairment is more or less severe. In actual experience, these impairments assume importance in combination with increased body requirements of nutrients such as accompany surgery, trauma, infection, or other disease, and then the deficiencies may be devastating. In the U.S. ascorbic acid deficiency is largely limited to elderly male alcoholics usually living alone, where intake is diminished and alcohol use decreases it even further. The possible relation of absorption to the bone disease of the alcoholic and the elderly will be presented in a later section on bone.

B. Lipid and Carbohydrate Metabolism[45]

The substitution of large amounts of alcohol for ordinary macronutrients in the diet

Table 3
METABOLIC IMPAIRMENTS PRODUCED BY ALCOHOL

Absorptive defects	Vitamins C, A, D, thiamine, pyridoxine, folate
	Metals — Zn, Ca, Mg
	Macronutrients
	Fat
	Amino acids
Carbohydrate abnormalities	Oral diabetic glucose tolerance 20—40%
	Potentiated insulin release — 70%
	Decreased insulin release — 20%
	Decreased glucose absorption — 60%
Lipid abnormalities	Increased liver synthesis of fat and cholesterol
	— fatty liver
	Increased serum lipids Type IV
	Increased HDL (high density lipoproteins)
Alcohol metabolism	NAD/NADH decrease
	Acidosis, increased lactate, increased urate
	Limited folate mobilization
	Impaired removal of drugs
	Acetaldehyde formation
	Aberrant behavior
	Liver fibrosis
Diuresis of Mg, Zn	Losses from body
Increased requirement for vitamins	Folate, thiamine, nicotinic acid

alters both carbohydrate metabolism and lipid metabolism. The metabolism of ethanol seems obligate and the two carbon particles that result from its partial oxidation cannot be incorporated into storage glycogen, but can only go to fat.

In normal persons, alcohol levels up to 80 mg/dℓ (safe driving levels) do not alter blood sugar, but insulin secretion is potentiated and under the correct experimental conditions of limited food intake, reactive hypoglycemia can occur. Thus the plasma insulin response to glucose, arginine, or tolbutamide[46,47] is approximately twice as high in a person who has had alcohol present for 4 hr or longer.

In chronic alcoholism at all ages, there is an increased incidence of glucose intolerance that mimics diabetes. Many of these studies are performed immediately upon cessation of drinking (12 to 24 hr later at a time all ethanol has left the system), but before the person has reaccommodated to the intake of carbohydrate and, therefore may be of limited value.

Voegtlin and co-workers[48] found 40% of chronic alcoholics with impaired glucose tolerance. Lundquist found the impairment was less after intravenous glucose, suggesting a substantial role of intestinal glucagon.[49] Insulin, glucagon, and growth hormone release are all impaired in the chronic alcoholic.[50] Although alcoholic liver disease seems regularly associated with hyperglucagonemia, the majority of these patients do not have liver disease. Since the elderly have impaired glucose metabolism compared to younger patients, it seems clear that the defects in chronic alcoholism and the defects in aging will be additive. In the alcoholic there is "reactive hypoglycemia" due to insulin over-release; the early senile diabetic is similar. Although alcohol in the well-nourished person does not cause an under-release or delayed release of insulin, it certainly does in the chronic alcoholic — both growth hormone and insulin are delayed in release. With aging there is a similar delayed release of insulin and it could be fully expected that these will be additive. Although the diabetes of both the elderly and the alcoholic is brought out by the stress of infection, usually ketoacidosis is infrequent. Pancreatitis in the alcoholic is often associated with diabetes.

Alcohol is a precursor of cholesterol and in the Type IV hyperlipidemia of Levy,[51] it is responsible for major rises in the lipid level. The caloric deficit found in many alcoholics leads to lowered levels of cholesterol in the serum that often rise as the patient eats more normally and remains abstinent. High density lipoproteins are considered beneficial by aiding the clearance of cholesterol from tissue, inhibiting the uptake of low-density lipoprotein (which in turn induces all cells of the body to form more cholesterol). It is now clear in a number of well-designed epidemiological studies that alcohol consumption is associated with an increase in high-density lipoprotein. Thus Castelli and co-workers[52] correlated alcohol intake and the blood lipids in multiple studies throughout the U.S. and found that alcohol consumption was positively associated with increasing high-density lipoprotein cholesterol levels. This response was present even at very low levels of alcohol consumption. In similar studies in one center, Barboriak, et al.[53,54] found that HDL values were both positively associated with alcohol intake and inversely related to coronary occlusion. Williams found this also applied to men in Great Britain.[55]

C. Consequences of Alcohol Metabolism

Alcohol is metabolized to acetaldehyde by a soluble enzyme requiring NAD as a cofactor. The enzyme is present in the intestine, in the retina, and in the liver and oxidizes alcohol at a rate limited by the availability of NAD in the cell. As a result, during ethanol oxidation the level of NADH in the liver cell increases profoundly, and traces of acetaldehyde are possible. A variety of reactions in the liver cell requiring NAD are slowed or stopped completely. Among those of some importance is the formation of pyruvate and the reaction that releases liver stores of folate into folate in the blood.[3] The extra lactate in the blood raises the uric acid and can contribute to gouty arthritis in the elderly.

Acetaldehyde is a highly active intermediate. In the brain, one postulate has it combine with norepinephrine to a morphinelike material.[56] In the liver, it is postulated to promote organelle injury,[57] particularly of the mitochondrion. Both the brain and the liver repair themselves less readily in the elderly.

D. Nutrient Loss or Increased Requirements in the Alcoholic

Alcohol produces a diuresis of magnesium and zinc whenever the blood level of ethanol changes. Both metals may be profoundly depleted. The chronic acidosis of alcoholism leads to increased urinary loss of K and Ca which contribute to bone dissolution.

Folate requirements are higher in the drinking person than in the nondrinking person. Sullivan and Herbert[58] demonstrated that dietary levels of folate sufficient to maintain normal marrow led to macrocytic anemia when alcohol was added. Alcohol prevents the maintenance of folate from liver stores and the amount in the urine and bile decrease. A recent study indicates declining folate stores with age and this is aggravated by alcohol.[59] Thiamine, riboflavin, and pyridoxine also seem to have higher requirements during drinking — ring sideroblasts — a pyridoxine deficiency is more prevalent in the drinking elderly.[60]

VII. MYOCARDIAL AND CORONARY DISEASE

The prevalences of vascular disease adversely affecting the heart increases with ageing.[61,62] The effects of alcohol interacting with age have clear benefits and clear adverse effects on myocardial and coronary artery diseases. Alcohol is a mild vasodilator and at all ages increases acutely the cardiac output, the heart rate and produces a mild elevation of the blood pressure all combining to increase the work of the heart. There is clear decrease in cardiac contractility, at alcohol blood levels of 100 to 200 mg/dℓ

in dogs.[63] These findings have been almost always confirmed in man.[64] In chronic studies there is convincing evidence of functional myocardial abnormalities in man with a long history of large alcoholic intakes, but little or no evidence of clinical cardiac disease.[65] Despite this effect on myocardial function, there is little evidence of decrease in coronary blood flow (Regan and co-workers).[66]

There is statistically strong association between blood pressure and known drinking habits in the study by Klatsky and co-workers[67] of 83,947 men in the Kaiser-Permanente clinics. Persons taking more than six drinks daily had significantly higher blood pressure. Kannell and Sorlie[68] found similarly in the Framingham heart study that hypertension was more prevalent among those who drank more than 60 oz of alcohol monthly.

Klatsky has provided multiple studies on the Kaiser-Permanente clinic populations demonstrating that nondrinkers are at a significantly greater risk of myocardial infarction than users of alcohol. These differences indicating a beneficial effect of alcohol were present at both one and two drinks each day and at three or more drinks. These data were corrected for smoking, obesity, psychological traits and hypertension and a beneficial effect of alcohol still emerged.[69-70] Stason[71] and associates found a lower rate of coronary artery disease in the 4,263 persons in the Framingham study among those drinking an average of at least 1 oz of ethanol daily. A case-control study of 399 hospitalized patients with nonfatal myocardial infarction showed fewer cases than expected among those who averaged six or more drinks daily.

Similar beneficial effects of alcohol were noted by Hennekens and co-workers[72] in an analysis of death from coronary artery disease among 568 married white men in Florida with appropriately selected controls. Information was obtained on alcohol consumption for 3 months prior to death. After controlling for most variables the risk ratio was significantly lower for those drinking five drinks per day than for abstainers. In a subsequent paper,[73] the protective effect of beer, wine, and spirits was comparable. Barboriak, et al.[74] has measured the degree of coronary artery involvement on arteriography and compared these findings with the drinking history. The patients who were abstainers or consumed less than an equivalent of 180 mℓ of absolute alcohol per week, had higher coronary artery occlusion scores than the group consuming more than that amount.

It seems clear that alcohol has mild but definite adverse effects on the myocardium but beneficial effects on coronary artery disease. The beneficial effects seem to occur with more than two and less than six portions of alcohol daily; the adverse myocardial effect seems to occur in those who drink in excess of six portions daily. The benefit to the elderly of one or two drinks daily probably outweigh any harmful effects in this range.

VIII. CANCER AND ALCOHOLISM

Cancer increases in prevalence in the elderly and a number of specific cancers are positively associated with alcoholism. In a highly valuable epidemiological study[75] the effect of alcohol, tobacco, and age were separately and together related to the incidence of cancer. These studies indicated clearly that carcinoma of the tongue and larynx were positively correlated with alcohol and age; alcohol positively correlated with carcinoma of the tongue, buccal cavity, oropharynx, hypopharynx, larynx, and esophagus as well as liver. In many studies, primary cancer of the liver in adults relates positively to the incidence of alcoholism (Tuyns and Audigier).[76] The majority of heavy drinkers are also smokers and the smoking acts in additive conjunction with alcohol in carcinoma of the mouth, pharynx, and the esophagus.[77] On the other hand, though carcinoma of the lung is more prevalent in alcoholics, this is entirely due to the high association with smoking.[78]

The mechanism of this increase problem may be any of several. Alcohol is rarely ingested in pure form; the complex chemicals in alcoholic beverages (congeners) may be carcinogens. Alcoholism is associated with altered immunological status and this may be an important effect. Alcoholics frequently have diminished vitamin A content.[79] Normal vitamin A status in some way prevents the emergence of epithelial malignancies.

IX. SKELETAL PROBLEMS IN THE ALCOHOLIC AND IN THE ELDERLY

Alcoholics have an increased incidence of aseptic necrosis of the hip, and the cause is generally held to be ischemia from fat embolism.[80] The elderly are not more prone to this lesion. Thinning of bone mineral content is a prominent feature of both alcoholics and the elderly. Our own studies show clearly that alcoholic males of all ages have thin bones as measured by the isotopic absorption method in the radius and the ulna using the Cameron Bone densitometer, but the cause is unclear. With aging, loss of bone mineral mass begins between age 25 and 35 in all individuals, progresses rapidly in the 5th and 6th decade. In both the elderly and the alcoholic, the decalcification may be sufficiently severe to produce fractures. Frequent fractures are a prominent feature of both alcoholics[81] and the elderly, but the high incidence of trauma in the former is of greater importance.

In the elderly, the principal bone disease is osteoporosis and this rises either from a loss of the matrix in which the bone is layed down or from a very long-standing slow negative calcium balance, largely brought about by diminished intake. There is little or no evidence of vitamin D deficiency or impaired conversion of dietary D to the active forms used in the body. In the alcoholic, there are many additional problems that may be involved. Biopsies obtained show both osteoporosis and osteomalacia,[82] and therefore show elements of profound interference with vitamin D or calcium metabolism as well as laying down of the protein matrix. Nearly all active alcoholics have mild malabsorption of fat and the absorption of fat soluble vitamins is even more deranged. The fatty acids in the stool bind calcium which prevents its absorption. The mild acidosis resulting from the chronic metabolism of alcohol produces increased excretion of calcium in the urine. Protein synthesis is impaired in nearly all systems in which it has been measured in the alcoholic, and this may contribute to osteoid problems, and to problems in the formation of hormones.

There are conflicting points on the total bone mass in alcoholics. Roginsky et al., measured total body bone mass by neutron activation.[83] He found a modest *increase* in his 12 alcoholics compared to 24 normals, no patient was over age 50. In contrast, Dalén[84] compared seven alcoholics and seven controls average age 56 by X-ray spectrophotometry 43 months apart, the alcoholics heavily drinking. They had significant loss of bone during this time, most prominent in the lower extremities suggesting an age factor.

Nilsson and Westlin[85] studied 58 alcoholics without fractures and 35 with fractures and compared them with 56 age-matched normals. The bone densitometry by gamma absorption showed no difference between the normal and the alcoholics, or those with fractures, but after age 50 there were marked differences with a progressively enlarging difference with increasing age. The oldest patients were in their mid-70s. A followup study of this problem by the same authors[86] suggested that alcoholics following gastrectomy had the most severe demineralization of all.

It seems clear that alcoholism promotes calcium malabsorption and calcium loss as well as dissolution of bone from many different causes. This aggravates the normal development of osteoporosis in the elderly and many accentuate it. I did not locate data suggesting that the increased losses of calcium in the urine led to the floation of more stones.

X. SUMMARY

Chronic alcoholism and aging produce similar impairments that seem additive in memory loss, loss of myocardial function, and propensity to diabetes. Both promote calcium loss from bone and impairments of vitamin D function. Chronic disease combined with alcoholism and aging profoundly magnifies deficiencies of trace nutrients both vitamins and minerals. Alcohol seems to have a modest beneficial effect on coronary artery disease and on behavior in the elderly confined to institutions.

REFERENCES

1. **Mezey, E. and Santora, P. B.,** Liver abnormalities in alcoholism: alcohol consumption and nutrition, in *Fermented Food Beverages in Nutrition,* Gastineau, G. F., Darby, W. J., and Turner, T. B., Eds., Academic Press, New York, 1979, 303.
2. **Hurt, R. D., Nelson, R. A., Dickson, E. R., Higgins, J. A., and Morse, R. M.,** Nutritional status of alcoholics before and after admission to an alcoholism treatment unit, in *Fermented Food Beverages in Nutrition,* Gastineau, G. F., Darby, W. J., and Turner, T. B., Eds., Academic Press, New York, 1979, 397.
3. **Eichner, E. R. and Hillman, R. S.,** The evolution of anemia in alcoholic patients, *Am. J. Med.,* 50, 218, 1971.
4. **Hillman, R. S., McGuffin, R., and Campbell, C.,** Alcoholic interference with the folate enterohepatic cycle, *Trans. Assoc. Am. Physician,* 90, 145, 1977.
5. **Katz, P. C.,** National patterns of consumption and production of beer, in *Fermented Food Beverages in Nutrition,* Gastineau, G. F., Darby, W. J., and Turner, T. B., Eds., Academic Press, New York, 1979, 143.
6. **Cahalan, D., Cisin, I. H., and Crossley, H. M.,** *American Drinking Practices: a National Study of Drinking Behavior and Attitudes,* College and University Press, New Haven, CT., 1969.
7. **Schuckit, M. A.,** *Drug and Alcohol Abuse: A Clinical Guide to Diagnosis and Treatment,* Plenum Press, New York, 1979.
8. **Cahalan, D. and Cisin, I. H.,** American drinking practices: summary of findings from a national probability sample. I. Extent of drinking by population subgroups, *Q. J. Stud. Alcoholism,* 29, 130, 1968.
9. **McCarroll, J. R., and Haddon, W., Jr.,** A controlled study of fatal automobile accidents in New York City, *J. Chron. Dis.,* 15, 811, 1962.
10. **Wechsler, H.,** Alcohol level and home accidents, *Public Health Rep.,* 84, 1043, 1969.
11. **Waller, J. A.,** Nonhighway injury fatalities. I. The role of alcohol and problem drinking, drugs, and medical impairment, *J. Chron. Dis.,* 25, 33, 1972.
12. **Terris, M.,** The medical costs of excessive use of alcohol, in *Fermented Food Beverages in Nutrition,* Gastineau, G. F., Darby, W. J., and Turner, T. B., Eds., Academic Press, New York, 1979.
13. Advance Report, Final Mortality Statistics, 1975, *Mon. Vital Stat. Rep.,* 25 (11), Suppl., 1977.
14. **Eagleton, T. F. and Hathaway, W. D. (chm),** Subcommittees on Aging and on Alcoholism and Narcotics of the Committee on Labor and Public Welfare, U.S. Senate, Joint Hearings: Examination of the Problems of Alcohol and Drug Abuse among the Elderly, Comm. Print No. 75-687 0, U.S. Government Printing Office, Washington, D.C., 1975.
15. **Gitlow, S. E. and Peyser, H. S., Eds.,** *Alcoholism — A Practical Treatment Guide,* Grune & Stratton, New York, 1980.
16. **Schuckit, M. A.,** A treatment of alcohol in office and out-patient settings, in *Diagnosis and Treatment of Alcoholism,* Mendelson, J. H. and Mello, N. K., Eds., McGraw-Hill, New York, 1979, chap. 6.
17. **Halsted, C. H., Robles, E. A., and Mezey, E.,** Intestinal malabsorption in folate deficient alcoholics, *Gastroenterology,* 64, 526, 1973.
18. **Dutta, S. K., Mobarhan, S., and Iber, F.,** Associated liver disease in alcoholic pancreatitis, *Am. J. Dig. Dis.,* 23 (7), 618, 1978.

19. **Lelbach, W. K.**, Epidemiology of alcoholic liver disease, in *Progress in Liver Disease,* Vol. 5, Popper, H. and Schaffner, F., Eds., Grune & Stratton, New York, 1976, 494.
20. **Sarles, H., Sarles, J. C., and Camatte, R.**, Observations on 205 confirmed cases of acute pancreatitis, recurring pancreatitis, and chronic pancreatitis, *Gut,* 6, 545, 1965.
21. **Hibbs, H. G., Ferrans, V. J., and Black, W. C.**, Alcoholic cardiopathy, an electron microscope study, *Am. Heart J.,* 69, 766, 1965.
22. The HANES Survey, National Center for Health Statistics, 1971 to 73, Vital and Health Statistics Series 1-NOS 10A 10B DHEW, Publication 73 — 1310 U.S. Government Printing Office, Washington, D.C., February, 1973.
23. Food and Nutrition Board, *Recommended Dietary Allowances,* 9th ed., Food and Nutrition Board, National Research Council, National Academy of Sciences, Washington, D.C., 1980.
24. **Baum, R. and Iber, F.**, Initial treatment of the alcoholic patient, in *Alcoholism,* Gitlow, S. and Peyser, H. S., Eds., Grune & Stratton, New York, 1980.
25. **Sellers, B. M., Naranjo, C. A., Giles, H. G., Frecker, R. C., and Beeching, M.**, Intravenous diazepam and oral ethanol interaction, *Clin. Pharmacol. Ther.,* 28 (5), 638, 1980.
26. **Koltz, U., Avant, G. R., Hoyumpa, A., Schenker, S., and Wilkinson, G. R.**, The effect of age and liver disease on the disposition and elimination of diazepam in adult man, *J. Clin. Invest.,* 55, 347, 1975.
27. **Roberts, R. K., Wilkinson, G. R., Branch, R. A., and Schenker, S.**, Effect of age and parenchymal liver disease on the disposition and elimination of chlordiazepoxide, *Gastroenterology,* 75 (3), 479, 1978.
28. **Lang, A. R., Goechner, D. J., Adesso, V. J., and Marlatt, G. A.**, Effects of alcohol on aggression in male social drinkers, *J. Abnorm. Psychol.,* 84, 508, 1975.
29. **Wolff, H. G., Hardy, J. D., and Goodell, H.**, Studies on pain: measurement of the effect of ethyl alcohol on the pain threshold and on the alarm reaction, *J. Pharmacol. Exp. Ther.,* 75, 38, 1942.
30. **Carpenter, J. A.**, Effects of alcoholic beverages on skin conductance: an exploratory study, *Q. J. Stud. Alcohol,* 18, 1, 1957.
31. American Bible Society, Genesis 9: 21, 1975.
32. **Damrau, F., Liddy, E., and Damrau, A. M.**, Value of stout as a sedative and relaxing soporific, *J. Am. Geriatr. Soc.,* 11, 238, 1963.
33. **Farkas, G. M. and Rosen, R. C.**, Effect of alcohol on elicited male sexual response, *J. Stud. Alcohol,* 37 (3), 265, 1976.
34. **Wilson, G. T. and Lawson, D. M.**, Expectancies, alcohol and sexual arousal in male social drinkers, *J. Abnormal Psychol.,* 85 (6), 587, 1976.
35. **Wilson, G. T. and Lawson, D. M.**, Expectancies, alcohol and sexual arousal in women, *J. Abnormal Psychol.,* 87 (3), 358, 1978.
36. **Seltzer, B. and Sherwin, I.**, Organic brain syndrome: an empirical study and critical review, *Am. J. Psychol.,* 135 (1), 13, 1978.
37. **Davies, G. V.**, The differential diagnosis of the mental disorders of late life, *Med. J. Aust. Sydney,* 1, 242, 1969.
38. **Cutting, J.**, Patterns of performance in amnesic subjects, *J. Neurology Neurosurg. Psychiatry,* 41 (3), 278, 1978.
39. **Freund, G.**, Physical dependence on ethanol: conceptual considerations, *Drug Alcohol Dependence,* 4(1,2), 173, 1979.
40. **Ryan, C. and Butters, N.**, Further evidence for a continuum-of-impairment encompassing male alcoholic Korsakoff patients and chronic alcoholic men, *Alcoholism,* 4(2), 190, 1980.
41. **Kastenbaum, R. and Slater, P. E.**, Effects of wine on the interpersonal behavior of geriatric patients: an exploratory study, in *New Thoughts on Old Age,* Kastenbaum, R., Ed., Spring, New York, 1964, 191.
42. **Black, A. L.**, Altering behavior of geriatric patients with beer. II, *Northwest Med.,* 68(5), 453, 1969.
43. **Mishara, B. L. and Kastenbaum, R.**, Wine in the treatment of long-term geriatric patients in mental institutions, *J. Am. Geriatr. Soc.,* 22, 88, 1974.
44. **Mishara, B. L., Kastenbaum, R., Baker, F., and Patterson, R. D.**, Alcohol effects in old age: an experimental investigation, *Soc. Sci. Med.,* 9, 535, 1975.
45. **Marks, V.**, Alcohol and carbohydrate metabolism, *Clin. Endocrinol. Metabol.,* 7 (2), 333, 1978.
46. **Arky, R. A. and Freinkel, N.**, Alcohol hypoglycemia. V. Alcohol infusion to test gluconeogenesis in starvation, with special reference to obesity, *N. Engl. J. Med.,* 274, 426, 1966.
47. **Arky, R. A., Veverbrants, E., and Abramson, E. A.**, Irreversible hypoglycemia: a complication of alcohol and insulin, *JAMA,* 206, 575, 1968.
48. **Voegtlin, W. L., O'Hollaren, L. P., and O'Hollaren, N.**, The glucose tolerance of alcohol addicts: study of 303 cases, *Q. J. Alcoholism,* 4, 163, 1943.
49. **Lundquist, G. A. R.**, Glucose tolerance in alcoholism, *Br. J. Addiction,* 61, 51, 1965.

50. Joffe, B. I., Shires, R., Seftel, H. C., and Heding, L. G., Plasma insulin, C-peptide, and glucagon levels in acute phase of ethanol-induced hypoglycaemia, *Br. Med. J.*, 2 (6088), 678, 1977.

51. Ginsberg, H., Olefsky, J., and Farquhar, J. W., Moderate ethanol ingestion and plasma triglyceride levels. A study in normal and hypertriglyceride persons, *Am. Int. Med.*, 80, 443, 1974.

52. Castelli, W. P., Doyle, J. T., Gordon, T., and Hames, C. G., Alcohol and blood lipids: the cooperative lipoprotein phenotyping study, *Lancet*, 2, 153, 1977.

53. Barboriak, J. J., Anderson, A. J., and Hoffmann, R. G., Interrelationship between coronary artery occlusion, high-density lipoprotein cholesterol, and alcohol intake, *J. Lab. Clin. Med.*, 94(2), 348, 1979.

54. Barboriak, J. J., Anderson, A. J., Rimm, A. A., and Tristani, F. E., Alcohol and coronary arteries, *Alcoholism*, 3, 29, 1979.

55. Williams, P., Robinson, D., and Bailey, A., High-density lipoprotein and coronary risk factors in normal men, *Lancet*, 1(8107), 72, 1979.

56. Walsh, M. J., Jr. and Truitt, E. B., The CNS effect of acetaldehyde and ethanol and interactions with catecholamines and psychotropic drugs, *Pharmacologist*, 11, 279, 1969.

57. Truitt, E. B. and Walsh, M. J., The role of acetaldehyde in the action of ethanol, in *The Biology of Alcoholism*, Vol. 1, Kissin, B. and Begliter, H., Eds., Plenum Press, New York, 1971, 161.

58. Sullivan, L. W. and Herbert, V., Symposium of hematopiesis by ethanol, *J. Clin. Invest.*, 43, 2048, 1964.

59. Rosenauerová-Ostra, A., Hilgertová, J., and Sonka, J., Urinary foraminoglutamite in man — normal values related to sex and age — effects of low calorie intake and alcohol consumption, *Clin. Chim. Acta*, 73, 39, 1976.

60. Pierce, H. I., McGuffin, R. G., and Hillman, R. S., Clinical studies in alcoholic sideroblastosis, *Arch. Int. Med.*, 136(3), 283, 1976.

61. Turner, T. B., Mezey, E., and Kimball, A. W., Measurement of alcohol-related effects in man: chronic effects in relation to levels of alcohol consumption, parts A & B, *Johns Hopkins Med. J.*, 141(5), 235 and 141(6), 273, 1977.

62. LaPorte, R. E., Cresanta, J. L., and Kuller, L. H., The relationship of alcohol consumption to atherosclerotic heart disease, *Prev. Med.*, 9(1), 22, 1980.

63. Wendt, V. E., Ajeluni, R., and Bruce, T. A., Acute effects of alcohol in the dog and human myocardium, *Am. J. Cardiol.*, 17, 804, 1966.

64. Regan, T. J., Weisse, A. D., and Moschos, C. B., The myocardial effect of acute and chronic usage of ethanol in man, *Trans. Assoc. Am. Phys.*, 78, 82, 1965.

65. Klatsky, A. L., Effects of alcohol on the cardiovascular system, in *Fermented Food Beverages in Nutrition*, Gastineau, C. F., Darby, W. J., and Turner, T. B., Eds., Academic Press, New York, 1979.

66. Regan, T. J., Khan, M. I., Ettinger, P. O., Haider, B., and Lyons, M. M., Myocardial function and lipid metabolism in the chronic alcoholic animal, *J. Clin. Invest.*, 54, 740, 1974.

67. Klatsky, A. L., Friedman, G. D., and Siegelaub, M. S., Alcohol consumption before myocardial infarction: results from the Kaiser-Permanente epidemiologic study of myocardial infarction, *Ann. Int. Med.*, 81, 294, 1974.

68. Kannell, W. B. and Sorlie, P., Hypertension in Framingham, in *Epidemiology and Control of Hypertension*, Paul, O., Ed., Yearbook Medical Publishers, Chicago, 1974.

69. Klatsky, A. L., Friedman, G. D., and Siegelaub, A. B., Alcohol use, myocardial infarction, sudden cardiac death, and hypertension, *Alcoholism Res.*, 3, 33, 1979.

70. Hennekens, C. H., Rosner, B., and Cole, D. S., Daily alcohol consumption and fatal coronary heart disease, *Am. J. Epidemiol.*, 107, 196, 1978.

71. Stason, W. B., Neff, R. K., Miettinen, O. S., and Jick, H., Alcohol consumption and nonfatal myocardial infarction, *Am. J. Epidemiol.*, 104, 603, 1976.

72. Hennekens, C. H., Rosner, B., and Cole, D. S., Daily alcohol consumption and fatal coronary heart disease, *Am. J. Epidemiol.*, 107, 196, 1978.

73. Hennekens, C. H., Willett, W., Rosner, B., Cole, D. S., and Mayrent, S. L., Effects of beer, wine, and liquor in coronary deaths, *JAMA*, 242, 1973, 1979.

74. Barboriak, J. J., Rimm, A. A., Anderson, A. J., and Schmidhoffer, M., Coronary artery occlusion and alcohol intake, *Br. Heart J.*, 39(3), 289, 1977.

75. Schottenfeld, D., Alcohol as a co-factor in etiology of cancer, *Cancer*, 43 (5 Suppl.), 1962, 1979.

76. Tuyns, A. J. and Audigier, J. C., Double wave cohort increased for esophageal and laryngeal cancer in France in relation to reduced alcohol consumption during the second world war, *Digestion*, 14(3), 197, 1976.

77. Gitlow, S. E. and Peyser, H. S., Alcoholism — A Practical Treatment Guide, in *The Medical Complications of Alcoholism*, Seixas, F. A., Ed., 165, Grune & Stratton, New York, 1980.

78. Wynder, E. L. and Stellman, S. D., Impact of long term filter cigarette usage on lung and larynx cancer risk — a case control study, *J. Natl. Cancer Inst.*, 62, 471, 1979.

79. Russell, R. M., Morrison, S. A., and Smith, F. R., Vitamin A reversal of abnormal dark adaptation in cirrhosis. Study of effects on the plasma retinol transport system, *Ann. Int. Med.*, 88, 622, 1978.

80. Solomon, L., Drug-induced arthropathic and necrosis on the femoral neck, *J. Bone Jt. Surg.*, 55B, 246, 1973.

81. Nilsson, B. E., Conditions contributing to fracture of the femoral neck, *Acta Chir. Scand.*, 136, 383, 1970.

82. Saville, P. D., Changes in bone mass with age and alcoholism, *J. Bone Jt. Surg.*, 47 (A), 492, 1965.

83. Roginsky, M. S., Zanzi, I., and Cohn, S. H., Skeletal and lean body mass in alcoholics with and without cirrhosis, *Calcif. Tiss. Res.*, 21, 386, 1976.

84. Dalén, J. H., *Acta Orthop. Scand.*, 47, 469, 1976.

85. Nilsson, B. E. and Westlin, N. E., The fracture incidence after gastrectomy, *Acta Chir. Scand.*, 137, 533, 1971.

86. Nillson, B. E. and Westlin, N. E., Femur density in alcoholism and after gastrectomy, *Calcif. Tiss. Res.*, 10, 167, 1972.

Chapter 12

DIETARY RESTRICTION AND LIFE EXTENSION — BIOLOGICAL MECHANISMS

Charles H. Barrows, Jr., and Gertrude C. Kokkonen

TABLE OF CONTENTS

I. INTRODUCTION

Because life span extension has not always been considered a desirable goal of research, gerontologists have suggested that efforts should be made to add life to years rather than years to life. Whether aging research will be successful in increasing either life to years or years to life remains to be seen. However, experiments designed to increase life span through dietary manipulations are continuing. It is the aim of this article to review and discuss those nutritional manipulations which have been indicated to increase the life span of laboratory animals.

Life extension due to dietary restriction is observed in a variety of species and may likely represent a very basic biological process. Unfortunately, the mechanisms responsible remain unknown. However, there are a number of studies which have measured various physiological and biochemical variables, as well as disease incidence, in normal animals as well as in those whose life span has been increased by dietary restriction. From such data, working models may evolve which would be useful in proposing various testable hypotheses related to this phenomenon. Therefore, it would be of interest to examine these data.

II. RESTRICTION OF CALORIES OR DIETARY PROTEINS

Any increase in life span associated with dietary manipulations is generally believed to be due to a restriction of dietary calories. However, most studies in an attempt to accomplish caloric restriction have restricted the intake of a nutritionally adequate diet so that not only has the caloric intake been reduced but also the protein and other dietary components as well. It must be recognized that it is experimentally difficult to hold all dietary components constant and reduce only calories. In order to achieve only caloric restriction under *ad libitum* conditions, there must be adjustments in the diets according to an animal's intake which changes markedly with growth and is dependent upon dietary composition. Thus far, caloric restriction has been successfully accomplished only once and the data indicated that restriction of calories indeed increased the life span of C_3H mice.[1]

The *ad libitum* feeding of a diet containing insufficient amounts of protein to support maximal growth has been shown to increase the life span of animals.[2] However, it is not clear the degree to which caloric restriction occurs under these experimental conditions. For example, it has been reported that reducing dietary protein did not affect the caloric intake of adult rats.[3] However, Ross reported that the caloric intake of growing rats fed a synthetic diet containing 8% casein was reduced when compared to that of animals fed a commercial diet.[4] Barrows et al. reported an 11% decrease in the intake of young rats fed a 10%, as compared to a 20%, protein diet.[5]

In contrast, Stoltzner has reported a marked increase in the caloric intake of BALB/c mice fed *ad libitum* diets containing low amounts of protein.[6] Therefore, on the basis of data presently available, it is not possible to conclude that calories are the sole dietary component which influence life span.

III. INFLUENCE OF AGE

It has been generally believed that nutritional manipulations which increase life span had to be imposed during growth. This concept originated as a result of the early work of Minot postulating that senescence follows the cessation of growth.[7-8] In addition, McCay et al. showed that an increased life span was associated with growth retardation.[9-10] Furthermore, Lansing indicated that aging in the rotifer involved a cytoplasmic factor the appearance of which coincided with the cessation of growth.[11] How-

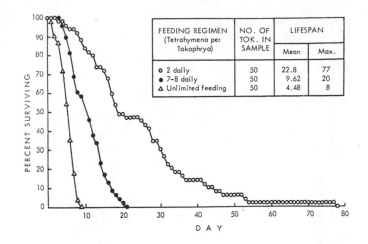

FIGURE 1. The percent survivorship of *Tokophrya lemnarum*.

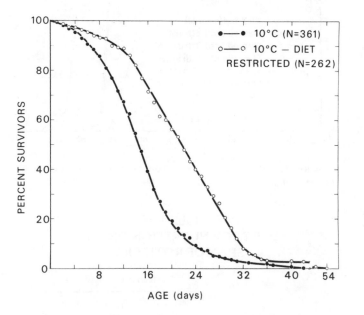

FIGURE 2. The percent survivorship of *Campanularia flexuosa* fed artemia daily or every third day.

ever, more recently, studies have indicated that dietary restriction imposed in adult life was effective in increasing life span.

Increased life span associated with underfeeding has been reported in the following growing animal model systems: *Tokophyra* (Figure 1),[12] *Campanularia flexuosa* (Figure 2),[13] *Daphnia* (Figure 3),[14] rotifers (Table 1),[15] *Drosophila*,[16] and fish (Figure 4).[17] In addition, a number of laboratory experiments have been carried out on rodents. McCay et al. carried out a series of three studies that supported the observation that nutritional deprivation increases life span.[18-20] Since these early studies, the increased life span associated with underfeeding has been reported in rats by Berg and Simms (Table 2),[21] Ross (Table 3),[4] Masoro et al.,[22] Leveille (Figure 5),[23] and Reisen et al.,[24] and in mice by Leto et al. (Figure 6).[25]

The life expectancy of adult animals can be increased by dietary manipulations as has been shown by Stuchlikova et al., (Figure 7)[26] Beauchene et al. (Table 4),[27] Fanestil

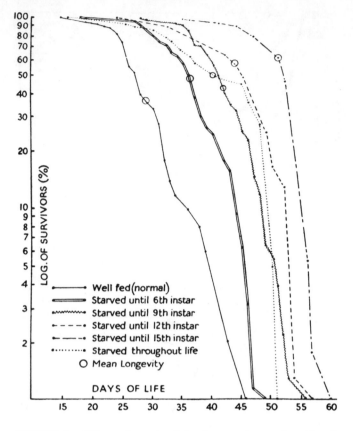

FIGURE 3. Effect of restricted food upon the survivorship of *Daphnia longispina.*

Table 1
EFFECT OF NUTRITION ON LIFE
SPAN OF ROTIFERS

		Mean life span (days)		
Experiment		Diet I[a]	Diet II[b]	Diet III[c]
1	Mn	35.7	43.8	58.6
	± SEM	±2.1	±3.0	±1.9
2	Mn	36.0	45.6	56.5
	± SEM	±1.2	±2.5	±2.2
3	Mn	29.0	46.2	49.1
	± SEM	±2.8	±3.2	±2.2
Mean	Mn	34.0	45.3	54.7
	± SEM	±1.1	±1.7	±1.3

[a]   Algae and fresh pond water daily.
[b]   Fresh pond water daily.
[c]   Fresh pond water—Mon., Wed., and Fri.

and Barrows (Table 5),[15] Ross (Table 6),[28] Nolen (Table 7),[29] Miller and Payne (Table 8),[30] and Barrows and Kokkonen (Table 9).[3] It is obvious from these data that there are a number of inconsistencies regarding the effect of dietary restriction on the exten-

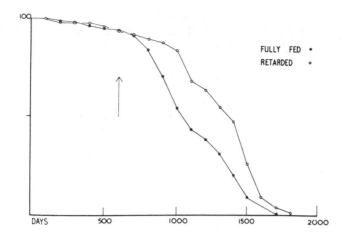

FIGURE 4. Survivorship curve of female *Lebistes reticulatus* fed live *Tubifex* worms weekly (●) or biweekly (O). Arrow indicates re-alimentation of the restricted fish. The animals were maintained at 23°C.

Table 2
THE EFFECT OF REDUCED DIETARY INTAKE ON LIFE SPAN OF MALE SPRAGUE-DAWLEY RATS

Diet[a]	N[b]	Survivorship at 799 days (%)	Max. body wt. (g)
Ad libitum	50	48	448
33% Restriction	48	87	342
46% Restriction	76	81	275

[a] Rockland "D free" pellets.
[b] Number of rats at start.

sion of life span in adult animals. Unfortunately, the limited amount of data does not allow for a critical evaluation of the variables which may be influencing the ability of a mature organism to respond to dietary manipulation. However, the age at which dietary manipulations are initiated is important. This is clearly indicated by the data of Dunham shown in Figure 8.[31] Daphnia adequately fed up to the sixth instar, then subjected to dietary restriction, showed an increase in life span. However, a shortening in life span was observed if this dietary manipulation was imposed later in life. A shortening of life span due to dietary restriction imposed in 19-month-old rats has been observed by Barrows and Roeder.[32] In these experiments, restricted animals were offered 50% of the diet consumed by the *ad libitum* fed controls and their life spans were 20.5 ± 0.44 and 22.3 ± 0.43 months, respectively. It is also apparent from the studies of Kopec[33] and David et al. (Figure 9)[34] that the degree of dietary restriction imposed on an adult organism may influence the life span of Drosophila.

The sex of an adult animal may also influence its response to dietary restriction in terms of life span. For example, the life-shortening effect of dietary restriction in adult drosophila was more marked in males (33%) than in females (17%).[34] In addition, the life span of 445-day-old female, but not male rats, was increased by decreasing the dietary protein.[35] Thus it is apparent that further studies must be carried out to define effective ways of consistently increasing the life span of adult organisms.

Table 3
THE EFFECT OF DIETARY INTAKES AND PROTEIN LEVELS ON LIFE SPAN OF MALE SPRAGUE-DAWLEY RATS

Unrestricted Dietary Intake

Diets	Commercial	A	B	C	D
N[a]	150.0	25.0	25.0	25.0	25.0
Casein (%)	23.0	30.0	50.8	8.0	21.6
Caloric value (Cal/g)	3.1	4.1	4.2	4.1	4.2
Food intake (g/day)	25.0	17.4	18.8	15.0	19.6
Max. body wt (g)	610.0		(not available)		
Mean life span (days)	730.0	305.0	595.0	825.0	600.0
Max. life span (days)	1072.0	347.0	810.0	1251.0	895.0

Restricted Dietary Intake

Diets	A	B	C	D
N[a]	150.0	60.0	150.0	135.0
Casein (%)	30.0	50.8	8.0	21.6
Caloric value (Cal/g)	4.1	4.2	4.1	4.2
Food intake (g/day)	14.3	8.5	14.3	5.3
Max. body weight (g)	420.0	287.0	390.0	162.0
Mean life span (days)	904.0	935.0	818.0	929.0

[a]   Number of rats at start.

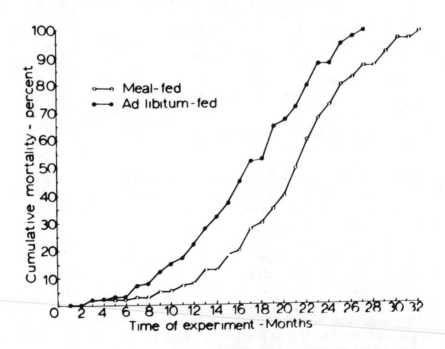

FIGURE 5.   Cumulative mortality for male Sprague-Dawley rats offered food for periods of two hours (O—O, meal-fed) or 24 hours (●—●, *ad libitum*-fed) daily.

IV. PHYSIOLOGICAL AND BIOCHEMICAL CHARACTERISTICS OF RESTRICTED ANIMALS

Figure 10 shows that animals whose life span has been increased by low protein feeding (4%) have a lower rectal temperature than do those fed the control diet (24%

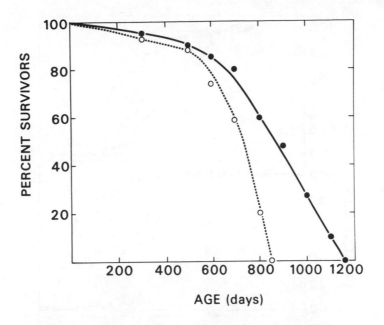

FIGURE 6. Survivorship curve of female C57BL/6J mice fed *ad libitum* either a 26% casein diet (O) or 4% casein diet (●); the mean lifespans and SEMS were 685 ± 22.8 and 852 ± 27.4 days respectively.

protein).[25] In addition, the low body temperatures of these mice were associated with an increased oxygen consumption (Figure 11).[25] Although the incidence of many diseases increases with age, the relationship between diseases and aging remains unknown. The data of Saxton et al. (Figure 12),[36] Ross and Bras (Figure 13),[37] Visscher et al. (Table 10),[1] Berg and Simms (Table 11),[21] and Bras (Table 12)[38] clearly indicate that dietary restriction which increased life span delayed the onset of a variety of diseases in mice and rats. However, the data are not consistent regarding the relationship between dietary restriction and disease prevalence. Furthermore, there are no indications as to the mechanisms responsible for this delay in onset.

There have been reports on the effects of long-term dietary restriction on immunological functions. In one study, Stoltzner et al.[39] fed BALB/C male mice *ad libitum* a diet that contained either 24, 8, or 4% protein derived from casein. In another study, Gerbase-DeLima et al.[40] fed C57BL/6J female mice a nutritionally adequate diet (21.6% casein) *ad libitum* or every other day. Stoltzner et al.[39] reported that there were no differences in mitogenic response after 125 days of age between restricted and non-restricted animals when lymphocytes were cultured with various mitogens. The data of Gerbase-DeLima et al.,[40] however, indicate marked differences in these immunological indices especially after middle age, 52 to 55 weeks. A diminished primary antibody response to sheep red blood cells was also reported by Stoltzner et al.[39] On the other hand, the data of Gerbase-DeLima et al.[40] indicate this immunological function is markedly greater in middle-aged, restricted animals than in controls. These apparent discrepancies between the two reports may be explained by differences in strain, sex and/or dietary manipulation. Walford et al.[41] proposed that the initial suppression of the immunological responses was followed by a maturation of a normal response pattern later in life. The peak response was then carried on into later life whereas control animals showed their age-related decline in immunological responses.

The life span of rotifers transferred to fresh pond water daily and given algae (Diet I) was 34 days. Rotifers deprived of algae and given fresh pond water daily (Diet II) lived 45 days. When the animals were deprived of algae and transferred to fresh pond

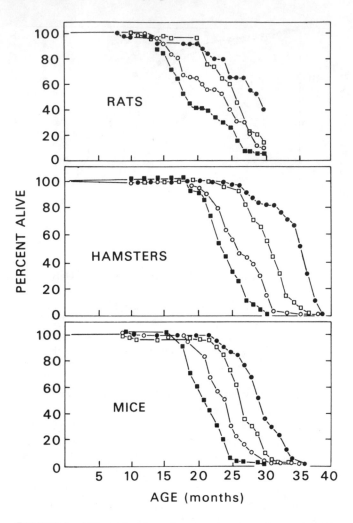

FIGURE 7.   Effect of various dietary regimens on the survivorship of rats, hamsters, and mice. Group 1 (■) was fed *ad libitum* throughout life; Group 2 (O) was fed one half the amount of food consumed by Group 1 throughout their life; Group 3 (□) was fed *ad libitum* until 1 year of age and then restricted thereafter; Group 4 (●) was restricted until 1 year of age and then fed *ad libitum* thereafter.

water only on Monday, Wednesday, and Friday (Diet III), the life span was increased to 54 days.[15] Data presently available indicate that the pattern of change of most enzymatic activities throughout the life span is characterized by an increasing concentration during early life, a period of relatively stable values during adulthood, and a decreased activity during senescence.[42] In Figure 14 it can be seen that this normal age-associated pattern of change was observed in the lactic dehydrogenase (LDH) activity of rotifers under all three dietary regimes. However, dietary restriction delayed the time of occurrence of the change.[15] Figure 15 shows a similar effect when malic dehydrogenase (MDH) activity was measured. The enzymatic activities are expressed as the total amount of enzyme per rotifer.[15] In order to minimize the influence of changes in body mass on changes in the enzymatic activities, a ratio of malic dehydrogenase to lactic dehydrogenase (MDH/LDH) was calculated in individual animals and is presented in Figure 16. In control rotifers the ratio decreased markedly at the age of 13 days. Reduced dietary intake, which increased the life span to 54 days, delayed this

Table 4
THE EFFECT OF INTERMITTENT FEEDING[a] ON LIFE SPAN OF MALE WISTAR RATS

Diet[b]	N[c]	Mean life span + SEM (weeks)
Ad lib.[d]	25	133.1 ± 4.1
Ad lib.-restricted[e]	30	150.0 ± 4.6
Restricted-ad lib.[e]	30	149.2 ± 3.6
Restricted[d]	25	163.4 ± 3.9

[a] Fed every other day.
[b] Wayne Lab Blox Diet.
[c] Number of rats at start.
[d] Throughout life span.
[e] Dietary regimen changed at 1 year of age.

Table 5
THE EFFECT OF CHANGES IN NUTRITION FOLLOWING CESSATION OF EGG PRODUCTION ON THE LIFE SPAN OF ROTIFER (PHILODINA ACUTICORNIS)

N[a]	Interval A—C[b]	Interval C—E[b]	Mean life span + SEM (days)
30	I[c]	I	33.4 ± 1.27
28	I	III	41.8 ± 2.62
22	III	III	53.4 ± 3.65
29	III	I	57.7 + 1.13

[a] Number at start.
[b] A = day hatched; C = end of egg production; E = death.
[c] I = algae and fresh pond water daily; III = fresh pond water Mon., Wed., and Fri., animals maintained at 25°C.

decrement until the 33rd day of life.[15] Similar data on the delay in time of occurrence of changes in enzymatic activities have been reported by Ross for the enzymes adenosine triphosphatase and alkaline phosphatase in the livers of rats (Figure 17).[43]

On the other hand, when enzymatic activities were expressed either per unit DNA or per cell a different pattern of change with age due to dietary restriction is observed. For example, feeding ad libitum a diet containing 4% protein increased the life span of female mice. The activities of various enzymes calculated on the basis of DNA were low in these restricted animals (Figures 18-20).[44] In addition, it has been reported that hepatocytic alkaline phosphatase, histidase, adenosine triphosphatase, as well as catalase (Figure 21) activities were markedly lower in animals whose life span was increased by dietary restriction as compared to control rats.[45]

It is of interest to establish whether the various dietary manipulations which increase life span do so by a common biological mechanism. A recent series of studies measuring various biochemical, immunological, and morphological variables were carried out in mice fed two dietary regimes reported to increase life span; namely, low protein and intermittent feeding.[4,25,27,46,47] The activities of succinoxidase, cholinesterase, and malic

Table 6

DAILY DIETARY ALLOTMENTS AND MORTALITY RISK AFTER 300
DAYS OF AGE

Diet (% casein)	Level of allotment %	Total food (g)	Casein (g)	Sucrose (g)	Corn oil (g)	Total calories (kcal)	Mortality[b] index (×100)
Commercial[a]	100	25.0				85.51	105
	80	20.0				68.4	106
	70	17.5				59.9	83
	60	15.0				51.3	79
A (30.0%)	100	18.0	5.40	10.98	0.90	73.6	5550
	90	16.2	4.86	9.88	0.81	66.3	1180
	80	14.4	4.32	8.78	0.72	58.9	1940
	71.5	12.9	3.86	7.85	0.64	52.6	723
B (50.9%)	100	19.0	9.66	6.44	1.61	78.9	178
	78	14.8	7.53	5.02	1.25	61.4	122
	55.9	10.6	5.40	3.60	0.90	44.1	115
	40	7.6	3.86	2.58	0.64	31.6	675
C (8.0%)	100	15.0	1.20	12.45	0.75	61.4	2103
	96	14.4	1.15	11.95	0.72	58.9	2882
	86.8	13.0	1.04	10.81	0.65	53.3	3195
	79.3	11.9	.95	9.88	0.60	48.7	3195
D (21.6%)	100	20.0	4.32	10.81	2.70	84.8	200
	80.7	16.1	3.49	8.72	2.18	68.4	126
	59.6	11.9	2.58	6.44	1.61	50.6	99
	52	10.4	2.25	5.62	1.41	44.1	68

[a]   Purina Lab Chow, 23% protein
[b]   Mortality ratio values less than 100 are indicative of the beneficial influences resulting from the change in dietary regimen; values more than 100, of the detrimental influences.

Table 7

THE EFFECT OF REDUCED DIETARY
INTAKE ON THE MEAN SURVIVAL
TIME OF SPRAGUE-DAWLEY RATS

Diet[a]	Mean survival time (days) Males[b]	Females[b]
Ad lib.	706	756
20% Restriction	856	872
40% Restriction	924	872
Ad lib. for 12 weeks, 20% restriction thereafter	801	871
Ad lib. for 12 weeks, 40% restriction thereafter	927	943
20% Restriction for 12 weeks, *Ad lib.* thereafter	723	788
40% Restriction for 12 weeks, *Ad lib.* thereafter	782	805

[a]   Natural products diet: lipid, 18.5%; protein, 23%; ash, 6.2%; 4.4 kcal/g.
[b]   50 rats at start; diets started just after weaning.

Table 8
THE EFFECT OF VARIOUS DIETARY REGIMENS ON LIFE SPAN OF FEMALE RATS

Dietary regimen[a]	Life expectancy ± SE (days)	Significant differences
A	763 ± 94	$P<0.001$
B	980 ± 50	$P<0.001$
C	828 ± 73	
D	282 ± 40	
E	<100	

[a]   A — stock diet throughout life; B — stock diet for 120 days, then 20% stock diet and 80% starch; C — 30% stock diet and 70% starch throughout life; E — protein free diet. All diets were *ad libitum*.

Table 9
THE EFFECT OF DIETARY PROTEIN LEVELS ON THE SURVIVAL OF 16-MONTH FEMALE WISTAR RATS

Dietary protein levels (%)	N	Survival (weeks)
24	44	29.5 ± 2.28[a]
12	44	37.0 ± 2.00[b]
8	44	30.0 ± 2.30
4	44	31.6 ± 1.70

[a]   Mean ± SEM
[b] $P = .001$

dehydrogenase were decreased in the 4%-protein groups and intermittent-fed animals (sacrificed following a 24-hr fast period) and increased in intermittent-fed animals (sacrificed following a 24-hr feeding period) (Table 13).[48] Furthermore, the mean values of the enzymatic activities per mg of DNA of the intermittent-fed and intermittent-fasted animals were essentially the same as that of the 24% *ad libitum* controls. Therefore, these data did not indicate the existence of a common biochemical alteration to explain the phenomenon of increased life span due to dietary restriction. However, the morphological data showed that microvilli present on the surface of podocytes and their processes of the kidney, vary according to age and dietary restriction. The results shown in Figure 22 clearly indicate that both types of dietary restriction produce the same effect, i.e., a lower amount of microvilli as compared to normal animals of the same age.[49] Similarly, the mitogenic activity of 3-week-old mice placed on these diets for a period of 1 month were lower in both animals fed the 4% protein diet and those intermittently fed as compared to control animals (Figure 23).[50] Therefore, this morphological and immunological data may represent evidence of a common biological alteration found in these dietarily restricted animals fed dietary regimes reported to increase life span.

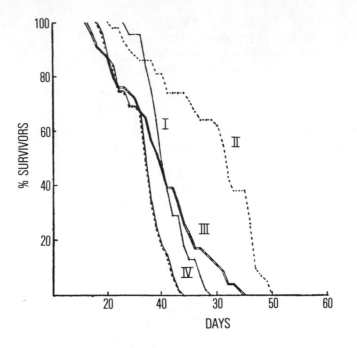

FIGURE 8.   The effect of dietary restriction on the survivorship curves of D. *longispina.* I — represents well-fed controls; II — semistarved controls; III — group well-fed to 6th instar and then semistarved; and IV — well-fed to 12th instar and then semistarved. Semistarvation was brought about by diluting normal medium some 30 to 40 times with pond water.

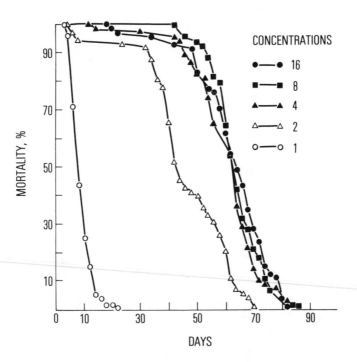

FIGURE 9.   Survival curves of adult *Drosophila* (both sexes). The usual axenic medium contained 8% brewer's yeast and 8% cornflour. This medium was diluted with an agar solution in order to produce concentrations ranging from 16 to 1%.

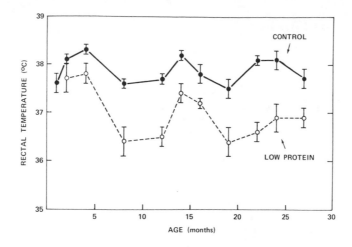

FIGURE 10.   Effect of low-protein feeding on rectal temperature of female C57BL/6J mice. Vertical bars represent SEM. The mean life span and SEM of the animals fed either the low-protein or control diet was 852 ± 27.4 days, and 685 ± 22.8 days, respectively.

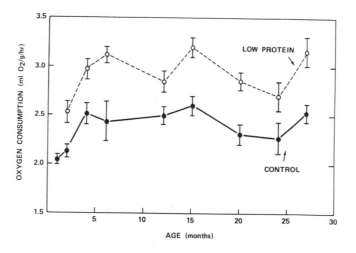

FIGURE 11.   Effect of low-protein feeding on oxygen consumption of C57BL/6J female mice. Vertical bars represent SEM. The mean life span and SEM of the animals fed either the low-protein or control diet was 852 ± 27.4 days and 685 ± 22.8 days, respectively.

V. BIOLOGICAL MECHANISMS

Efforts will be made to relate physiological and biochemical differences between normal and dietarily restricted animals to concepts regarding the causes of biological aging. Unfortunately, little information is available on the effect of body temperature on the life span of homeothermic animals. Nevertheless the life span of poikilothermic animals increases with decreased environmental temperature.[51] It is generally assumed that this latter finding is a result of a decreased metabolic rate due to the lowering of the rates of biochemical reactions at the reduced temperatures. However, the low body temperatures of the mice described by Leto et al.[25] were associated with an increased oxygen consumption. Furthermore, studies of Clark and Kidwell[52] and Clarke and Smith,[53] in which poikilotherms had been exposed to different temperatures at various

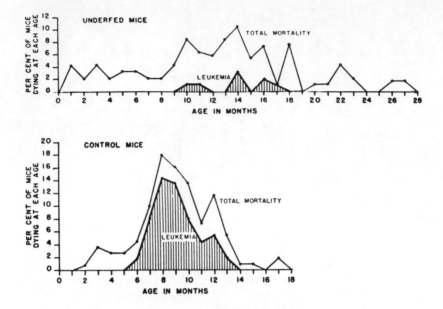

FIGURE 12.   Effect of underfeeding on the mortality and incidence of leukemia in AKR mice. The underfed (47 males, 47 females) mice were offered 1.5 g of Wayne Fox Food Blox® daily; controls (52 males, 59 females) were given the same diet *ad libitum*.

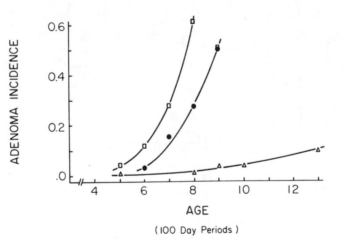

FIGURE 13.   Influence of dietary regimen on the incidence of adenomas in male COBS (Charles River) rats. (□) Rats fed *ad libitum* throughout postweaning life; (△) rats fed a restricted amount of diet throughout postweaning life; (●) rats fed a restricted amount of diet 21 to 70 days of age, and then fed *ad libitum*. Composition of diet: casein, 22.0%; sucrose, 58.5%; Mazola® oil, 13.5%; salt mixture (USP XII), 6.0%; vitamins, and trace elements.

times in the life cycle, suggest a more complicated mechanism which may be independent of basal metabolic rate. Complete agreement on the effects of oxygen uptake on the life span of animals is not found in data presently available. For many years an inverse correlation has been described among various species of mammals, i.e., the higher the oxygen uptake per unit of body weight, the shorter the life span.[54] Indeed Kibler and Johnson showed that rats exposed to cold temperatures throughout their

Table 10
THE EFFECT OF DIETARY RESTRICTION
ON THE INCIDENCE OF SPONTANEOUS
MAMMARY CARCINOMA AND THE
SURVIVAL OF C₃H MICE

	Restricted	Unrestricted
N[a]	44	51
Caloric intake/day[b]	8.4	11.5
Protein intake/day[b]	0.64	0.65
Max. body weight (g)	15.5	32.0
% Survival at 16 months	57.0	29.0
Cumulative tumors[c] (%) at 16 months	0	63.0

[a]   Number of mice at start.
[b]   After 100 days of age.
[c]   Spontaneous mammary carcinoma.

Table 11
THE EFFECT OF DIETARY RESTRICTION ON THE
INCIDENCE OF THREE MAJOR DISEASES IN MALE
SPRAGUE-DAWLEY RATS

		% Incidence[b]		
	N[a]	Glomerularnephritis	Periarteritis	Myocardial degeneration
Unrestricted	24	100	63	96
33% Restricted	42	36	17	28
46% Restricted	38	13	3	24

[a]   Number of rats at start.
[b]   At 800 days of age.

life experienced a marked decrease in longevity and a 40% increase in oxygen consumption.[55] However, Weiss reported that although the life span of the F-1 generation was higher and the BMR lower than either parental strains (AXC and Fisher), the BMR of the parents were essentially the same in spite of marked differences in longevity.[56,57] Finally, Storer has reported a direct relationship between oxygen consumption and life span among 18 strains of mice.[58] Should the longevity of individuals within a strain vary inversely with basal metabolic rate, the increased oxygen consumption due to dietary restriction would shorten life span, whereas, should the converse relationship exist, the increased oxygen consumption of these mice would result in an increased life span. Therefore the interrelationship among life span, body temperature, and basal metabolic rate provides no information toward an understanding of the mechanism responsible for the increased life span associated with dietary restriction.

It has been proposed that the fertilized egg contains all the genetic information necessary for the orderly sequence of events occurring during the life of an organism. The coded information of the DNA is transcribed to messenger RNA and translated into proteins. It is obvious that new information must be transmitted at different ages in order to account for the various changes seen in an organism throughout its life.[59] It is possible that the rate of occurrence of these programmed events is influenced by the rate of synthesis of specific regulatory RNAs and proteins. Thus it may be proposed

Table 12
PROGRESSIVE
GLOMERULONEPHROSIS
INDEX OF MALE SPRAGUE-
DAWLEY RATS FED
SEMISYNTHETIC DIETS

Dietary groups[a]	Number of cases		Disease index[b]
	Expected	Observed	
A	186.4	46	24.7
B	88.2	1	1.1
C	152.5	16	10.5
D	10.5	4	1.9

[a]   The intakes of animals fed diet A, B, C, or D were restricted (See Table 3).

[b]   Computed from rats dying from natural death only. Disease index expressed as percentage (computed as number of actual against expected cases). Expected cases equals disease rate at each age period of "control" population times exposure of experimental population. A value of the index of less than 100 indicates a beneficial effect of the experimental diet.

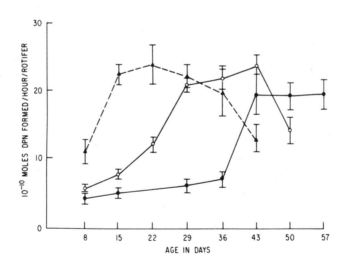

FIGURE 14.   Effect of nutrition on lactic dehydrogenase activity in rotifers *(Philodina acuticornis)*. (▲) Diet I (algae and fresh pond water daily; mean life span = 34.0 ± 1.1 days); (O) Diet II (fresh pond water daily; mean life span = 45.3 ± 1.7 days); and (●) Diet III (fresh pond water Mon., Wed., and Fri.; mean life span = 54.7 ± 1.3 days). Vertical bars represent SEM.

that a possible way to retard the rate of aging would be to decrease the rates of syntheses of specific RNAs and proteins during the life of an organism. The studies cited regarding the changes in enzymatic activities throughout the life span of rotifers and rats may support this concept. For example, in these studies the typical pattern of

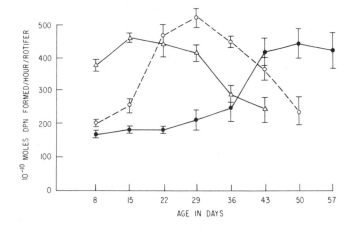

FIGURE 15.   Effect of nutrition on malic dehydrogenase activity in
rotifers *(Philodina acuticornis).* (△) Diet I (algae and fresh pond water
daily; mean life span = 34.0 ± 1.1 days); (O) Diet II (fresh pond
water daily; mean life span = 45.3 ± 1.7 days); and (●) Diet III (fresh
pond water Mon., Wed., and Fri.; mean life span = 54.7 ± 1.3 days).
Vertical bars represent SEM.

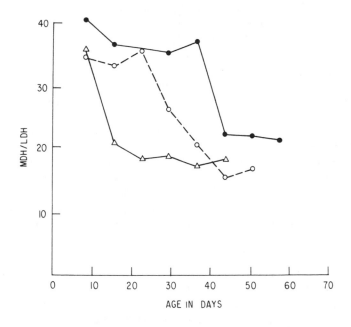

FIGURE 16.   Effect of nutrition on MDH/LDH. (△) Diet I (algae
and fresh pond water daily; mean life span = 34.0 ± 1.1 days); (O)
Diet II (fresh pond water daily; mean life span = 45.3 ± 1.7 days);
and (●) Diet III (fresh pond water Mon., Wed., and Fri.; mean life
span = 54.7 ± 1.3 days).

changes observed in most enzymatic activities throughout the life span, i.e., an increase
in concentration during early life, a period of relatively stable values during adulthood,
and decreased activity during senescence, were found regardless of the life span. However, dietary restriction which increased life span delayed the time of occurrence of
these changes. This concept may also be supported by the immunological studies of

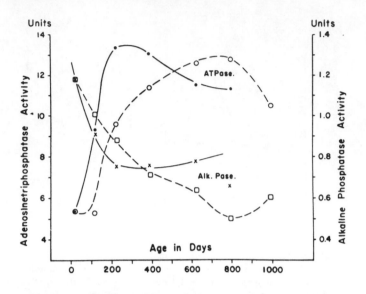

FIGURE 17.   Effect of diet and age on the activity of hepatic adenosinetriphosphatase and alkaline phosphatase in male Sprague-Dawley rats. Enzymatic activities are expressed as activity per milligram
wet weight of tissue. Rats maintained on commercial diet *ad libitum:*
(×) alkaline phosphatase activity; (●) adenosinetriphosphatase activity. Rats whose daily food allotment of Diet C was restricted (see Table 3): (□) alkaline phosphatase activity; (○) adenosinetriphosphatase
activity.

Walford[41] who proposed that the initial suppression of the immunological responses
of restricted animals was followed by a maturation of a normal response pattern later
in life. This peak response was then carried on into later life whereas control animals
showed their age-related decline in immunological responses. If disease is an integral
part of aging and is genetically controlled, then it seems to follow that dietary restriction should delay the onset of specific diseases as well as increase life span. Indeed, it
has been previously pointed out that the onset of many diseases found in rats and mice
is delayed in animals whose life span has been increased by dietary restriction. Therefore, there are many studies which support the concept that dietary restriction which
increases life span also delays the occurrence of specific programmed events at least
during early life.

At present there is no evidence to support the concept that aging results from the
expression of deleterious genes in late life. In addition the ability to increase the life
span of adult organisms indicates that another mechanism must exist independent of
alterations in the readout of the genetic code. It has been proposed that dietary restriction results in limited amounts of amino acids which result in decreased protein synthesis and consequent decreased use of the genetic code. It was further proposed that
the age changes observed in tissue proteins are the result of selective errors caused by
use of the genetic code.[48] In addition, studies previously cited suggest a reduced use
of the genetic code in the tissues of restricted animals. For example, feeding *ad libitum*
a diet containing 4% protein increased the life span of female C57BL/6J mice. The
activities of various enzymes calculated on the basis of DNA were low in these restricted animals. In addition, Ross has reported that hepatocytic catalase, alkaline
phosphatase, histidase, and adenosine triphosphatase activities were markedly lower
in animals whose life span was increased by dietary restriction as compared to control
rats.[45] The work of Schimke supports the premise that reduced enzymatic activity per

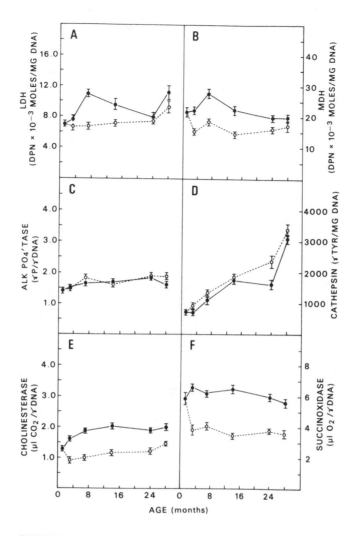

FIGURE 18. Effect of age and diet on the enzymatic activities of liver of female C57BL/6J mice fed (●) 26% casein diet or (O) 4% casein diet. Vertical bars represent SEM. The mean life span and SEM of the animals fed either the low-protein or control diet was 852 ± 27.4 days and 685 ± 22.8 days, respectively.

DNA or per cell represents a reduced enzyme synthesis.[60] For example, Figure 24 shows that when rats were fed diets in which the protein was decreased from 70 to 8%, the animals reduced their total liver arginase from approximately 9 mg to 2 mg and the rates of both synthesis and degradation decreased from 0.7 mg arginase per gram of protein per 3 days to 0.2 mg arginase per gram of protein per 3 days. Therefore, a reduction in cellular enzymatic activity due to a reduction in dietary protein is the result of a decreased rate of protein synthesis when steady state conditions are reached. A decreased rate of protein synthesis is most likely to result in a reduced use of the genetic code.

VI. SUMMARY

Dietary restriction has been shown to increase the life span of a variety of species. The beneficial effects of dietary restriction can be brought about when underfeeding

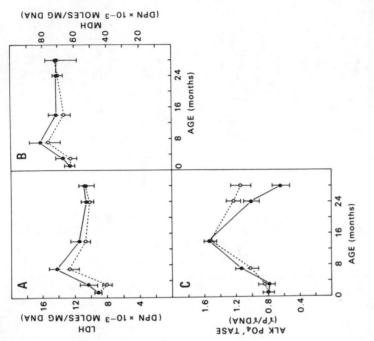

FIGURE 20.   Effect of age and diet on the enzymatic activities of hearts of female C57BL/6J mice fed (●) 26% casein diet or (○) 4% casein diet. Vertical bars represent SEM. The mean life span and SEM of the animals fed either the low-protein or control diet was 852 ± 27.4 days and 685 ± 22.8 days, respectively.

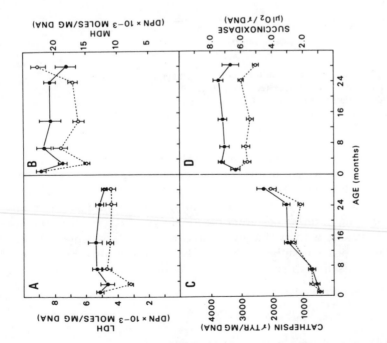

FIGURE 19.   Effect of age and diet on the enzymatic activities of kidneys of female C57BL/6J mice fed (●) 26% casein diet or (○) 4% casein diet. Vertical bars represent SEM. The mean life span and SEM of the animals fed either the low-protein or control diet was 852 ± 27.4 days and 685 ± 22.8 days, respectively.

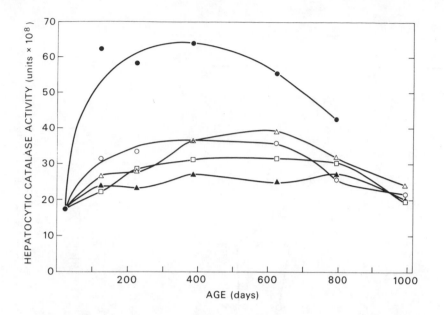

FIGURE 21.   Effect of diet and age on the activity of hepatic catalase in male Sprague-Dawley rats. Rats maintained on commercial diet *ad libitum* (●); rats whose daily food allotment was restricted (see Table 3): (○) Diet A; (△) Diet B; (□) Diet C; (▲) Diet D.

Table 13
THE EFFECT OF VARIOUS DIETARY REGIMENS ON ENZYMATIC ACTIVITIES IN LIVERS OF FEMALE MICE

	24% Protein	4% Protein	Intermittent[a] fed	Intermittent[b] fasted
Malic dehydrogenase (mmol DPNH/hr/mg DNA)				
2 month-old[c]	10.211 ± 0.293[d]	7.344 ± 0.148[e]	11.578 ± 0.178[e]	10.371 ± 0.506
7 month-old[c]	7.998 ± 0.343	5.543 ± 0.383[e]	9.714 ± 0.409[e]	7.009 ± 0.218[e]
22 month-old[f]	8.377 ± 0.601	6.427 ± 0.404[e]	9.916 ± 0.778	—
Succinoxidase (u 10_2/hr/γDNA)				
2 month-old	6.71 ± 0.37	4.00 ± 0.12[e]	7.53 ± 0.20	6.73 ± 0.21
7 month-old	5.96 ± 0.26	3.21 ± 0.16[e]	6.99 ± 0.22[e]	5.87 ± 0.20
22 month-old	7.29 ± 0.32	3.39 ± 0.22[e]	7.41 ± 0.47	—
Cholinesterase (u $1CO_2$/hr/λDNA)				
2 month-old	7.34 ± 0.31	5.02 ± 0.30[e]	9.79 ± 0.49[e]	6.36 ± 0.32[e]
7 month-old	6.82 ± 0.44	3.95 ± 0.32[e]	8.47 ± 0.27[e]	6.06 ± 0.31
22 month-old	6.29 ± 0.46	4.69 ± 0.31[e]	8.35 ± 0.83[e]	—

[a]   Fed *ad libitum* a 24% protein diet on Mon., Wed., and Fri.; sacrificed Tues. or Thurs.
[b]   Fed *ad libitum* a 24% protein diet Mon., Wed., and Fri.; sacrificed Wed. or Fri.
[c]   C57BL/6J mice fed dietary regimes from weaning.
[d]   Mean ± SEM.
[e]   p<05 when compared to values obtained for animals fed the 24% protein diet.
[f]   CBA mice fed dietary regimes from 17 months of age.

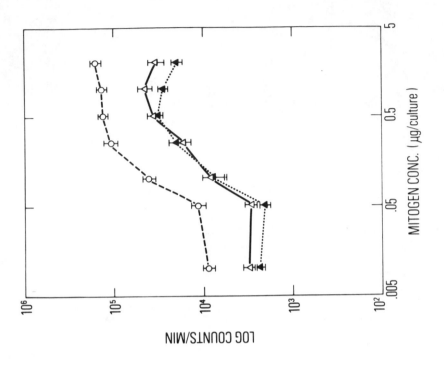
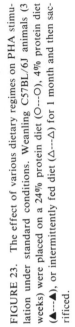

FIGURE 23. The effect of various dietary regimes on PHA stimulation under standard conditions. Weanling C57BL/6J animals (3 weeks) were placed on a 24% protein diet (O---O), 4% protein diet (▲--▲), or intermittently fed diet (△--△) for 1 month and then sacrificed.

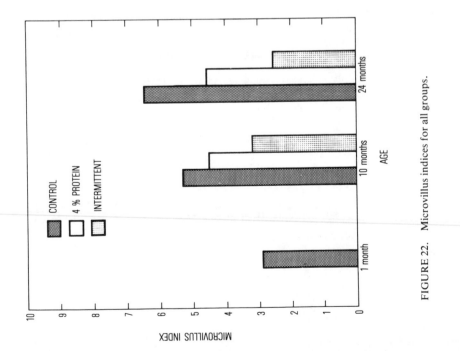

FIGURE 22. Microvillus indices for all groups.

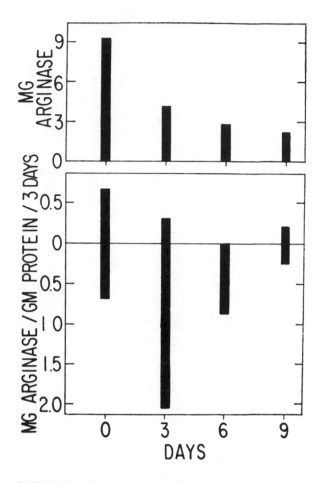

FIGURE 24.   Rates of synthesis and degradation of rat liver arginase when dietary protein is reduced from 70 to 8% casein. The upper set of bars indicates the total milligrams of arginase in the pooled sample of livers at the end of the specified experimental period. The lower set of bars shows the rates of synthesis and degradation expressed as milligrams of arginase synthesized and degraded per gram of total liver protein per observational period.

is initiated in adult as well as young growing animals. Dietary restriction has been shown to reduce body temperature; increase basal metabolic rate; delay the onset of a variety of diseases; delay age-associated changes in biochemical, immunological, and morphological variables; as well as reduce the enzymatic activities of cells. Attempts to relate these changes to current concepts regarding the causes of biological aging have failed to establish a biological mechanism responsible for the increased life span associated with dietary restriction.

REFERENCES

1. Visscher, M. B., Barnes, Z. B., and Sivertsen, I., The influence of caloric restriction upon the incidence of spontaneous mammary carcinoma in mice, *Surgery*, 11, 48, 1942.
2. Barrows, C. H. and Kokkonen, G. C., Relationship between nutrition and aging, in *Advances in Nutritional Research*, Vol. 1, Draper, H. H., Ed., Plenum Press, New York, 1977, 253.

3. Barrows, C. H. and Kokkonen, G. C., Protein synthesis, development, growth, and life span, *Growth,* 39, 525, 1975.

4. Ross, M. H., Length of life and nutrition in the rat, *J. Nutr.,* 75, 197, 1961.

5. Barrows, C. H., Roeder, L. M., and Fanestil, D. D., The effects of restriction of total dietary intake and protein intake, and of fasting interval on the biochemical composition of rat tissues, *J. Gerontol.,* 20, 374, 1965.

6. Stoltzner, G., Effects of life-long dietary protein restriction on mortality, growth, organ weights, blood counts, liver aldolase, and kidney catalase in BALB/C mice, *Growth,* 41, 337, 1977.

7. Minot, C. S., The problem of age, growth, and death; a study of cytomorphis based on lectures at the Lovell Institute, March, 1907, Lovell Institute, London, 1908.

8. Minot, C. S., *Moderne Probleme der Biologie,* Jena, 1913.

9. McCay, C. M., Ellis, G. H., Barnes, L. L., Smith, C. A. H., and Sperling, G., Chemical and pathological changes in aging and after retarded growth, *J. Nutr.,* 18, 15, 1931.

10. McCay, C. M., Dilley, W. E., and Crowell, M. F., Growth rates of brook trout reared upon purified rations, upon dry skim milk diets, and upon feed combinations of cereal grains, *J. Nutr.,* 1, 233, 1929.

11. Lansing, A., Evidence of aging as a consequence of growth cessation, *Proc. Natl. Acad. Sci.,* 34, 304, 1948.

12. MacKeen, P. C. and Mitchell, R. B., personal communication, 1976.

13. Brock, M. A., personal communication, 1976.

14. Ingle, E., Wood, T. R., and Banta, A. M., A study of longevity, growth, reproduction, and heart rate in *Daphnia longispina* as influenced by limitations in quantity of food, *J. Exp. Zool.,* 76, 325, 1937.

15. Fanestil, D. D. and Barrows, C. H., Aging in the rotifer, *J. Gerontol.,* 20, 462, 1965.

16. Loeb, J. and Northrop, J. H., On the influence of food and temperature upon the duration of life, *J. Biol. Chem.,* 32, 103, 1917.

17. Comfort, A., Effect of delayed and resumed growth on the longevitiy of a fish (*Lebistes reticulatus* Peters) in captivity, *Gerontologia,* 8, 150, 1963.

18. McCay, C. M., Crowell, M. F., and Maynard, L. A., The effect of retarded growth upon the length of life span and upon the ultimate body size, *J. Nutr.,* 10, 63, 1935.

19. McCay, C. M., Maynard, L. A., Sperling, G., and Barnes, L. L., Retarded growth, life span, ultimate body size, and age changes in the albino rat after feeding diets restricted in calories, *J. Nutr.,* 18, 1, 1939.

20. McCay, C. M., Sperling, G., and Barnes, L. L., Growth, ageing, chronic diseases, and life span in rats, *Arch. Biochem.,* 2, 469, 1943.

21. Berg, B. N. and Simms, H. S., Nutrition and longevity in the rat. II. Longevity and onset of disease with different levels of food intake, *J. Nutr.,* 71, 255, 1960.

22. Masoro, E. J., Bertrand, H., Liepa, G., and Yu, B. P., Analysis and exploration of age-related changes in mammalian structure and function, *Fed. Proc.,* 38, 1956, 1979.

23. Leveille, G. A., The long-term effects of meal-eating on lipogenesis, enzyme activity, and longevity in the rat, *J. Nutr.,* 102, 549, 1972.

24. Reisen, W. H., Herbst, E. J., Walliker, C., and Elvehjem, C. A., The effect of restricted caloric intake on the longevity of rats, *Am. J. Physiol.,* 148, 614, 1947.

25. Leto, S., Kokkonen, G. C., and Barrows, C. H., Dietary protein, lifespan, and physiological variables in female mice, *J. Gerontol.,* 31, 149, 1976.

26. Stuchlikova, E., Juricova-Horakova, M., and Deyl, Z., New aspects of the dietary effect of life prolongation in rodents. What is the role of obesity in aging?, *Expl. Gerontol.,* 10, 141, 1975.

27. Beauchene, R. E., Bales, C. W., Smith, C. A., Tucker, S. M., and Mason, R. L., The effect of food restriction on body composition and longevitiy of rats, *Physiologist,* 22, 4, 1979.

28. Ross, M. H., Life expectancy modification by change in dietary regimen of the mature rat, in *Proc. 7th Int. Cong. Nutr.,* 5, 35, 1967.

29. Nolen, G. A., Effect of various restricted dietary regimes on the growth, health, and longevity of albino rats, *J. Nutr.,* 102, 1477, 1972.

30. Miller, D. S. and Payne, P. R., Longevity and protein intake, *Exp. Gerontol.,* 3, 231, 1968.

31. Dunham, H. H., Abundant feeding followed by restricted feeding and longevity in Daphnia, *Physiol. Zool.,* 11, 399, 1938.

32. Barrows, C. H. and Roeder, L. M., The effect of reduced dietary intake on enzymatic activities and lifespan of rats, *J. Gerontol.,* 20, 69, 1965.

33. Kopec, S., On the influence of intermittent starvation on the longevity of the imaginal stage of *Drosophila melanogaster,* *Br. J. Exp. Biol.,* 5, 204, 1928.

34. David, J., Van Herrewege, J., and Fouillet, P., Quantitative underfeeding of Drosophila: effects on adult longevity and fecundity, *Exp. Gerontol.,* 6, 249, 1971.

35. McCay, C., Maynard, L. A., Sperling, G., and Osgood, H., Nutritional requirements during the latter half of life, *J. Nutr.*, 21, 45, 1941.

36. Saxton, J. A., Boon, M. C., and Furth, J., Observations on the inhibition of development of spontaneous leukemia in mice by underfeeding, *Cancer Res.*, 4, 401, 1944.

37. Ross, M. H. and Bras, G ., Lasting influence of early caloric restriction on prevalence of neoplasms in the rat, *J. Natl. Cancer Inst.*, 47, 1095, 1971.

38. Bras, G., Age-associated kidney lesions in the rat, *J. Infect. Dis.*, 120, 131, 1969.

39. Stoltzner, G. H. and Dorsey, B. A., Life-long dietary protein restriction and immune function: responses to mitogens and sheep erythrocytes in BALB/C mice, *Am. J. Clin. Nutr.*, 33, 1264, 1980.

40. Gerbase-DeLima, M., Lui, R. K., Cheney, K. E., Mickey, R., and Walford, R. L., Immune function and survival in a long-lived mouse strain subjected to undernutrition, *Gerontologia*, 21, 184, 1975.

41. Walford, R. L., Lui, R. K., Gerbase-DeLima, M., Mathies, M., and Smith, G. S., Longterm dietary restriction and immune function in mice: response to sheep red blood cells and to mitogenic agents, *Mech. Ageing Dev.*, 2, 447, 1974.

42. Barrows, C. H. and Roeder, L. M., Effect of age on protein synthesis in rats, *J. Gerontol.*, 16, 321, 1961.

43. Ross, M. H., Protein, calories, and life expectancy, *Fed. Proc.*, 18, 1190, 1959.

44. Leto, S., Kokkonen, G. C., and Barrows, C. H., Dietary protein, lifespan, and biochemical variables in female mice, *J. Gerontol.*, 31, 144, 1976.

45. Ross, M. H., Aging, nutrition, and hepatic enzyme activity patterns in the rat, *J. Nutr.*, 97, 565, 1969.

46. Carlson, A. J. and Hoelzel, F., Apparent prolongation of the lifespan of rats by intermittent fasting, *J. Nutr.*, 31, 363, 1946.

47. Tucker, S. M., Mason, R. L., and Beauchene, R. E., Influence of diet and feed restriction on kidney function of aging male rats, *J. Gerontol.*, 31, 364, 1976.

48. Barrows, C. H. and Kokkonen, G. C., The effect of various dietary restricted regimes on biochemical variables in the mouse, *Growth*, 42, 71, 1978.

49. Johnson, J. E. and Barrows, C. H., Effects of age and dietary restriction on the kidney glomeruli of mice: observations by scanning electron microscopy, *Anat. Rec.*, 196, 145, 1980.

50. Mann, P. L., The effect of various dietary restricted regimes on some immunological parameters of mice, *Growth*, 42, 87, 1978.

51. Strehler, B. L., Studies on the comparative physiology of aging. II. On the mechanism of temperature life-shortening in *Drosophila melanogaster*, *J. Gerontol.*, 16, 2, 1961.

52. Clark, A. M. and Kidwell, R. N., Effects of developmental temperature on the adult lifespan of *Mormoniella vitripenuis* females, *Exp. Gerontol.*, 2, 79, 1967.

53. Clarke, J. M. and Smith, J. M., Independence of temperature on the rate of aging in *Drosophila subobscura*, *Nature*, 190, 1027, 1961.

54. Rubner, M., *Das Problem der Lebensdauer und seine Beziehungen zu Wachstum und Ernahrung*, R. Oldenbourg, Munchen, 1908.

55. Kibler, H. H. and Johnson, H. D., Metabolic rate and aging in rats during exposure to cold., *J. Gerontol.*, 16, 13, 1961.

56. Weiss, A. K., Metabolism during aging in highly inbred and F_1 hybrid rats, *Fed. Proc.*, 21, 219, 1962.

57. Weiss, A. K., A lifespan study of rat metabolic rates, in *Proc. 7th Int. Cong. Gerontol.*, Vienna, Viennese Medical Academy, 1, 215, 1966.

58. Storer, J. B., Relation of lifespan to brain weight, body weight, and metabolic rates among inbred mouse strains, *Exp. Gerontol.*, 2, 173, 1967.

59. Barrows, C. H., Nutrition, aging, and genetic program, *Am. J. Clin. Nutr.*, 25, 829, 1972.

60. Schimke, R. R., The importance of both synthesis and degradation in the control of arginase levels in rat liver, *J. Biol. Chem.*, 239, 3808, 1964.

Chapter 13

NUTRITION AND THE HYPOTHALAMIC-PITUITARY INFLUENCE ON AGING

Arthur V. Everitt

TABLE OF CONTENTS

I. INTRODUCTION

It is well known that long-term food restriction begun in the young rodent will prolong life, delay the onset of a number of diseases, and retard several physiological aging processes.[1-4] However, the mechanism of the life-prolonging and anti-aging actions of food restriction is unknown. One theory suggests that food restriction slows the rate of aging because it reduces the secretion of a pituitary aging factor.[1,5]

II. UNDERNUTRITION AND AGING

A. Life Duration

Caloric restriction (up to 50%) begun in the young rat and maintained throughout life has been shown by many investigators[2-4,6-18] to significantly extend both the mean and maximum life duration. A reduced intake of calories also prolongs the life of the mouse[19-22] and fish[23] as well as that of invertebrates such as the protozoan *Tokophyra*,[24] the rotifer,[25] the crustacean *Daphnia*,[26] the silk worm,[27] and the fruit fly *Drosophila*.[28-30] Such studies suggest that the life-prolonging action of food restriction begun in early life may be a general biological phenomenon acting by a common mechanism.

B. Disease

Autopsy studies of food restricted rats reveal a reduced incidence of many diseases of old age[31] such as chronic renal disease (nephrosis, glomerulonephritis),[32-34] tumors,[18,35,36] periarteritis,[33] myocardial degeneration,[33] skeletal muscle degeneration,[33] and skeletal disease.[37] Dietary restriction delays the age of onset of these diseases.[31,33] It is tempting to suggest that food restriction prolongs life by delaying the onset of diseases which terminate life. Immune-associated diseases such as tumors and renal disease may be delayed in onset because caloric restriction slows the age-related decline in immune function.[22,38]

C. Physiological Aging

Reduced food intake retards several physiological age changes. Long term caloric restriction in the rat or mouse retards the rate of aging in tail tendon collagen fibres,[39-41] delays the age of onset of puberty,[42-45] prolongs the duration of reproductive life,[14,42,46-48] and delays age related changes in serum lipids.[49] Food restriction in the young rat appears to delay the development and maturation of neuroendocrine functions.[50]

III. UNDERNUTRITION AND ORGAN FUNCTION

The food-restricted rat lives longer than its fullyfed control largely because of increased resistance to the diseases of old age. However, changes in organ function may also improve survival.[1,49] When food intake is reduced metabolic rate falls.[51-54] The lowered metabolic rate may contribute to the increased survival of food-restricted animals as forecast by the rate of living theory of Pearl.[29] An organ working at a slow rate would be expected to last longer than the same organ working at a fast rate.

The physiological effects of undernutrition have been studied extensively in human subjects and are summarized in the monograph *The Biology of Human Starvation*.[55] Undernutrition slows gastric emptying, reduces vital capacity and other lung volumes, drops both systolic and diastolic blood pressure, decreases heart rate, lowers glomerular filtration rate, diminishes creatinine and urea clearance, and decreases muscular work capacity. With less energy available from the diet, the body adapts by reducing the level of many organ functions including the capacity for physical work. If wear and tear are significant factors in aging then a low level of organ function must be associated with increased life span of the organ.

It is not clear whether these decrements in organ function are due directly to a lack of nutrients acting at the tissue level or indirectly to reduced secretion of pituitary and other hormones. The level of many cardiovascular, renal, and metabolic functions are decreased by hypophysectomy.[56,57]

IV. UNDERNUTRITION AND HYPOTHALAMIC-PITUITARY FUNCTION

In the food-restricted rat, retarded growth, maturation, and aging may be partly due to the reduced secretion of pituitary and other hormones which are necessary for these processes. In 1925 Jackson[58] studied the inhibitory action of undernutrition on growth and structural changes and postulated that these changes were due to reduced pituitary function. In 1940 Mulinos and Pomerantz[59] found that food restriction depressed many pituitary functions in the rat, and described the state of undernutrition as a 'pseudo-hypophysectomy'. Later studies confirmed these observations showing that food restriction not only depressed growth and the endocrine functions of the pituitary, thyroid, adrenal cortex and gonads, but also reduced the corresponding blood hormone levels.

With the advent of radioimmunoassay techniques it became possible to demonstrate a decline in the blood levels of almost all anterior pituitary hormones in the fasted rat. The work of Campbell et al.[60] showed that either acute starvation (no food) for 7 days or chronic severe food restriction for 3 weeks (no food for 1 week, followed by 1/4 *ad libitum* food intake for 2 weeks) significantly depressed the circulating levels of luteinizing hormone (LH), thyroid stimulating hormone (TSH), growth hormone (GH), and prolactin (PRL); follicle stimulating hormone (FSH) was depressed only in acutely starved rats. Thus severe reductions in food intake result in decreased secretion of at least five anterior pituitary hormones. These workers found that serum LH, FSH, TSH, and PRL are increased by hypothalamic releasing hormones (LH releasing hormone [LRH] and thyrotropin releasing hormone [TRH]) in acutely starved or chronically food restricted rats. Their data indicate that the decreased secretion of anterior pituitary hormones in food-restricted rats is due primarily to reduced hypothalamic stimulation, rather than to the inability of the pituitary to secrete hormones.

V. UNDERNUTRITION, HYPOTHALAMIC-PITUITARY FUNCTION, AND AGING

Food restriction has been shown to depress certain hypothalamic-pituitary functions leading to reduced pituitary hormone secretion. It has been postulated[1,5] that the anti-aging action of food restriction is due to the reduced secretion of an aging factor by the pituitary. This is supported by the observation of similar anti-aging actions of food restriction and hypophysectomy (with cortisone replacement therapy only) (Table 1) in retarding collagen aging, inhibiting the onset of certain diseases of old age, and prolonging life in the rat.[18] Compared with intact fully fed controls, both hypophysectomized and food restricted rats are remarkably free of pathological lesions except for respiratory disease which is common to all conventional rats.

The physiology of both groups of rats is remarkably similar. Both procedures have similar depressing effects on body functions (Table 2) such as heart rate, hemoglobin, white cell count, and creatinine excretion.

The anti-aging action of food restriction may have a hormonal rather than nutri-

Table 1
COMPARISON OF THE ANTI-AGING ACTIONS OF HYPOPHYSECTOMY (AT 70 DAYS) AND FOOD RESTRICTION (BEGUN AT 70 DAYS) IN CONVENTIONAL MALE WISTAR RATS.

Parameter	Controls	Hypophysectomized at 70 days	Food restricted from 70 days
Collagen breaking time (min)	135 ± 16	25 ± 3.2	30 ± 3.0
Proteinuria (mg/day)	18.5 ± 2.9	2.1 ± 0.3	2.2 ± 0.3
Renal enlargement	8%	0%	0%
Total tumor incidence	64%	5%	15%
Cardiac enlargement	21%	0%	0%
Hind limb paralysis	71%	0%	0%
Mean life duration (days ± SE)	785 ± 34	916 ± 46	858 ± 38
Maximum life duration (days)	1120	1342	1282

Note: Incidence of disease is derived from autopsy data on 88 controls, 40 hypophysectomized, and 36 food-restricted rats aged 800 days or more. Collagen and proteinuria tests were performed at 850 days. Data are Means ± SE, or percentage incidence of disease.

From Everitt, A. V., Seedsman, N. J., and Jones, F., *Mech. Age Dev.*, 12, 161, 1980. With permission.

Table 2
COMPARISON OF THE EFFECTS OF HYPOPHYSECTOMY AND OF FOOD RESTRICTION BEGUN AT 70 DAYS ON ORGAN FUNCTION TESTS IN MALE WISTAR RATS AGED 700 TO 750 DAYS

Parameter	Controls	Hypophysectomized at 70 days	Food restricted from 70 days
Number of rats	10	7	6
Body weight	485 ± 8	174 ± 6	187 ± 6
Food intake (g/day)	19.1 ± 1.3	6.8 ± 0.5	7
Heart rate (/min)	352 ± 21	246 ± 18	275 ± 22
Hemoglobin (g/100 mℓ)	14.8 ± 0.3	12.8 ± 0.4	13.3 ± 0.2
White cell count (10^3 cells/$\mu\ell$)	8.5 ± 0.7	4.1 ± 0.5	5.2 ± 0.6
Creatinine excretion (mg/day)	21.4 ± 1.0	6.5 ± 0.4	7.4 ± 0.6

Note: Data are means ± SE.

tional basis. Doubling the food intake of hypophysectomized rats by means of hypothalamic lesions does not increase the aging of tail tendon collagen fibers significantly (Figure 1) nor increase proteinuria.[61] It has also been shown that proteinuria development in old age in hypophysectomized rats is increased by chronic growth hormone injections begun early in life (Table 3) and the proteinuria is significantly greater than in intact rats eating the same quantity of food. However, in the case of thyroidectomy (which also retards collagen and renal aging) the anti-aging effects have been related to the lowered food intake rather than the loss of thyroid hormone (Table 4), since thyroxine does not increase collagen aging in food restricted thyroidectomized rats.[40]

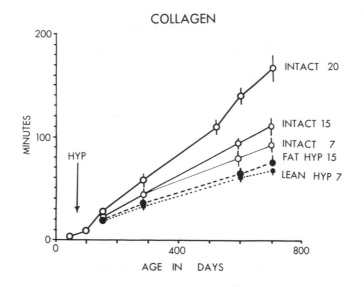

FIGURE 1. The failure of increased food intake to accelerate the aging of tail tendon collagen in the hypophysectomized male Wistar rat. The food intake in hypophysectomized rats of 7 g/day was increased to 15 g by hypothalamic lesions. Intact rats eating 7, 15, and 20 g of food per day had significantly greater rates of collagen aging than hypophysectomized rats. Collagen fiber aging was measured as the breaking time of isolated fibers in 7 M urea at 40°C. l(From Everitt, A. V., manuscript in preparation.)

Table 3
EFFECT OF CHRONIC GROWTH HORMONE REPLACEMENT THERAPY ON PROTEIN EXCRETION AT 640 DAYS IN HYPOPHYSECTOMIZED MALE WISTAR RATS COMPARED WITH FOOD-RESTRICTED RATS

	No. of rats	Food intake (g/day)	Body weight (g)	Protein excretion (mg/day)
Controls	10	18.5 ± 0.9	505 ± 9	22.2 ± 2.3
Hypophysectomized	7	6.8 ± 0.6	142 ± 8	2.8 ± 0.5
Hypophysectomized + growth hormone	5	10.3 ± 0.7	232 ± 8	6.9 ± 0.7
Food restricted	6	7	163 ± 6	3.3 ± 0.4
Food restricted	6	10	254 ± 10	4.2 ± 0.3

Note: Protein excretion is a measure of age-related renal disease. The kidneys of growth hormone treated rats showed more thickening of the basement membranes of glomeruli and tubules than either hypophysectomized or food restricted rats. Treatments were begun at age 70 days. Data are Means ± SE.

It has been proposed that the beneficial effects of early food restriction on aging and longevity are due to biochemical changes in the brain,[4] particularly in the hypothalamus.[62-63] Certain nutrients such as amino acids are necessary for neurotransmitter formation. A lack of tryptophan has a similar anti-aging action in the rat as caloric restriction.[64] Finch[62] has suggested that physiological aging is due to changes in the metabolism of catecholamines in the hypothalamus. Acute studies[65] of food-restricted rats reveal a shift in the time of peak catecholamine concentration. However, in a

Table 4

EFFECTS OF THYROIDECTOMY, THYROXINE
AND FOOD RESTRICTION ON THE BREAKING
TIME OF COLLAGEN FIBERS FROM RAT TAIL
TENDON AT AGE 250 DAYS

Group	No. of rats	Food intake (g/day)	Collagen breaking time (min)
Sham control	9	19.9±0.8	18.6±0.9
Thyroidectomized	8	12.6±0.7	11.1±0.5
Thyroidectomized + thyroxine	7	19.3±1.2	20.3±1.7
Sham food restricted	9	14	11.7±0.3
Thyroidectomized + thyroxine + food restriction	9	14	11.8±0.6

Note: Treatments were begun at 85 days. Data are Means ± S.E.

From Giles, J. S. and Everitt, A. V., *Gerontologia,* 13, 65, 1965.

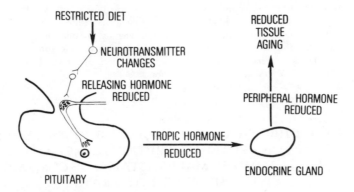

FIGURE 2.   Model to explain the anti-aging action of undernutrition. It is proposed that undernutrition produces changes in neurotransmitter metabolism in the hypothalamus, which lead in turn to decreases in secretion of releasing hormone, pituitary tropic hormone, and finally the corresponding peripheral hormone. Since the peripheral hormone has an aging action on tissues, a fall in its secretion would slow the rate of tissue aging.

chronic developmental study[50] caloric restriction failed to alter brain catecholamine levels in female rats. Further data are urgently required to assess the long term effects of food restriction on age changes in catecholamine metabolism in the hypothalamus.

A model to explain the anti-aging action of undernutrition is shown in Figure 2. Undernutrition by altering neurotransmitter metabolism in the hypothalamus reduces the secretion of releasing hormones and thence pituitary tropic and peripheral hormones; the lack of hormones then slows tissue aging. In a modification of this model a hypothalamic clock or center[66] has been proposed whose working depends on the actions of neurotransmitters. The clock is thought to time the program of development and aging by means of peripheral hormones and neurosecretions. Hormones[67] are believed to affect tissue development and aging by altering the expression of genes in the tissues. Nutrients and metabolites also affect the expression of genes, but the hormonal action is probably more important in higher animals.[68] The relative contributions of the direct aging action of nutrients and metabolites on tissue cells and the indirect action via hypothalamic-pituitary complex are unknown.

VI. OVERNUTRITION, HYPOTHALAMIC-PITUITARY FUNCTION, AND AGING

A. Life Duration, Aging, and Disease

Overnutrition leading to overweight and obesity is associated with shortened life in man,[69-74] rat,[75] and mouse.[76] Life span is shortened due to increased mortality from degenerative diseases[70,72-75] of the cardiovascular system and kidneys, and from diabetes mellitus and liver disorders. The only evidence of accelerated physiological aging in obesity is the reported early onset of puberty in obese children[77,78] and the overfed rat.[44]

B. Organ Functions

The physiology of overnutrition and obesity is not well documented.[1] In human subjects obesity is associated with increased blood pressure,[72,79] cardiac output,[80] and glomerular filtration,[81] but there is evidence of impaired pulmonary function[82] and reduced capacity for physical work.[83] The major metabolic changes[84-86] are elevated blood glucose and triglyceride levels.

C. Pituitary and Endocrine Function

The effects of overnutrition on pituitary and other endocrine functions have been incompletely investigated.[1] In obese subjects there is evidence of increased secretion of cortisol[87,88] and insulin.[89,90] Hypothalamic obesity in experimental animals[91,92] is accompanied by hyperinsulinemia and reduced secretion of most pituitary and target gland hormones.

D. Hypothalamic-Pituitary Function and Aging

Apart from the increased secretion of cortisol and presumably pituitary ACTH, there is no evidence of hypersecretion of pituitary hormones in the overnutrition of obesity. The hyperadrenocorticism of Cushing's disease is associated with accelerated cardiovascular aging[93] in the form of hyperlipidemia, hypertension, arteriosclerosis, myocardial infarction, and cerebrovascular accidents. The extent to which the raised cortisol secretion in obese patients contributes to cardiovascular pathophysiologic derangements is not known.

Activation of the hypothalamic-pituitary-thyroid axis in rats exposed to low temperatures produces a large rise in food intake.[94-96] In such cold-acclimated rats, life span is diminished and there is a premature onset of certain diseases of old age such as nephritis and periarteritis.[96,97] The hormonal mechanism is complicated by the concurrent hypersecretion of corticosteroids and catecholamines in cold-adapted rats.[98] Nonetheless, this is a case where high food intake and hypersecretion of pituitary, thyroid, and adrenal hormones are associated with accelerated aging and shortened life span.

The hyperinsulinemia of obesity appears to be due to the high calorie intake alone, since the feeding of high calorie diets to nonobese subjects elevates the plasma insulin level.[84] Hyperinsulinemia is then believed to lead to hypertriglyceridemia, obesity, diabetes mellitus, and atherosclerosis.[84,99,100]

Thus, in states of overnutrition, a number of studies associate high secretion rates of pituitary, thyroid, adrenocortical, and pancreatic B cell hormones with the development of age-related diseases. However, the aging effects of high food intake and hypersecretion of hormones have not been separated.

VII. PROBLEMS AND IMPLICATIONS

A. Nutrition Studies in Hypophysectomized Rats

At this stage it is not known if nutrients directly affect tissue aging or if they act indirectly via some central regulatory mechanism such as the hypothalamic-pituitary complex. In order to demonstrate an indirect action via the pituitary, it will be necessary to investigate the effects of nutrition on aging in hypophysectomized rats.

In such nutrition studies hypophysectomized rats will require some form of hormone replacement therapy. Without replacement therapy hypophysectomized rats cannot withstand starvation and nutrient deprivation. The hormones most essential for survival appear to be the adrenocortical hormones normally controlled by pituitary ACTH. In our laboratory, weekly subcutaneous injections of cortisone acetate prolong the life of hypophysectomized rats[18] and provide resistance to the normal day-to-day stresses of community life in a cage. Denckla et al.[103] administers corticosterone, deoxycorticosterone, and thyroxine in the drinking water of hypophysectomized rats.

The strict control of nutrition demands individual housing of animals. Such isolation[104] affects the physiology of the animal by increasing food intake, body weight, blood pressure, corticosteroid secretion, and catecholamine metabolism. Some of these changes are dependent on pituitary hormone secretion and thus complicate the interpretation of nutrition studies in the isolated hypophysectomized rat.

B. Nutrition and Brain Function

Nutrients which are precursors of neurotransmitters may be able to compensate for the loss of neurons in old age.[63,105] It is shown that certain amino acids are able to increase the synthesis of neurotransmitters in the remaining neurons and so alleviate the effects of declining brain function. Studies of this type may be of great benefit to the elderly, but may not yield much information about the more basic mechanisms of aging.

The search for the putative central regulator[64,66] of aging may be difficult and require many decades of research because of the long-term nature of aging research. Such a regulator would be expected to modulate processes such as the onset of puberty, collagen aging in tail tendon, the onset of reproductive senescence, the decline of immunological functions, the onset of age-related diseases, and the duration of life. In studying short-term phenomena such as sleep, a lesion experiment to localize a sleep center could demonstrate an effect within a week in a rat. However, in studying long-term phenomena such as aging the corresponding lesion experiment to localize an aging center could take 6 months to yield an answer. Similarly nutrition studies on such a center would require a corresponding delay before demonstrating a significant effect.

VIII. CONCLUSIONS

Both food restriction and hypophysectomy (with corticosteroid replacement therapy) have similar anti-aging actions in the rat. Since chronic food restriction reduces the secretion of most anterior pituitary hormones, it is postulated that food factors accelerate aging by promoting the secretion of a pituitary aging factor. There are several studies which support this hypothesis. However, to obtain unequivocal proof of this indirect aging action of nutrients via the pituitary it will be necessary to conduct many nutrition-aging studies on hypophysectomized rats.

ACKNOWLEDGMENTS

I am especially grateful to Mr. Frank Jones, who performed most of the hypophysectomies, and to Roussel Pharmaceuticals, Sydney, who generously supplied the cortisone acetate used in these studies. The hypophysectomy studies reported here were supported, in part, by grants from the Consolidated Medical Research Fund of the University of Sydney and the University Research Grant.

REFERENCES

1. Everitt, A. V. and Porter, B., Nutrition and aging, in *Hypothalamus, Pituitary, and Aging,* Everitt, A. V. and Burgess, J. A., Eds., Charles C Thomas, Springfield, Ill., 1976, chap. 30.
2. Ross, M. H., Nutrition and longevity in experimental animals, in *Nutrition and Aging,* Winick, M., Ed., John Wiley and Sons, New York, 1976.
3. Barrows, C. H., Jr. and Kokkonen, G. C., Diet and life extension in animal model systems, *Age,* 1, 131, 1978.
4. Young, V. R., Diet as a modulator of aging and longevity, *Fed. Proc.,* 38, 1994, 1979.
5. Everitt, A. V., The hypothalamic-pituitary control of aging and age related pathology, *Exp. Gerontol.,* 8, 265, 1973.
6. Osborne, T. B., Mendel, L. B., and Ferry, E. L., The effect of retardation of growth upon the breeding period and duration of life of rats, *Science,* 40, 294, 1917.
7. McCay, C. M., Crowell, M. F., and Maynard, L. A., The effect of retarded growth upon the length of the life span and upon ultimate body size, *J. Nutr.,* 10, 63, 1935.
8. McCay, C. M., Maynard, L. A., Sperling, G., and Barnes, L. L., Retarded growth, life span, ultimate body size, and age changes in the albino rat after feeding diets restricted in calories, *J. Nutr.,* 18, 1, 1939.
9. McCay, C. M., Sperling, G., and Barnes, L. L., Growth, ageing, chronic diseases, and life span in rats, *Arch. Biochem.,* 2, 469, 1943.
10. Carlson, A. J. and Hoelzel, F., Apparent prolongation of the life span of rats by intermittent fasting, *J. Nutr.,* 31, 363, 1946.
11. Riesen, W. H., Herbst, E. J., Walliker, C., and Elvehjem, C. A., The effect of restricted caloric intake on the longevity of rats, *Am. J. Physiol.,* 148, 614, 1947.
12. Ross, M. H., Length of life and nutrition in the rat, *J. Nutr.,* 75, 197, 1961.
13. Ross, M. H., Length of life and caloric intake, *Am. J. Clin. Nutr.,* 25, 834, 1972.
14. Berg, B. N., Nutrition and longevity in the rat. I. Food intake in relation to size, health, and longevity, *J. Nutr.,* 71, 242, 1960.
15. Nolen, G. A., Effect of various restricted regimens on the growth, health and longevity of albino rats, *J. Nutr.,* 102, 1477, 1972.
16. Stuchlíková, E., Jǔricová-Horoková, M., and Deyl, Z., New aspect of the dietary effect of life prolongation in rodents. What is the role of obesity in aging? *Exp. Gerontol.,* 10, 141, 1975.
17. Drori, D. and Folman, Y., Environmental effects on longevity in the male rat: exercise, mating, castration, and restricted feeding, *Exp. Gerontol.,* 11, 25, 1976.
18. Everitt, A. V., Seedsman, N. J., and Jones, F., The effects of hypophysectomy and continuous food restriction, begun at ages 70 and 400 days, on collagen aging, proteinuria, incidence of pathology and longevity in the male rat, *Mech. Age Dev.,* 12, 161, 1980.
19. Lee, Y. C. P., Visscher, M. B., and King, J. T., Life span and causes of death in inbred mice in relation to diet, *J. Gerontol.,* 11, 364, 1956.
20. Lane, P. W. and Dickie, M. M., The effect of restricted food intake on the life span of genetically obese mice, *J. Nutr.,* 64, 549, 1958.
21. Silberberg, R., Jarrett, S. R., and Silberberg, M., Life span of mice fed enriched or restricted diets during growth, *Am. J. Physiol.,* 200, 332, 1961.
22. Gerbase-DeLima, M., Liu, R. K., Cheney, K. E., Mickey, R., and Walford, R. L., Immune function and survival in a long-lived mouse strain subjected to undernutrition, *Gerontologia,* 21, 184, 1975.
23. Comfort, A., Effect of delayed and resumed growth on the longevity of a fish (*Levistes reticulatus,* Peters) in captivity, *Gerontologia,* 8, 150, 1963.
24. Rudzinska, M., The use of a protozoan for studies on aging, *Gerontologia,* 6, 206, 1962.
25. Fanestil, D. D. and Barrows, C. H., Jr., Aging in the rotifer, *J. Gerontol.,* 20, 462, 1965.
26. Ingle, L. T., Wood, T. R., and Banta, A. M., A study of longevity, growth, reproduction, and heart rate in *Daphnia longespina* as influenced by limitations in quantity of food, *J. Exp. Zool.,* 76, 325, 1937.
27. Kellogg, V. L. and Bell, R. G., Variations induced in larval, pupal, and imaginal stages of *Bombyx mori* by controlled variations in food supply, *Science,* 18, 741, 1903.

28. Northrop, J., The effect of prolongation of the period of growth on the total duration of life, *J. Biol. Chem.,* 32, 123, 1917.

29. Pearl, R., *The Rate of Living,* Knopf, New York, 1928.

30. Greiff, D., Longevity in *Drosophila melanogaster* and its ebony mutant in the absence of food, *Am. Naturalist,* 74, 363, 1940.

31. Berg, B. N., Pathology and aging, in *Hypothalamus, Pituitary, and Aging,* Everitt, A. V. and Burgess, J. A., Eds., Charles C Thomas, Springfield, Ill., 1976, chap. 3.

32. Saxton, J. A., Jr. and Kimball, G. C., Relation of nephrosis and other diseases of albino rats to age and to modifications of diet, *Arch. Pathol.,* 32, 951, 1941.

33. Berg, B. N. and Simms, H. S., Nutrition and longevity in the rat. II. Longevity and onset of disease with different levels of food intake, *J. Nutr.,* 71, 255, 1960.

34. Bras, G. and Ross, M. H., Kidney disease and nutrition in the rat, *Toxicol. Appl. Pharmacol.,* 6, 247, 1964.

35. Saxton, J. A., Jr., Sperling, G., Barnes, L. L., and McCay, C. M., The influence of nutrition upon the incidence of spontaneous tumors of the albino rat, *Acta Unio Int. Contra Cancrum,* 6, 423, 1948.

36. Ross, M. H. and Bras, G., Tumor incidence patterns and nutrition in the rat, *J. Nutr.,* 87, 245, 1965.

37. Silberberg, M. and Silberberg, R., Diet and life span, *Physiol. Rev.,* 35, 347, 1955.

38. Weindruch, R. H., Kristie, J. A., Cheney, K. E., and Walford, R. L., Influence of controlled dietary restriction on immunological function and aging, *Fed. Proc.,* 38, 2007, 1979.

39. Chvapil, M. and Hruza, Z., The influence of aging and undernutrition on chemical contractility and relaxation of collagen fibres in rats, *Gerontologia,* 3, 241, 1959.

40. Giles, J. S. and Everitt, A. V., The role of thyroid and food intake in the aging of collagen fibres. I. In the young rat, *Gerontologia,* 13, 65, 1967.

41. Everitt, A. V., Food intake, growth, and ageing of collagen in rat tail tendon, *Gerontologia,* 17, 98, 1971.

42. Merry, F. J. and Holehan, A. M., Onset of puberty and duration of fertility in rats fed a restricted diet, *J. Reprod. Fert.,* 57, 253, 1979.

43. Lintern-Moore, S. and Everitt, A. V., The effect of restricted food intake on the size and composition of the ovarian follicle population in the Wistar rat, *Biol. Reprod.,* 19, 688, 1978.

44. Kennedy, G. C. and Mitra, J., Body weight and food intake as initiating factors for puberty in the rat, *J. Physiol.,* 166, 408, 1963.

45. Glass, A. R. and Swerdloff, R. S., Nutritional influences on sexual maturation in the rat, *Fed. Proc.,* 39, 2360, 1980.

46. Holecková, E. and Chvapil, M., The effect of intermittent feeding and fasting and of domestication on biological age in the rat, *Gerontologia,* 11, 96, 1965.

47. Carr, C. J., King, J. T., and Visscher, M. B., Delay of senescence infertility by dietary restriction, *Fed. Proc.,* 8, 22, 1949.

48. Visscher, M. B., King, J. K., and Lee, Y. C. P., Further studies on influence of age and diet upon reproductive senescence in strain A female mice, *Am. J. Physiol.,* 170, 72, 1952.

49. Liepa, G. V., Masoro, E. J., Bertrand, H. A., and Yu, B. P., Food restriction as a modulator of age-related changes in serum lipids, *Am. J. Physiol.,* 238, E253, 1980.

50. Segall, P. E., Ooka, H., Rose, K., and Timiras, P. S., Neural and endocrine development after chronic tryptophan deficiency in rats. I. Brain monoamine and pituitary responses, *Mech. Age Dev.,* 7, 1, 1978.

51. Lea, M. and Lucia, S. B., Some relationships between caloric restriction and body weight in the rat. I. Body composition, liver lipids, and organ weights, *J. Nutr.,* 74, 243, 1961.

52. Taylor, H. L. and Keys, A., Adaptation to caloric restriction, *Science,* 112, 215, 1950.

53. Hansen-Smith, F. M., Maksud, M. G., and Van Horn, D. L., Effect of dietary protein restriction or food restriction on oxygen consumption and mitochondrial distribution in cardiac and red and white skeletal muscle of rats, *J. Nutr.,* 107, 525, 1977.

54. Tung, J. G. V., Heat production of lean and obese mice in response to fasting, food restriction, and thyroxine, *Proc. Soc. Exp. Biol. Med.,* 160, 266, 1979.

55. Keys, A., Brozek, J., Henschel, A., Mickelson, D., and Taylor, H. L., *The Biology of Human Starvation,* University of Minnesota Press, Minneapolis, 1950.

56. Kovacs, K. and Horvath, E., Pituitary control of cardiovascular and renal function, in *Hypothalamus, Pituitary, and Aging,* Everitt, A. V. and Burgess, J. A., Eds., Charles C Thomas, Springfield, Ill., 1976, chap. 13.

57. Everitt, A. V., Hypophysectomy and aging in the rat, in *Hypothalamus, Pituitary, and Aging,* Everitt, A. V. and Burgess, J. A., Eds., Charles C Thomas, Springfield, Ill., 1976, chap. 4.

58. Jackson, C. M., *The Effects of Inanition and Malnutrition upon Growth and Structure,* Blakiston, Philadelphia, 1925.

59. Mulinos, M. G. and Pomerantz, L., Pseudo-hypophysectomy, a condition resembling hypophysectomy produced by malnutrition, *J. Nutr.,* 19, 493, 1940.

60. Campbell, G. A., Kurcz, Marshall, S., and Meites, J., Effects of starvation in rats on serum levels of follicle stimulating hormone, luteinizing hormone, thyrotropin, growth hormone, and prolactin; response to LH-releasing hormone and thyrotropin releasing hormone, *Endocrinology*, 100, 580, 1977.
61. Everitt, A. V., The anti-aging action of hypophysectomy in hypothalamic obese rats, manuscript in preparation.
62. Finch, C. E., Physiological changes of aging in mammals, *Q. Rev. Biol.*, 51, 49, 1976.
63. Samorajski, T., Central neurotransmitter substances and aging: a review, *J. Am. Geriatr. Soc.*, 25, 337, 1977.
64. Segall, P. E., Interrelations of dietary and hormonal effects in aging, *Mech. Age Dev.*, 9, 515, 1979.
65. Krieger, D. T., Crowley, W. R., O'Donohue, and Jacobowitz, D. M., Effects of food restriction on the periodicity of corticosteroids in plasma and on monoamine concentrations in discrete brain nuclei, *Brain Res.*, 188, 167, 1980.
66. Everitt, A. V., The genetic clock-hormone theory of aging, seminar on Biological and Social Aspects of Mortality and Length of Life, International Union for the Scientific Study of Population, Fiuggi Terme, Italy, May 13 to 16, 1980.
67. Adelman, R. C., Age-dependent hormonal regulation of mammalian gene expression, in *Hypothalamus, Pituitary, and Aging*, Everitt, A. V. and Burgess, J. A., Eds., Charles C Thomas, Springfield, Ill., 1976, chap. 33.
68. Maclean, N., *Control of Gene Expression*, Academic Press, New York, 1976.
69. Armstrong, D. B. I., Dublin, I., Wheatley, M., and Marks, H., Obesity and its relation to health and disease, *J. Am. Med. Assoc.*, 147, 1007, 1951.
70. Marks, W. H., Influence of obesity on morbidity and mortality, *Bull. N.Y. Acad. Med.*, 36, 296, 1960.
71. Watanabe, T., Yukawa, K., and Sakamoto, A., Nutritional intake and longevity; international comparative study, *Acta Med. Nagasaki*, 13, 44, 1968.
72. *1979 Build and Blood Pressure Study*, Society of Actuaries, Chicago, 1980.
73. Mann, C. V., The influence of obesity on health, *N. Engl. J. Med.*, 291, 178, 1974.
74. Van Itallie, T. B., Obesity: adverse effects on health and longevity, *Am. J. Clin. Nutr.*, Suppl. 32, 2723, 1979.
75. Koletsky, S., Pathologic findings and laboratory data in a new strain of obese hypertensive rats, *Am. J. Pathol.*, 80, 129, 1975.
76. Lane, P. W. and Dickie, M. M., The effect of restricted food intake on the life span of genetically obese mice, *J. Nutr.*, 64, 549, 1958.
77. Bruch, H., Obesity in relation to puberty, *J. Pediatr.*, 19, 365, 1941.
78. Wolff, O. H., Obesity in childhood, *Q. J. Med.*, 24, 109, 1955.
79. Chiang, B. N., Perlman, L. V., and Epstein, F. H., Overweight and hypertension: a review, *Circulation*, 39, 403, 1969.
80. Alexander, J. K., Obesity and the circulation, *Mod. Concepts Cardiovasc. Dis.*, 32, 799, 1963.
81. Gelman, A., Singulem, D., Sustovich, D. R., Ajzen, H., and Ramos, O. L., Starvation and renal function, *Am. J. Med. Sci.*, 263, 465, 1972.
82. Barrera, F., Reidenberg, M. M., and Winters, W. L., Pulmonary function in the obese patient, *Am. J. Med. Sci.*, 254, 785, 1967.
83. Dempsey, J. A., Relationship between obesity and treadmill performance in sedentary and active young men, *Res. Q.*, 35, 288, 1964.
84. Olefsky, J., Crapo, P. A., Ginsberg, H., and Reaven, G. M., Metabolic effects of increased caloric intake in man, *Metabolism*, 24, 494, 1975.
85. Bierman, E. L. and Glomset, J. A., Disorders of lipid metabolism, in *Textbook of Endocrinology*, Williams, R. H., Ed., W. B. Saunders, Philadelphia, 1974, chap. 18.
86. Vaughan, R. W., Gandolfi, A. J., and Bentley, J. B., Biochemical considerations of morbid obesity, *Life Sci.*, 26, 2215, 1980.
87. Schteingart, D. E., Characteristics of increased adrenocortical function observed in obese persons, *Ann. N.Y. Acad. Sci.*, 131, 388, 1965.
88. Jackson, I. M. D. and Mowat, J. I., Hypothalamic-pituitary-adrenal function in obesity and the cortisol secretion rate following prolonged starvation, *Acta Endocrinol.*, 63, 415, 1970.
89. Bagdade, J. D., Basal insulin and obesity, *Lancet*, 2, 630, 1968.
90. Rabinowitz, D., Some endocrine and metabolic aspects of obesity, *Ann. Rev. Med.*, 21, 241, 1970.
91. Bray, G. A. and York, D. A., Hypothalamic and genetic obesity in experimental animals: an autonomic and endocrine hypothesis, *Physiol. Rev.*, 59, 719, 1979.
92. Nosadini, R., Ursini, F., Tessari, P., Garotti, M. C., de Biasi, F., and Tiengo, A., Hormonal and metabolic characteristics of genetically obese Sprague-Dawley rats, *Eur. J. Clin. Invest.*, 10, 113, 1980.

93. Wexler, B. C., Comparative aspects of hyperadrenocorticism and aging, in *Hypothalamus, Pituitary, and Aging,* Everitt, A. V. and Burgess, J. A., Eds., Charles C Thomas, Springfield, Ill., 1976, chap. 17.

94. Hsieh, A. C. L. and Ti, K. W., The effects of L-thyroxine and cold exposure on the amount of food consumed and absorbed by male albino rats, *J. Nutr.,* 72, 283, 1960.

95. Johnson, H. D., Kibler, H. H., and Silsby, H., The influence of ambient temperature of 9°C and 28°C on thyroid function of rats during growth and aging, *Gerontologia,* 9, 18, 1964.

96. Johnson, H. D., Kintner, and Kibler, H. H., Effects of 48F (8.9C) and 83F (28.4C) on longevity and pathology of male rats, *J. Gerontol.,* 18, 29, 1963.

97. Heroux, O. and Campbell, J. S., A study of the pathology and lifespan of 6°C and 30°C acclimated rats, *Lab. Invest.,* 9, 305, 1960.

98. Heroux, O., Catecholamines, corticosteroids, and thyroid hormones in nonshivering thermogenesis under different environmental conditions, in *Physiology and Pathology of Adaptation Mechanisms,* Bajusz, E., Ed., Pergamon Press, Oxford, 1969, 347.

99. Dilman, V. M., The hypothalamic control of aging and age-associated pathology. The elevation mechanism of aging, in *Hypothalamus, Pituitary, and Aging,* Everitt, A. V. and Burgess, J. A., Eds., Charles C Thomas, Springfield, Ill., 1976, chap. 32.

100. Nestel, P. J., Carroll, K. F., and Havenstein, N., Plasma triglyceride response to carbohydrates, fats, and caloric intake, *Metabolism,* 19, 1, 1970.

101. Boros-Farkas, M. and Everitt, A. V., Comparative studies of age tests on collagen fibres, *Gerontologia,* 13, 37, 1967.

102. Everitt, A. V. and Cavanagh, L. M., The aging process in the hypophysectomized rat, *Gerontologia,* 11, 198, 1965.

103. Scott, M., Bolla, R., and Denckla, W. D., Age related changes in immune function of rats and the effect of long term hypophysectomy, *Mech. Age Dev.,* 11, 127, 1979.

104. Bennett, T. and Gardner, S. M., Corticosteroid involvement in the changes in noradrenergic responsiveness of tissues from rats made hypertensive by short term isolation, *Br. J. Pharmacol.,* 64, 129, 1978.

105. Lytle, L. D. and Altar, A., Diet, central nervous system, and aging, *Fed. Proc.,* 38, 2017, 1979.

INDEX

A

B